W 20.55

NHS Blood and Transplant

00002344

KV-338-386

The Limits of Consent

The Limits of Consent

A Socio-ethical Approach to Human Subject Research in Medicine

Edited by

Oonagh Corrigan, John McMillan,

Kathleen Liddell,

Martin Richards and
Charles Weijer

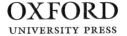

OXFORD
UNIVERSITY PRESS

OXFORD
UNIVERSITY PRESS

Great Clarendon Street, Oxford OX2 6DP

Oxford University Press is a department of the University of Oxford.
It furthers the University's objective of excellence in research, scholarship,
and education by publishing worldwide in

Oxford New York

Auckland Cape Town Dar es Salaam Hong Kong Karachi
Kuala Lumpur Madrid Melbourne Mexico City Nairobi
New Delhi Shanghai Taipei Toronto

With offices in

Argentina Austria Brazil Chile Czech Republic France Greece
Guatemala Hungary Italy Japan Poland Portugal Singapore
South Korea Switzerland Thailand Turkey Ukraine Vietnam

Oxford is a registered trade mark of Oxford University Press
in the UK and in certain other countries

Published in the United States
by Oxford University Press Inc., New York

© Oxford University Press 2009

The moral rights of the authors have been asserted
Database right Oxford University Press (maker)

First published 2009

All rights reserved. No part of this publication may be reproduced,
stored in a retrieval system, or transmitted, in any form or by any means,
without the prior permission in writing of Oxford University Press,
or as expressly permitted by law, or under terms agreed with the appropriate
reprographics rights organization. Enquiries concerning reproduction
outside the scope of the above should be sent to the Rights Department,
Oxford University Press, at the address above

You must not circulate this book in any other binding or cover
and you must impose this same condition on any acquirer

British Library Cataloguing in Publication Data

Data available

Library of Congress Cataloging in Publication Data

Data available

Typeset by Cepha Imaging Private Ltd., Bangalore, India
Printed in Great Britain
on acid-free paper by
the MPG Books Group

ISBN 978–0–19–923146–1

1 3 5 7 9 10 8 6 4 2

Whilst every effort has been made to ensure that the contents of this book are as complete,
accurate and up-to-date as possible at the date of writing, Oxford University Press is not
able to give any guarantee or assurance that such is the case. Readers are urged to take
appropriately qualified medical advice in all cases. The information in this book is
intended to be useful to the general reader, but should not be used as a means of
self-diagnosis or for the prescription of medication.

Foreword

We live with the legacy of persons unwittingly and/or unwillingly made subjects of research. In the name of science, prisoners of war, mentally impaired adults, poor people in need of medical care, children, and ordinary, competent men and women have been frozen, radiated, punctured, left untreated, and exposed to infectious agents without explanation or permission. This shameful-legacy-in-need-of-a-solution has given us – by means of long deliberations of several commissions and committees in different locations around the world – the noble idea of informed consent.

How else could we have responded? Informed consent is a clear and logical answer to the abuses of mid-twentieth century medical research: no experimenting on humans without their consent. Those who participate in research projects must be competent to decide for themselves, must be told what they are getting into, and must give their voluntary, uncoerced consent.

So far so good. Informed consent is arguably the most important product of bioethics – a concrete and explicit procedure built on the practical moral theories of this 40-something year-old interdiscipline. But, as the authors of the articles collected here so convincingly show, informed consent has not done, nor can it do, all the ethical work it is asked to do.

Why have the problems with informed consent so well-described in this anthology – problems of indiscriminate use, ignorance of community and family interests, displacement of trust, diminishment of the obligation to participate in research, and lack of consideration of different cultural traditions – escaped notice for so long? Largely because, until recently, the interdiscipline of bioethics has been dominated by medicine, law, and moral philosophy. In the early years of bioethics, social science was seen as interesting but irrelevant because, after all, 'you can't get an *ought* from an *is*'. Only gradually have social scientists been able to convince bioethicists that it is also true that 'you can't get an *is* from an *ought*'.

The work and organization of bioethics is not exempt from normal social processes: social policies (like informed consent), even those formulated with legal precision and based on sound moral philosophy, do not always produce the desired ethical outcome.

It comes as no surprise to social scientists schooled in the working of bureaucracies that informed consent has become routinized, that "consent" has become a transitive verb ("The researcher consented Mrs. Jones") where the research subject becomes the object of another's action rather than a thinking, deliberating person.

A bit late (some 60 years after the Nuremberg Code), but better than never, *The Limits of Consent* shows us how informed consent works on the ground, revealing where it does important ethical work, where it adds nothing to the protection of research subjects and patients, and where it promotes less than ethical outcomes. By putting the noble idea of informed consent in its historical and social context the authors of this volume move us closer to realizing the respect for persons that is required to protect those who entrust themselves to medicine and medical research.

Raymond De Vries
Ann Arbor, Michigan
September 2008

Acknowledgements

The book's editors are extremely grateful to the Wellcome Trust, the Institute of Applied Ethics at Hull University and Cambridge Genetics knowledge Park for their support in funding the initial workshop that has led to this volume. We also express our thanks to those who attended for their contribution to our debate. Last but not least, we are indebted to the patients and research subjects who participated in the research written about in this volume and hope that issues raised and the recommendations authors have made will improve the experience of future research subjects and the development of structures that facilitate high quality ethical research for patient benefit.
We dedicate this book to our former colleague Peter Lipton, Professor of History and Philosophy of Science at the University of Cambridge, who died suddenly aged 53. A great scholar and orator his humility and conviviality were evident to all who encountered him. His recent contribution to ethical debate as a member of the Nuffield Council on Bioethics was another example of his ability to bring clarity and insight to complex issues affecting us all. We hope that this book in some small way does the same.

Oonagh Corrigan
2008

Contents

List of contributors

Phil Bielby
Law School and
Institute of Applied Ethics,
The University of Hull,
United Kingdom

Michael Burgess
Principal, College for
Interdisciplinary Studies, Professor,
W. Maurice Young Centre for
Applied Ethics, and Department of
Medical Genetics,
University of British Columbia,
Canada

Joanna Collerton
Principal Clinical Research Fellow,
Institute for Ageing and Health,
Campus for Ageing and Vitality
Newcastle University,
United Kingdom

Oonagh Corrigan
Senior Lecturer,
Peninsula Medical School,
University of Plymouth,
United Kingdom

Karen Davies
Clinical Research Nurse Manager,
Institute for Ageing and Health,
Campus for Ageing and Vitality
Newcastle University,
United Kingdom

Angus Dawson
Senior Lecturer in Ethics and
Philosophy,
Centre for Professional Ethics,
School of Law,
Keele University,
United Kingdom

Diana Elbourne
Professor of Health Care Evaluation,
London School of Hygiene and Tropical
Medicine,
University of London,
United Kingdom

Jo Garcia
Senior Research Officer,
Social Science Research Unit,
University of London,
United Kingdom

Erica Haimes
Professor of Sociology and Professorial
Fellow,
Director of Policy, Ethics and Life
Sciences (PEALS) Research Institute,
Newcastle University,
United Kingdom

Nina Hallowell
Reader in Social Sciences
and Public Health,
Public Health Sciences,
University of Edinburgh,
United Kingdom

Søren Holm
Professorial Fellow in Bioethics,
Cardiff Law School, United Kingdom;
Section for Medical Ethics
University of Oslo,
Norway

Julian C. Hughes
Consultant and Honorary Clinical
Senior Lecturer
Institute for Ageing and Health
Newcastle University,
United Kingdom

Stephen John
Hughes Hall Centre for Biomedical
Science in Society, Hughes Hall,
University of Cambridge,
UK

Josephine Johnston
Research Scholar,
Director of Research Operations,
The Hastings Center,
New York,
U.S.A.

Thomas B.L. Kirkwood
Professor of Medicine,
Director,
Institute for Ageing and Health,
Campus for Ageing and Vitality
Newcastle University,
United Kingdom

Kathleen Liddell
University Lecturer,
Faculty of Law,
University of Cambridge,
United Kingdom

John McMillan
Senior Lecturer, Hull/York Medical
School and Philosophy Department,
University of Hull,
United Kingdom

Søren Madsen
Consultant Gastro-enterologist,
Køge University Hospital,
Denmark

Paul B. Miller
Assistant Professor,
Faculty of Law,
Queen's University,
Canada

Margaret Ponder
Research Associate,
Centre for Family Research,
University of Cambridge,
United Kingdom

Martin Richards
Emeritus Professor of Family Research,
Centre for Family Research,
University of Cambridge,
United Kingdom

Claire Snowdon
Lecturer London School of Hygiene and
Tropical Medicine, University of London
and Centre for Family Research,
University of Cambridge,
United Kingdom

Helen Statham
Deputy Director,
Centre for Family Research,
University of Cambridge,
United Kingdom

Lorraine Summerville
Doctoral Researcher,
School of Geography,
Politics and Sociology,
Newcastle University,
United Kingdom

James Tansey
Chair in Business Ethics,
W. Maurice Young Centre for Applied
Ethics and the Faculty of Commerce,
University of British Columbia,
Canada

Charles Weijer
Professor and Canada Research
Chair in Bioethics,
Department of Philosophy,
University of Western Ontario,
Canada

Introduction

Oonagh Corrigan, John McMillan,
and Charles Weijer

Informed consent has come to play a central role in research involving patients and non-patient-subjects. Since its appearance as the first principle of the Nuremberg Code in 1947 and particularly following renewed impetus during the 1960s, a plethora of ethics guidelines, policy mandates, legislation, and academic discussions have ensued (Faden and Beauchamp 1986). Indeed, one may wonder if there is need for 'yet another book' on informed consent. But this volume is not merely another collection of essays on the subject. The impetus for the book arose out of a concern among the editors that despite its ubiquitous nature, neither the nuances, complexities, and limitations of consent nor the implications of these had been fully explored. While there has been a growing awareness that gaining a research subject's authentic, fully informed consent is not easy to achieve in practice, solutions to the problem have tended to focus on ways to enhance the consent gaining process by improving the information given to prospective subjects and by allowing them sufficient time to consider such information (Flory and Emanuel 2004). Problems with consent are thus thought to be solved by improving consent. Furthermore, while there is a substantial established body of academic literature on consent and, more recently, on the experiences of patients in clinical research, such work often adopts a single disciplinary perspective.

One of the unique features of this book is that it explores issues related to consent from an interdisciplinary perspective and does so by situating them within the context of the various relationships where they take place. Specific features of the relationships within the context of medicine, such as those between researcher and patient, researcher and community, researcher and special population, and research institutions and the public are studied. The aim is not merely to analyse the 'limits of consent' but to examine issues beyond consent that too often the narrow focus on consent overlooks. Most importantly, we present a distinctive interdisciplinary perspective with contributions from the fields of moral philosophy, law, and the social sciences. In doing so, the book draws upon a diverse set of approaches and methodologies, including moral theorizing, legal analysis, and qualitative research. Interdisciplinarity has been fostered throughout. Initial chapters were redrafted following their presentation during a two-day workshop where they were discussed by the contributing authors and other experts. So while the contributors are experts within their respective disciplines, their work has also been influenced by feedback

and literature from other disciplines. The book's editors specialize in moral philosophy, law, and social science and have long-running commitments to an interdisciplinary bioethics endeavour and have worked collectively to ensure a cogent integration
of individual chapters. Furthermore, as the issue of consent has an international
standing in law, with North America often laying doing down paths in policy and
ethics that other counties have later followed, this volume presents work from the UK,
the United States, and Canada. However, while the book renders problematic many
issues associated with consent and urges consideration of ethical principles and
additional aspects other than consent, we do not advocate in any way a discarding or
diminishing of its significance. Indeed, we are very mindful of the historical lesson of
the importance of informed consent and the need to pay careful attention to the
welfare of human subjects in research.

History of consent

History shows us not only the necessity for consent but that the adoption of consent
practices in biomedical research was a hard fought battle. Following The Nuremberg
War Crime Trials where details of horrific experiments carried out on prisoners by
Nazi physicians were revealed, the Nuremberg Code (1947) was established as the first
international ethical statement of the principles that should regulate research. The
code was developed with the intention 'to ensure medical research could never again
be abused' (Porter 1997, 651). The first principle, which hitherto was to become the
primary bioethical consideration for all clinical research, stipulated 'the voluntary
consent of the human subject is absolutely essential' (Nuremberg Code 1947). Despite
what we now recognize as the historic nature of the document, the initial impact of
the Nuremberg Code on the conduct of medical research was minimal. In the first
two decades following the war, clinical researchers interpreted the document as an
indictment of Nazi atrocities and not as a guide relevant to their own activities
(Rothman 1991). It was further believed that the adoption of informed consent
would be an intrusion to the clinician/patient-subject relationship and would undermine medical authority (Katz 1996).

Medical organizations though were persistent and in 1964 the World Medical
Association produced the Declaration of Helsinki (World Medical Association 2004),
a more comprehensive set of guidelines that further emphasized the role of informed
consent.[1] However, the importance of consent really rose to the fore following revelations that emerged during the 1960s where it came to light that patients were often
taking part in research without adequate informed consent. Details of many such
cases were revealed by two whistleblowers, Maurice Pappworth (Pappworth 1967) in
the UK and Henry Beecher (Beecher 1970; Beecher 1966) in the US. Beecher, an
anaesthesiologist and respected clinical researcher, detailed in the *New England
Journal of Medicine* 22 examples of 'unethical or questionably ethical procedures' in
the medical literature (Beecher 1966).

---

[1] The Declaration of Helsinki was later updated and revised in 1975, 1983, 1989, 1996, 2000,
2002, and 2004.

In one study identified by Beecher, researchers at the Jewish Chronic Disease Hospital in Brooklyn, New York injected elderly patients with live cancer cells in order to test whether their immune systems would destroy the cells. According to the researchers, consent was obtained verbally but not documented. However, none of the patients were told that the injections contained cancerous cells. In another study, mentally challenged children in the Willowbrook State School in Long Island, New York were infected intentionally with the hepatitis A virus in order to develop a vaccine. Children early in the course of the study were fed stool extract from infected children in order to transmit the virus; later subjects were injected with the virus. The validity of parental consent in the study was criticized because children who were study participants were preferentially admitted into an otherwise overcrowded institution.

More than any other scandal, the Tuskegee syphilis study has left an indelible mark on the American psyche (Reverby 2000). It was the longest running study conducted by the US Public Health Service, lasting 40 years (1932-72), and involving 399 black men from Tuskegee, Alabama, suffering from syphilis and 201 uninfected control subjects. Despite the existence of effective, but toxic, treatment, no treatment was given to study subjects. From its inception, the study was based on racist precepts.

> The doctors who devised and directed the Tuskegee Study accepted the mainstream assumptions regarding blacks and venereal disease. The premise that blacks, promiscuous and lustful, would not seek or continue treatment, shaped the study. A test of untreated syphilis seemed 'natural' because the USPHS presumed the men would never be treated; the Tuskegee Syphilis Study made that a self-fulfilling prophecy.

> (Brandt 1978)

No informed consent was sought for study enrolment. Beyond this, subjects were deceived repeatedly during the study. At one point, spinal taps (the withdrawal of fluid from the spinal canal with a long needle) done purely for research purposes were described as 'special free treatment'. Even after the widespread availability of penicillin in the late 1940s, study subjects were neither told of nor offered treatment. As a consequence it is estimated that 20 per cent of study subjects died prematurely. Cases such as these prompted media attention and raised public concern leading to the implementation of further mechanisms to ensure the adherence of informed consent procedures.

Institutions in the US in particular were at the forefront of the establishment of new initiatives to protect research subjects. Following the revelations of unethical studies at Willowbrook and the Jewish Chronic Disease Hospital, in 1966, US Surgeon General Stewart mandated local peer review for ethical acceptability for all Public Health Service studies. Later federal regulations made it a legal requirement that biomedical research involving human subjects be subject to institutional review board (IRB) review. The establishment of IRBs in the US was soon followed by similar establishments in Canada (where the committees are called research ethics boards or REBs), the UK (research ethics committees or RECs), and other Western countries (McNeill 1993). The principal mandate for these committees was, and continues to be, the review of proposals to carry out research on patients or healthy persons within the medical environment. These bodies act as gatekeepers to safeguard the welfare of subjects in trials and ensure that prior informed consent is obtained from patients taking part in biomedical research. Following this, most medical journals have introduced ethics policies demanding that the research has been formally approved by a research ethics committee as a prerequisite for publication (International Committee of Medical Journal Editors 2008).

The revelation of the Tuskegee syphilis study by Jean Heller of the Associated Press in 1972 led rapidly to Senate hearings, chaired by Senator Ted Kennedy, into ethical standards for research with human beings. The Senate hearings had two major consequences. First, in 1974, the US federal government promulgated the first federal regulations governing the conduct of research. Current regulations, revised most recently in 2005, set out protections for human subjects in research that is federally funded or carried out at institutions who accept federal funds (Department of Health and Human Services 2008).

Second, the National Commission for the Protection of Human Subjects of Biomedical and Behavioral Research was created to examine ethical issues in research in detail. Over its four-year lifespan from 1974 to 1978, the National Commission produced 10 volumes of reports on a wide variety of topics. In its last report, the Belmont Report (1979), the National Commission articulates three moral principles to govern the conduct of human subjects research (National Commission for the Protection of Human Subjects of Biomedical and Behavioral Research 1979). The now famous ethical principles of respect for persons, beneficence, and justice remain central in the research ethics literature today. The first principle, respect for persons, emphasizes the concept of the 'autonomous agent' or 'individual capable of deliberation about personal goals and of acting under the direction of such deliberation.' The Belmont Report goes on to explain that to 'respect autonomy is to give weight to autonomous persons' considered opinions and choices while refraining from obstructing their actions unless they are clearly detrimental to others.' The primary implication of the principle of respect for persons is the requirement that research subjects give informed consent. Informed consent was further articulated to include the voluntary agreement of the subject to enter the study based on a disclosure of 'adequate' information about the study to the subject by the investigator. In order to be considered sufficient, information disclosed to subjects must generally include the research procedure, its purpose, anticipated benefits and harms, alternative treatments (where applicable), an invitation to ask any questions, and a statement that the subject may withdraw from the study at any time. Information must be presented to study subjects in a way that is best suited to their educational background and investigators have an obligation for 'ascertaining that the subject has comprehended the information.' While the Belmont Report also established the principles of beneficence and justice, undoubtedly it is informed consent that has since achieved the most persistent attention.

Despite US federal regulations and oversight of research by IRBs, scandal continues to dog medical research in the United States and concerns often involve whether appropriate informed consent was obtained. Discussions of cases, such as the much publicized death of a patient, Jesse Gelsinger, in a gene therapy trial (FDA and NIH 2000) and the death of a healthy volunteer subject who died as a result of taking part in a trial involving the inhalation of a chemical compound as part of an asthma study (Steinbrook 2002), tend to focus on the lack of information given to subjects regarding inherent risks, and breaches of the informed consent process (FDA and NIH 2000). Policy responses to such cases are inclined to result either in a tightening up of existing informed consent procedures or in the introduction of informed consent procedures where hitherto none had existed.

Since the 1980s, UK bodies such as the Royal College of Physicians, the Medical Research Council, the Association of the British Pharmaceutical Industry, the Royal College of Psychiatrists, the Royal College of Nursing Research Advisory Group, and the Department of Health have all produced various research ethics guidelines to aid both those carrying out research and the ethical review of such research. While such guidelines might be specific in their orientation, as for example the Royal College of Physicians' guidelines on 'Research on Healthy Volunteers' (Royal College of Physicians 1986), the advice given is in accordance with the Nuremberg Code and the Declaration of Helsinki. Although such guidance is seldom simplistic and provides information on ways to consider weighing up the relative risk and harms of proposed research there is evidence that research ethics committees have increasingly come to regard their main duty as ensuring prospective subjects understand the implication of taking part in the study. A UK survey of research ethics committee members revealed that attention to the informed consent process was regarded as the most important aspect of their work: more important than their duty to protect subjects from harm (Kent 1997).

Further evidence of the cultural dominance of consent is found in responses to recent medical scandals in the UK. Solutions to recent medical controversies, such as the retention of children's organs at Alder Hey Children's Hospital, have concentrated on the need for patients to be fully informed about procedures and their potential risks/hazards (Dyer 2000). In the case of Alder Hey Hospital Inquiry where organs and tissue from children who had died had often been removed, stored and used without proper consent was focused upon as the key problem. This led to a subsequent census by the Chief Medical Officer for England (2000) and the Isaacs Report (Department of Health 2003) which showed that storage and use of organs and tissue from both adults and children without proper consent has been widespread in the past. Ultimately a new Human Tissue Act 2004 (UK) was formulated making it an offence to carry activities on storage and use of whole bodies and human material (organs, tissues, and cells) without appropriate consent. While, as Kathleen Liddell (see Chapter 5 of this volume) argues, the Act has not established the centrality of consent as rigidly as it may appear on first reading, it nevertheless is another example of the way in which consent has become something of an 'ethical panacea' (Corrigan 2003).

In Canada, the ethical standards for research involving human subjects are set out in the *Tri-Council Policy Statement* (TCPS). In 1994, Canada's three main federal funding agencies, the Medical Research Council, Social Sciences and Humanities Research Council, and Natural Sciences and Engineering Research Council established the Tri-Council Working Group to draft a single set of guidelines to replace the patchwork of guidelines in existence at the time. In 1998, the TCPS was released and all universities and other research institutions who receive funds from any of the funding councils must abide by its provisions. Informed consent is a key protection for research subjects in the document. In most cases, the informed consent of the prospective research subject must be obtained, unless detailed provisions for exceptions from consent are fulfilled. Like their counterparts in the United States and the UK, Canadian Research Ethics Boards expend a great deal of their effort to ensure the consent process is adequate and information presented in the consent form is complete and comprehensible.

Despite these protections, Canada has not been immune from research controversy. The right of patient-subjects to be informed of new risks that emerge during the conduct of clinical trials was dramatically highlighted in case of Nancy Olivieri (Olivieri 2003; Thompson *et al.* 2001). Controversy arose when Dr. Olivieri, lead local researcher in a multi-centre clinical drug trial, issued revised consent forms in the middle of the study informing patients about evidence of unforeseen liver toxicity. The sponsoring pharmaceutical company, Apotex, challenged her right to do so and the University of Toronto and Hospital for Sick Children, which had commercial involvement with the company, failed to support her decision and indeed took action against her. While there are many interesting facets to this story, not least the issue of institutional conflict of interest, it is interesting to our discussion on consent that the only course of action that appeared to be open to Dr Olivieri was to inform patients. This further illustrates the importance of consent in protecting patients' welfare but at the same time is somewhat troubling insofar as it appears to have been the only means to do so.

The challenges for informed consent

While informed consent has clearly been in the ascendancy and, as the brief history we have outlined shows, this is not without good reason, there have been growing concerns about the need to understand the ways in which it is experienced in practice. Furthermore, while the main function of consent as articulated in research ethics guidelines, is to facilitate an individual's freedom of choice, respect their autonomy, and thus ensure their welfare as research participants, as philosophers Søren Holm and Søren Madsen argue in Chapter One, the role of consent has become additionally burdened. Drawing upon the actual experiences of those taking part in research they argue that the increasing breadth of information relating not simply to medically related interventions but to issues such as data protection, make unnecessary demands of those taking part in research, and increase the complexity of their decision-making process.

One way of taking the ethics of clinical research forward and isolating the ethical obligations researchers have to participants is by analysing the nature of the physician-researcher and patient-subject relationship. In Chapter Two, lawyer and philosopher Paul Miller and philosopher and physician Charles Weijer argue that understanding the relationship as one of trust entails a set of beneficence obligations above and beyond requirements for informed consent.

In Chapter Three, Paul Miller and Josie Johnstone undertake a legal analysis of the law of consent in human experimentation in Canada and the United States and trace out potential avenues of liability. Just what the role of consent is legally, and what limits may be placed on its use as a defence by the researcher, turns on whether the question is posed as one of the law of negligence, law of contract, or law of fiduciary duty. Considerable uncertainty remains in the law as to which of these regimes is likely to be applied by the courts in a given case.

In Chapter Four, social scientist Clare Snowdon and colleagues examine the decisions of parents of critically ill babies who had not consented to take part in research. Their decisions were based on a misunderstanding of the information they had been given. This chapter suggests that patients may be overburdened with information and perhaps in this kind of case better decisions could be facilitated by providing less information rather than more.

Perhaps the most significant legal development for research ethics in England and Wales is the Human Tissue Act 2004. In Chapter Five, lawyer Kathleen Liddell explains the way that debate about the content of this Act was dominated by a preoccupation with the necessity of consent for the use of human tissue. She argues that while consent appeared to function as the legal panacea in fact the legal position that was adopted was more subtle than the initial debates would have suggested and uses methods of legitimation that go beyond consent.

In Chapter Six, philosopher Angus Dawson argues that moral arguments regarding consent must take seriously the evidence relating to the ways consent is experienced by those it sets out to consider. If consent is designed to promote autonomy and fails to do so in practice then moral arguments need to be refined. As we have argued, the principle of respect for persons the moral rule of informed consent have achieved a pre-eminent role in practice. Although the standard articulation of research principles does not privilege one principle over another, other principles such as beneficence and justice as articulated in the Belmont Report have in practice been trumped by respect for persons (Wolpe 1998).

One way to move research ethics forward is to think carefully about the reasons we have to take part in medical research. In Chapter Seven, philosopher Stephen John argues that given certain assumptions about the kind of research under consideration, citizens sharing the benefit of medical research have a moral obligation to take part in research themselves. This argument is important because, if cogent, it might provide reasons for not being unduly concerned about the difficulties in getting adequately informed consent.

The next three chapters consider some of the challenges for consent presented by conducting research within mental health. In Chapter Eight, physician Julian Hughes and colleagues argue that the virtues of the researcher are crucial when conducting research with people with dementia. Consent is often particularly problematic with this group and for research to proceed, it must occur within a caring relationship that is structured by appropriate professional virtues. In Chapter Nine, lawyer Philip Bielby argues that legal approaches need to go beyond neatly sorting agents into those who have the capacity to consent and those who do not. He presents a number of arguments for the importance of supporting those for whom consent may be particularly difficult. In Chapter Ten, social scientist Margaret Ponder and colleagues consider the ethical issues that arose in a qualitative study conducted with men who had an intellectual disability. They relate a number of practical difficulties that they faced and question the assumption that it was appropriate for this group of participants to be included in the study.

Chapters Eleven and Twelve illustrate the extent to which the individualist view that underlies standard conceptions of autonomy fails when research involves families or communities. Social scientist Nina Hallowell (Chapter Eleven) shows how individuals with breast cancer who consent to take part in genetic testing do so out of an overriding sense of obligation to other kin members. Similarly, drawing upon interviews with members of canada's first nation communities, philosophers Mike Burgess and James Tansay show that community interests often override an individual's autonomy and that the informed consent model can often not adequately account for collective interests.

In the book's conclusion, Kathleen Liddell and Martin Richards then draw together the threads of these various chapters and further develop analysis to encourage thinking beyond consent. One of the main aims of this book is to move beyond a reification of consent and to consider more fully the needs, rights, and indeed the obligations of the subjects or participants of research and the researchers. Research subjects or research participants (Corrigan and Tutton 2006) as they have recently been referred to, however expert and knowledgeable, are reliant on the expertise, integrity, and trustworthiness of those conducting research and on systems of governance. The consent process cannot be the only means by which the rights and welfare of patients and healthy volunteers are protected. The hope, trust, and willingness of those participating in research demands that those conducting research and the systems of governance relating to ethics and oversight ensure that participants are not exploited and are treated with the due respect they deserve.

References

Beecher, H. (1966). Ethics and clinical research. *New England Journal of Medicine*, **274**, 1354–60.

–ibid.– (1970). *Research and the Individual Human Studies*. Boston: Little Brown.

Brandt, A. (1978). The case of the Tuskegee syphilis experiment. *Hastings Center Report*, **8**, 21–9.

Corrigan, O. (2003). Empty ethics: The problem with informed consent. *Sociology of Health and Illness* **25**, 768–92.

Corrigan, O. and Tutton, T. (2006). What's in a name? Subjects, volunteers, participants and activists in clinical research. *Clinical Ethic*, **1**, 101–4.

Department of Health (2003). 'The Isaacs Report.' http://www.archive2.official-documents.co.uk/reps/isaacs00/isaacs00.htm [accessed 14/5/08].

Department of Health and Human Services (2008). 'Protection of Human Subjects.' Website: http://www.hhs.gov/ohrp/humansubjects/guidance/45cfr46.htm [accessed 11/5/08].

Dyer, C. (2000). Consent needed for organ retention, BMA says. *British Medical Journal* **321**,1098a.

Faden, R. and Beauchamp, T. (1986). *A History and Theory of Informed Consent*. New York: Oxford University Press.

FDA and NIH (2000). New initiatives to protect participants in gene therapy trials. *HHS News*, March 7, 2000.

Flory, J. and Emanuel, E. (2004). Interventions to improve research participants' understanding in informed consent for research. *Journal of American Medical Association*, **292**, 1593–1601.

International Committee of Medical Journal Editors (2008). Uniform requirements for manuscripts submitted to biomedical journals: Writing and editing for biomedical publication. Website http://www.icmje.org/ [accessed 11/5/08].

Katz, J. (1996). Human sacrifice and human experimentation: Reflections at Nuremberg. In *Occasional Papers* http://lsr.nellco.org/cgi/viewcontent.cgi?article=1006&context=yale/ylsop [accessed 11/05/08]. Yale Law School.

Kent, G. (1997). The views of members of Local Research Ethics Committees, researchers and members of the public towards the roles and functions of LRECs. *Journal of Medical Ethics*, **23**, 186–90.

McNeill, P. (1993). *The Ethics and Politics of Human Experimentation*. Cambridge: Cambridge University Press.

National Commission for the Protection of Human Subjects of Biomedical and Behavioral Research (1979). *The Belmont Report: Ethical Principles and Guidelines for the Protection of Human Subjects of Research*. Washington, DC: U.S. Government Printing Office.

Olivieri, N. (2003). Patients' health or company profits? The commercialisation of academic research. *Science and Engineering Ethics*, **9**, 29–41.

Pappworth, M. (1967). *Human Guinea Pigs*. Middlesex, England: Penguin Books.

Porter, R. (1997). *The Greatest Benefit to Mankind*. London: HarperCollins.

Reverby, S. (2000). *Tuskegee's Truths: Rethinking the Tuskegee Syphilis Study*. Chapel Hill, North Carolina: University of North Carolina Press.

Rothman, D. (1991). *Strangers at the Bedside*. USA: Basic Books.

Royal College of Physicians (1986). *Research on Healthy Volunteers*. London: The Royal College of Physicians.

Steinbrook, R. (2002). Protecting research subjects – the crisis at John Hopkins. *New England Journal of Medicine*, **346**, 716–20.

Thompson, J., Baird, P. and Downie, J. (2001). *The Olivieri Report: The Complete Text of the Report of the Independent Inquiry Commissioned by the Canadian Association of University Teachers*. Toronto: James Lorimer and Company Ltd.

Wolpe, P. (1998). The triumph of autonomy in American bioethics: a sociological view. In *Bioethics and Society*, Raymond DeVries and Janardan Subedi (Eds). New Jersey: Prentice Hall.

World Medical Association (2004). *Declaration of Helsinki: Ethical Principles for Medical Research Involving Human Subjects*. http://www.wma.net/e/policy/b3.htm

Chapter 1

Informed consent in medical research – a procedure stretched beyond breaking point?

Søren Holm and Søren Madsen

1.1 Introduction

In this chapter, we want to consider the question of whether the institutionalized and formalized practice of informed consent in the context of clinical research has been stretched beyond breaking point. Do we now ask participants for consent to so many very different things that it becomes unclear what we have actually got valid, informed consent for? The chapter will not discuss consent outside of the research context; it will give an ethical and not a legal analysis of the issues. When in some places we quote and interpret legal texts, the analysis provided is thus philosophical and aimed at making a philosophical point. It is not intended to settle or even illuminate legal questions in any particular jurisdiction.

We will focus on those kinds of research where the potential participants are patients (i.e., not healthy volunteers) and where they have some important health interest at stake, usually because they have a serious illness and the research project is a trial of a new therapy. This kind of research includes the standard, double blind, randomized trial, as well as a range of other trial designs. We have chosen this focus for two reasons: (1) our own empirical research concerns this kind of trial, triangulating questionnaires and long qualitative interviews with participants in cancer and inflammatory bowel disease trials (Madsen *et al.* 1999, 2000a and b, 2002, 2007a and b), and (2) we think that this kind of research raises specific problems for the process of informed consent.

We will first give a brief account of the concept of informed consent and of its possible philosophical justifications. In this section, we will also try to understand why informed consent has become such a popular way of transferring rights from research participants to researchers and why it has been extended to cover new areas of rights transfers and new research practices.

In the next section, we will analyse what is known about the way in which potential trial participants make their decisions concerning whether or not to participate and we will consider the implications of this knowledge for informed consent.

Finally, we will provide a more theoretical discussion of whether informed consent is the right kind of transfer mechanism for rights to control health information or tissue samples.

1.2 **Informed consent – a brief account**

The concept of informed consent is a cornerstone in modern medical research ethics and has almost reached the position of an infallible dogma (Faden and Beauchamp 1986). It was enunciated by the Nuremberg war crimes tribunal in their judgement of the Nazi doctors who had conducted experiments with prisoners in the concentration camps. It has been a foundational principle in all the versions of the Helsinki Declaration of the World Medical Association. The concept of informed consent is a part of most national legislation concerning medical research (although the French interestingly use the term 'enlightened consent') and it is used in the Oviedo Convention of the Council of Europe (Council of Europe 1997). This almost universal acceptance is not surprising since the principle of informed consent has roots in very old legal traditions concerning unconsented touchings of the body and it also seems to be intuitively plausible.

The basic idea of informed consent is that a researcher is only (ethically and/or legally) justified in using a research subject in a project if the research subject has consented to being so used.

For a consent to be a valid informed consent four elements must be present:

1. The relevant information has been given;
2. The relevant information has been understood;
3. The person is capable of consenting;
4. The person is uncoerced.

The two last elements make an, often tacit, assumption explicit by pointing out that a valid consent has to be voluntary, and it has to be given by somebody who is psychologically capable of consenting.

It is important to note that there are several quite different ethical justifications of the principle of informed consent. According to deontological ethics, informed consent is primarily a way of explicating the more basic duty of respect for autonomy in the research context. The principle of informed consent simply tells us what we should do if we want to respect the autonomy or right to self-determination of the research subjects. According to consequentialist theory, the principle of informed consent is justified as a rule of thumb or a lower level rule, because adhering to the principle will overall and in the long run lead to maximization of good consequences. A consequentialist could, for instance, point out: (1) that people want to have their self-determination respected and that respecting autonomy, therefore, leads to greater wellbeing, and (2) that public acceptance of medical research is important for the continuation of this kind of research and that such public acceptance would erode if people thought that they were being deceived by medical researchers.

According to both these justifications, informed consent can at most be a necessary condition for enrolling research subjects. If we also want informed consent to be a sufficient condition we will have to invoke a stronger principle of personal choice, where nothing can override the choices I make. This view is held by so-called 'libertarians', but it is not a principle that we usually accept in designing public policies.

Few would accept that healthy people should be allowed to consent to research projects with a major risk of death or disability, even if the outcomes of these projects are very important. It, therefore, seems safe to conclude that informed consent cannot be a sufficient condition for the acceptability of including subjects in a research project. Even those who argue that research ethics committees should not be paternalistic accept that there is some limit of the risk to which an individual can consent. Edwards *et al.*, for instance, argue against research ethics committee paternalism but state that '… there is no reason why RECs should be more restrictive than the "normal" constraints on people taking risks with themselves …' (Edwards *et al.* 2004, p. 89) thereby accepting some upper level on voluntarily assumed risk.

A supplementary justification for requiring informed consent is that through the consent process the individual prospective research subjects are able to apply their own values in the assessment of the benefits and burdens of the research. This is important because the idea that there is an 'objective' assessment of benefits and burdens applicable to all persons is problematic. There can legitimately be quite different ideas about whether the benefits outweigh the burdens, both when this is seen from a personal point of view and also seen from an impersonal point of view. This can be shown formally within the framework of rational choice theory, but can also be brought out by two banal examples. To a member of the religious society of Jehovah's Witnesses the fact that a project will improve blood transfusion techniques is not a positive benefit; and to a person with severe needle phobia (or a very low pain threshold) the fact that a project involves 'only' two extra blood samplings may be a major burden. A somewhat less banal example is that some persons may simply not value medical progress very highly. Some may simply be content with the present state of medical knowledge (as expressed in the dictum 'progress is an optional goal') and for them the balancing of benefits and burdens will again differ from that of medical researchers who usually value progress highly (Jonas 1969).

A more difficult problem in research ethics is whether informed consent is a necessary condition for the ethical acceptability of a research project. Or to put the converse question: 'Are there research projects where informed consent is not necessary?'.

It is obvious that if respect for autonomy is an absolute value or an absolute foundational moral principle, then there can be no ethically acceptable research projects without informed consent (at least if we accept the derivation of informed consent from respect for autonomy and this seems uncontroversial). However, no reasonable morality could hold respect for autonomy as an absolute principle, and most actual ethical systems encompass respect for autonomy as a value that can be balanced against other values. But from the general conclusion that informed consent *may not* always be necessary, we cannot infer the specific conclusion that informed consent *is not* necessary in a specific context without adducing further arguments.

A first attempt at providing such an argument could base itself on an assertion of equality between the treatment context and the research context. In the treatment context we in many cases give far less information than in the research context, and it could be claimed that there is not a sufficient difference between these two situations to warrant a difference in the consent process and in the information we should give.[1]

This assertion is, however, problematic. This is most easily seen if we consider randomized controlled trials, but the argument can be generalized to a range of other types of research. The testing of new therapies in randomized controlled trials does raise specific problems concerning informed consent. When we start a randomized trial, we are in a situation where we have reason to believe, but do not know for certain, that the new intervention will be effective (or more effective than the presently used treatment). The person asked to participate in a trial, therefore, has to make this decision in a context of larger uncertainty than in the normal therapeutic context. The experimental and the therapeutic context also differ with regard to the interests of the doctor/researcher. In the idealized therapeutic context, the doctor's only interest is the benefit of the patient. In the research context, the doctor is also interested in generating knowledge that may benefit future patients (even if the project shows that the new therapy is dangerous, this is a benefit to *future* patients, who may then avoid it).

These differences between research and treatment entail that we cannot just assume that the amount of information and the consent procedure should be the same in the two contexts. Why has informed consent become so important and popular in research ethics? There are probably a number of interrelated reasons. First, on the face of it, informed consent is a very simple device: 'I tell you what I want to do to you, you give me permission to do these things by your consent, and I am, therefore, absolved from a range of liabilities that would follow if I did not have your consent' (or alternatively some share of the responsibility for bad moral luck has been transferred from me to you (Dickenson 2003)[2] along the lines of the age-old principle of *volenti non fit injuria*.

Secondly, the informed consent mechanism does not involve any overt economic transaction: 'I do not give you anything of monetary value for your participation, and you do not give me anything of monetary value in order to participate'. By choosing informed consent as the mechanism for participation, the actual *quid pro quo* often involved in trial participation can be hidden from view and the crass world of commerce and contracts kept at bay (hence also the fiction that we only *compensate* healthy volunteers for their inconvenience).

Finally, informed consent conveniently obscures the power relationship between researchers and potential participants. Giving informed consent to research is often

---

[1] It is important not to conflate the issue of whether there should be a different consent process and more information in the research context with the separate issue of whether there should be specific ethical scrutiny of research projects (e.g., through an elaborate and often time-consuming research ethics committee system).

[2] Moral luck occurs when an agent may be treated as an object of moral judgment despite the fact that the actual occurrence of what he or she is assessed for depends on factors beyond his or her control. In the present case, the occurrence of severe side-effects of the trial medication is not under the investigator's control, but he or she is never the less morally responsible for it.

the only way in which a patient can get a treatment that he or she believes is the best, or can gain access to a more satisfactory follow-up regime (e.g., one where he or she will meet fewer and more well-informed doctors).

1.2.1 Extensions to the scope of informed consent

In recent decades, informed consent procedures have been 'chosen' as the mechanism for including participants in non-clinical research, involving very little bodily intervention e.g., epidemiological or most recently biobank research. This is not the focus of the present chapter. We focus on the considerable extension of the scope of informed consent in clinical research.

Today, informed consent may cover a wide range of issues in clinical research:

1. The permission for the researcher to perform certain interventions on the patient, to record data about the patient and his or her reaction to these interventions, and to obtain and analyse biological samples from the patient;

2. The permission to retain biological samples for later analysis;

3. The necessary permissions under the Data Protection Act 1998 (UK) or similar legislation in other jurisdictions for the retention of data and their analysis;

4. The necessary permissions under the Data Protection Act 1998 (UK) for data to be transferred to other jurisdictions;

5. The transfer of property rights in, and the assignment of intellectual property (IP) rights flowing from, the data and biological samples;

6. The necessary permissions for the transfer of information between the investigator and the sponsor;

7. The necessary permissions for the transfer of information between the investigator, the sponsor, and regulatory agencies, including the permissions for regulatory agencies to inspect patient records.

The involved actors either explicitly or implicitly taking part in the consent process may include:

a. The research participant;

b. The researcher in direct contact with the patient (e.g., a junior member of hospital staff);

c. The investigator (e.g., a senior member of staff);

d. The sponsor (e.g., a pharmaceutical firm);

e. A contract research organization;

f. The regulatory authorities (e.g., the authorities licensing health professionals, the authorities policing scientific fraud, and the drug licensing authorities).[3]

---

[3] All of these authorities are implicit participants in the consent process because they set the framework for consent (with regard to both content and process) and police transgressions of this framework.

Informed consent was initially developed to cover the set of permissions listed in 1 and 2 above, and was fairly similar to informed consent for diagnosis or treatment, although there was a greater emphasis on full information for reasons discussed above. Informed consent was something happening between a researcher and his or her research subjects and aimed at governing their relationship.

The extensions to cover permissions for information flow (3, 4, 6 and 7 in the list above) and for the transfer of potentially economically important rights (list item 5) are aimed at achieving very different purposes and [to govern] very different relationships (i.e., with parties outside the researcher – research subject relationship).

This raises problems of three kinds:

1. Certain of these permissions and transfers would usually not be governed by consent, but by other means of transfer or agreement if they took place between entities that were not situated as researcher and research subject.[4] If two entities want to exchange commercially valuable biological samples they would for instance usually sign a Materials Transfer Agreement which would be an often complicated, legal document stating the conditions of the transfer in great detail.

2. It is unlikely that medical doctors or other biomedical researchers are capable of explaining the meaning of the permissions and transfers to potential research subjects, thereby casting doubt on the idea of 'informed consent' for these parts of the consent (most doctors are probably not well versed in the intricacies of IP law or the potential for research records to be subpoenaed and are, therefore, for example unable to tell patients what they are actually giving up).

3. The conflation of all the permissions in one document may mislead the potential research subjects, who are likely to focus on the medical parts to the exclusion of what they might regard as add-ons of secondary importance.

The last of these problems is further compounded by the fact that the informed consent process almost always only gives the potential participant one choice to make, that is, the choice of whether to participate in one particular study, with no choice to opt out of specific components of the study, and no choice between different studies. The trial is thus presented as a complete package of different components that cannot be unbundled by the participant.

1.3 Patient decision-making in clinical research

In recent years, our knowledge about what happens during the informed consent process and how patients make decisions concerning whether to participate in clinical trials have grown considerably (Featherstone and Donovan 1998, 2002; Snowdon, Garcia, and Elbourne 1997; Elbourne, Snowdon, and Garcia 1997; Appelbaum *et al.* 1982, 1987; Jensen *et al.* 1993; Madsen *et al.* 1999, 2000, 2000a, b 2002).

---

[4] Any use of samples from UK Biobank by outside researchers will, for instance, require a Materials Transfer Agreement (UK Biobank 2006, section 2.8.4, 'Access agreements and fees').

Our own research, as well as the research of others, shows that patients who are asked to participate in a clinical trial engage in a complex decision-making process. Patients try to make sense of the trial itself, of the rationale for the trial, of the trial interventions and of the randomization process, and they try to make the decision that is right for them (Madsen, Holm, and Riis 2007a; Snowdon, Garcia, and Elbourne 1997; Featherstone and Donovan 1998, 2002). One of our respondents put it in the following way:

… What is this about, which consequences can there be, which side-effects are there for me, where is my disease related to the risks I'd put myself in … You need to know what you are opposing. At least, I am … If I face that situation at another time, and I cannot see that it specifically is better for me to choose one from the other, then I would say YES …

[Breast cancer, declined trial participation]

The research clearly shows that the parts of the whole trial set up that patients primarily focus on in this decision-making process are the trial treatments, their effectiveness and side-effects, and the allocation process. Other features of the trial are regarded as peripheral to the main decision: 'will participation in this trial maximize my personal chances of getting better?'. Our data on choice shows that this is the most important consideration both for those who participate (who tend to focus on the benefits of the new treatment) and those who decline participation (who tend to focus on the side-effects or on the uncertainty). Almost all patients actually develop a treatment preference during the information process and do not believe that there is equipoise (Madsen, Holm, and Riis 2007a; Snowdon, Garcia, and Elbourne 1997; Featherstone and Donovan 2002).

The decision is furthermore made in a context where most patients feel that they do not have all the necessary information (without necessarily being able to specify in detail what information they would like to have) and where many feel very lonely. In our grounded theory analysis of interviews with oncology trial participants and patients who have declined participation, the 'loneliness of autonomy' emerges as one of the core categories. The perceived informative insufficiency and the loneliness in the decision situation means that patients realize that they have to rely on the doctors and other health professionals, and that it becomes extremely important in their decision-making whether they trust the doctors, and whether they feel that the health professionals really care about them as persons (Figure 1.1 shows our model of the decision-making process) (Madsen, Holm, and Riis 2007a). In our interviews with cancer patients and patients with inflammatory bowel disease considerations of the eventual fate of the data and samples collected during the trial played only a negligible role in the constant weighing up of benefits and burdens of trial participation. A woman who declined trial participation despite being positive to trials in general described her reasoning in the following way, emphasizing the paramount importance of the immediate perceived clinical situation for her choice:

I see – using my common sense – the necessity of the trial, because that's the way you get things developed, get new knowledge and so forth, but in the situation, when it's yourself standing in it … It became entirely different for me … It was a shocking experience to realize that now it was personal and I couldn't participate. I was shocked that I couldn't

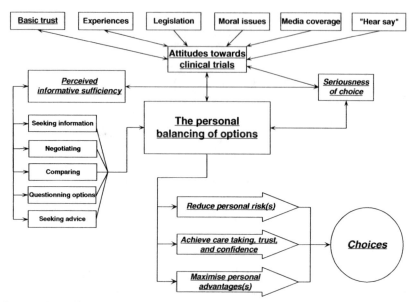

Fig. 1.1 The personal balancing of options performed by cancer patients in relation to choices throughout treatment courses inside and/or outside a clinical cancer trial (breast cancer and ovarian cancer).

contribute in helping others … I would very much have liked to do that, but I wasn't capable of it … I felt like a piece in a jigsaw … they were going to draw lots about whether I should have the best or the second best treatment … to compare and find out who survives and who dies … you see black and white only … For me it was about life and death also if you put it sharply … due to that, I wanted to choose myself. No drawing of lots should decide what should happen with my life …

[Breast cancer, declined trial participation]

And a woman who accepted participation put it as follows:

I don't think you realize, that your life is in a chaos, when you get such a diagnosis. I couldn't – if it was high or low or what, I could in no way figure it out at all. I just thought that it was all over … You don't know if you have said YES or NO, and you don't know what it is you've accepted …

[Breast cancer, accepted trial participation]

This focus on the clinical situation is not surprising. When a person has a serious or even life-threatening condition and a decision has to be made about trial participation, it is natural that the condition will take priority.

In summary, what patients focus on are the areas of the research that were core to the original concept of informed consent (the bodily interventions, the treatments, and the actual trial procedures). If we could find ways of dealing with the perceived insufficiency of information and with the loneliness experienced by many patients, there is good reason to believe that patients could give their fully informed and considered consent to participation and to the various procedures directly involved in the trial. We are not claiming that all potential research subjects can give informed consent or refusal if the informed consent process is optimized. We are only claiming that a substantial proportion of potential research subjects can give informed consent if the process is optimized. Our claim, furthermore, only applies in circumstances where there is sufficient time for the information process. It, therefore, does not apply to much research in emergency settings.

However, with regard to other areas of the research for which patients give consent as part of the whole bundled package of trial participation, the findings have clear negative implications for the empirical validity of the informed consent. We know that there are aspects of the trial that play no role in patients' decision-making about whether or not to participate and that these aspects are not trivial (e.g., because they are matters that in other contexts do interest people, influence their decisions, and are seen as very important) so we can put very little weight on the fact that the participants have signed a consent form where these aspects are mentioned. The consent is merely a convenient legal fiction.

Against this position it can be argued that it is a common occurrence in many other areas of life that we make agreements where only some part of the total consequences of our agreements is the focus for our decision-making, but that such agreements are nevertheless valid in their totality. Why should we, therefore, worry about this problem in the context of medical research? The main reason is in our view that informed consent for the kind of research we discuss here is often an agreement between parties of very unequal power.

Doctors possess various forms of power (Mechanic 1968; Brody 1993), including significant social power and status and this power does not disappear when doctors become researchers. It is in recognition of this fact that all research ethics regulations incorporate some version of article II.4 in the original 1964 version of the Helsinki Declaration: 'The refusal of the patient to participate in a study must never interfere with the physician–patient relationship.'

If the agreement concerning trial participation was a contract between parties of equal bargaining power, we might be inclined to think that we should uphold this legal fiction under some modified *caveat emptor* principle, but the informed consent device is very explicitly framed as not being a contract (see above) and the parties are usually not of equal bargaining power.

Furthermore, in standard contracts between consumers and firms, specific provisions in the contracts can be declared invalid even if the consumer has explicitly agreed to them, if they are deemed to be unfair and an abuse of the bargaining power of the firm. The 1993 EU directive on 'unfair terms in consumer contracts' (93/13/EEC of 5 April 1993), for instance, states in Articles 3.1 and 3.2:

Article 3

1. A contractual term which has not been individually negotiated shall be regarded as unfair if, contrary to the requirement of good faith, it causes a significant imbalance in the parties' rights and obligations arising under the contract, to the detriment of the consumer.

2. A term shall always be regarded as not individually negotiated where it has been drafted in advance and the consumer has, therefore, not been able to influence the substance of the term, particularly in the context of a pre-formulated standard contract.

The fact that certain aspects of a term or one specific term have been individually negotiated shall not exclude the application of this Article to the rest of a contract if an overall assessment of the contract indicates that it is nevertheless a pre-formulated standard contract.

Where any seller or supplier claims that a standard term has been individually negotiated, the burden of proof in this respect shall be incumbent on him.'

If this common contractual standard was applied to consent documents, many might be found to be unfair. Among the examples mentioned as unfair in an appendix to the Directive are, for instance, 'irrevocably binding the consumer to terms with which he had no real opportunity of becoming acquainted before the conclusion of the contract' or '… permitting the seller or supplier to retain the sums paid for services not yet supplied by him where it is the seller or supplier himself who dissolves the contract'. In consent documents, both these examples occur. In pharmaceutical trials under Good Clinical Practice guidelines, consent is often given to unspecified future access to personal data for regulatory authorities and that consent is usually taken to be irrevocable. Even if the research subject chooses to exercise her right to withdraw from the trial she cannot revoke her permission to allow this access to her data. And promises to provide the trial drug after the end of the trial can be revoked by the sponsor, without having to ask the former research subjects whether they then want some of their data back.

1.4 Informed consent and the transfer of rights

As part of informed consent to clinical research the patient does, as noted above, usually waive or transfer a number of rights to the researcher, to the sponsor of the research, and/or to the regulatory authorities responsible for regulating pharmaceutical products or therapeutic devices. The rights that are waived or transferred almost always include rights to control certain kinds of health information in order to make it lawful for the various parties to obtain, store, export and process sensitive data concerning the participants ('information rights'). But other rights may also be transferred, including rights concerning the control and use of tissue or blood samples collected during the trial ('tissue rights'), and the transfer of tissue also involves physical transfer of material.

Above we have discussed the issue of whether potential participants really consent to these transfers of rights, but here we want to discuss a more basic theoretical problem, that is, whether informed consent is the right process for the transfer of these rights and materials. It may be objected that there is no transfer of rights in the consent situation, but only a temporary or permanent waiver of rights or a giving of permission. However, nothing in our arguments below hinge on whether one or the other of these descriptions is correct.

Outside of the biomedical context the transfer of information rights from individuals to organisations is often handled by informed consent, partly because this is required by data protection legislation for all kinds of sensitive personal information, whereas transfer of materials or rights to the use of materials are most often handled by other transfer mechanisms (e.g., a gift does not involve informed consent), and between strangers the most common of these is probably contract (written or oral). Any further transfer of both kinds of rights between organizations usually involves contracts.

Is there any reason why a contract between the participant and the relevant party, who will often not be the researcher but the sponsor, could not govern the transfer of information and tissue rights in clinical research? One problem could be that contracts often involve money or a bilateral exchange of valuable goods and that that could be seen as inimical to the relationship between the researcher and the patient.[5] But as already noted there is a *quid pro quo* in many kinds of clinical research, and the relationship that such a contract would govern would be between the participant and the real beneficiary of the transfer of rights (i.e., often the sponsor). A contract would thus just make the real state of affairs transparent.

What kind of advisor would be suitable to give impartial, comprehensive, and accurate advice concerning the transfer of these kinds of rights? We will not dwell on the long-standing discussion of whether or not researchers can give impartial information concerning participation in their own research projects. Because even if we accept that researchers can give impartial advice, we would not have answered the question of whether they are likely to be able to give comprehensive and accurate advice about the transfer of information or tissue rights. There are reasons to doubt that the average medical doctor or other health professional is well suited to give comprehensive and accurate information concerning the full implications of consent to transfer information or tissue rights. Most health professionals are not well versed in the intricacies of data protection legislation, the parts of pharmaceutical regulations governing the access of regulators to primary data supporting licensing applications, or the various rules governing the transfer of and trade in biological samples. For instance, how many health professionals know under what conditions data and tissue samples can be transferred to other countries when there is initial consent to their collection and processing?

There are also specific situations where the biological materials that are transferred are or are likely to become valuable in themselves and not just valuable as part of a large biobank. Again it is unclear whether a health professional is the best person to ask about the implications of what is essentially a property transfer.[6] In any further transfer of this sample, there will most likely be a detailed material transfer

---

5 In some jurisdictions, the exchange of a 'consideration' is a necessary element of a legally valid contract.

6 We do not want to enter the very large discussion of whether there can be property rights in the human body as such or in tissue samples. We do, however, think that this issue is far less settled in principle than is usually assumed. Many institutions, firms and persons, for instance, own and trade human skeletons (see for instance http://www.skullsunlimited.com/humanskeletonnb.htm); and there is a simple way for any of us to gain legal ownership of our own tissue samples (apart from by making them part of a work of art). If you donate your tissue sample to a biobank and then buy it back from the bank, you will become the legal owner of your own sample.

agreement, or a contract of sale drawn up by the lawyers of the two parties to the transfer, and no-one would think that the best person to ask for information and advice is a health care professional.

Both from the point of view of the exchange in itself and from the point of view of information and advice concerning the exchange, there are thus good reasons why the standard practice of informed consent may not be the most suitable means of transaction concerning information and tissue rights.

It could, therefore, be argued that these parts of the clinical research package should be unbundled insofar as this is possible, and as a minimum made the subject of a completely independent informed consent process, or perhaps made part of a separate contractual or quasi-contractual agreement.

1.5 Conclusion

In this chapter, we have argued that although there are problems with informed consent even in its core function of providing permission for the bodily and other therapeutic interventions in a trial, and in some cases for randomization, these problems are not insurmountable and a proper informed consent process could be brought to work. However, there are both empirical and theoretical reasons to believe that informed consent is much less suited as a process for the transfer of information or tissue rights. It may, therefore, be time to cleanse the informed consent process of these more recent accretions and get back to basics.

How this can be done in practice is a complicated question. A modest suggestion is that the primary consent should only cover the core of the clinical trial (e.g., the randomization, the treatments, the additional tests, the strictly necessary future access to the patient's records). If the patient consents to this, the patient should be allowed to participate in the trial. Any consent to additional access to records or to long-term storage, and use of tissue samples should be optional. It should be discussed with the patient at a later stage when the patient is in a better position to decide and time is no longer an important factor, and refusal should not jeopardize trial participation.

Conflicts of interest

Both authors are medical doctors, but do not think that that in itself constitutes a conflict of interest.

Acknowledgements

The authors wish to acknowledge Professor Povl Riis, D.M.Sc., who has collaborated with us throughout our studies of the consent and trial process.

Our studies were made possible by grants from (alphabetically): Aage Louis-Hansen's Foundation; Anna and Jakob Jakobsen's Foundation; AstraZeneca Inc.; Beckett-Foundation; Danish Foundation of Cancer Research; Danish Medical Research Council; Danish Research Council for the Humanities; Desirée and Niels Yde's Foundation; Emil C. Hertz and spouse Inger Hertz' Foundation; Ferring Inc.; Glaxo Wellcome Inc.; Hede Nielsen's Foundation; Jacob Madsen's and Olga Madsen's

Foundation; Danish Hospital Foundation for Medical Research. Region of Copenhagen, the Faroe Islands and Greenland; Ove Villiam Buhl Olesen and Edith Buhl Olesen's Foundation; Sigrid Rigmor Moran's Foundation; The Foundation of 1870 and Vibeke Binder and Povl Riis' Foundation.

References

Appelbaum, P.S., Roth, L.H., and Lidz, C. (1982). The therapeutic misconception: informed consent in psychiatric research. *International Journal of Law and Psychiatry*, **5**, no. 3–4, 319–329.

Appelbaum, P.S., Roth, L.H., Lidz, C.W., Benson, P., and Winslade, W. (1987). False hopes and best data: consent to research and the therapeutic misconception. *Hastings Centre Report*, **17**, no. 2, 20–20.

Brody, H. (1993). *The Healer's Power*. Yale University Press: New Haven.

Council of Europe (1997). Convention for the Protection of Human Rights and Dignity of the Human Being with regard to the Application of Biology and Medicine: Convention on Human Rights and Biomedicine (ETS: 164). Strassbourg: Council of Europe.

Dickenson, D. (2003). *Risk and Luck in Medical Ethics*. Polity Press: Cambridge.

Edwards, S.J.L., Kirchin, S., and Huxtable, R. (2004). Research ethics committees and paternalism. *Journal of Medical Ethics*, **30**, 88–91.

Elbourne, D., Snowdon, C., and Garcia, J. (1997). Informed consent. Subjects may not understand concept of clinical trials. *British Medical Journal*, **315**, no. 7102, 248–249.

Faden, R.R. and Beauchamp, T. (1986). *A History and Theory of Informed Consent*. Oxford: Oxford University Press.

Featherstone, K. and Donovan, J. L. (1998). Random allocation or allocation at random? Patients' perspectives of participation in a randomized controlled trial. *British Medical Journal*, **317**, no. 7167, 1177–1180.

–ibid.– (2002). 'Why don't they just tell me straight, why allocate it?' The struggle to make sense of participating in a randomized controlled trial. *Social Science and Medicine* **55**, no. 5, 709–719.

Jensen, A.B., Madsen, B., Andersen, P., and Rose, C. (1993). Information for cancer patients entering a clinical trial – an evaluation of an information strategy. *European Journal of Cancer*, **29A**, 2235–2238.

Jonas, H. (1969). Philosophical reflections on experimenting with human subjects. *Daedalus*, **98**, 219–247.

Madsen, S.M., Holm, S., and Riis, P. (1999). Ethical aspects of clinical trials: the attitudes of the public and out-patients. *Journal of Internal Medicine*, **245**, 571–579.

Madsen, S.M., Holm, S., Davidsen, B., Munkholm, P., Schlichting, P., and Riis, P. (2000a). Ethical aspects of clinical trials: the attitudes of participants in two non-cancer trials. *Journal of Internal Medicine*, **248**, 461–473.

Madsen, S.M., Holm, S., and Riis, P. (2000b). The extent of written information: preferences among potential and actual trial subjects. *Bullet in of Medical Ethics*, **159**, 13–18.

Madsen, S.M., Mirza, M.R., Holm, S., Hilsted, K.L., Kampmann, K., and Riis, P. (2002). Attitudes towards clinical research of participants and non-participants. *Journal of Internal Medicine*, **251**, 156–168.

Madsen, S.M., Holm, S., and Riis, P. (2007a). Participating in a cancer clinical trial? The balancing of options in a loneliness of autonomy: a grounded theory interview study. *Acta Oncologica*, **46**, 49–59.

–ibid.– (2007b). Attitudes towards clinical research among cancer trial participants and non-participants: an interview study using a Grounded Theory approach. *Journal of Medical Ethics*, **33**, 34–40.

Mechanic, D. (1968). *Medical Sociology*. Free Press: New York.

Snowdon, C., Garcia, J., and Elbourne, D. (1997). Making sense of randomization; responses of parents of critically ill babies to random allocation of treatment in a clinical trial. *Social Science Medicine*, **45**, no. 9, 1337–1355.

–ibid.– (1998). Reactions of participants to the results of a randomized controlled trial: exploratory study. *British Medical Journal*, **317**, no. 7150, 21–26.

UK Biobank (2006). UK Biobank: protocol for a large-scale prospective epidemiological resource. Protocol No: UKBB-PROT-09–096 (Main Phase)

Chapter 2

Trust and exploitation in clinical research

Paul B. Miller and Charles Weijer

2.1 Beyond consent and back again

American bioethicists have long been known for their preoccupation with autonomy and informed consent. Founding members of the field have noted that bioethics emerged largely as a grass-roots movement advocating recognition of patient autonomy in medical decision-making (Rothman 1992; Jonsen 1998). Autonomy was a natural rallying point for newly minted bioethicists facing troubling implications of a deeply entrenched paternalistic model of the physician–patient relationship. Bioethicists have since worked hard to explain the meaning of autonomy and its philosophical basis (Beauchamp and Childress 2001). They have also done much to improve our understanding of the relationship between autonomy and informed consent and, in concert with leading courts around the world, to define the elements of valid informed consent (Faden and Beauchamp 1986).

Bioethicists working on the ethics of clinical research have historically been no less preoccupied with autonomy and informed consent. This should come as little surprise in light of the history of the field. Where bioethicists focusing on practice rallied against a traditional presumption that physicians were entitled to unilaterally make medical decisions in the best interests of their patients, bioethicists focusing on research faced a sordid history wherein the rights and interests of research subjects were disregarded, subordinated and often seriously compromised in the name of war, conquest, industry, and science. Informed consent became the cornerstone of academic and policy responses to successive revelations of abuse and exploitation of research subjects, beginning with the Nuremberg Code (Annas and Grodin 1992).

More recently, a number of prominent bioethicists have called upon their colleagues to broaden their horizons. It has increasingly been recognized that informed consent requirements often actually do little to serve patient-subjects' autonomy interests (O'Neill 2002). Moving beyond consent, some bioethicists have explored intensively the justice-based interests of patient-subjects in work on topics ranging from equitable selection of subjects to the demands of fairness in the development of research priorities. Others have engaged in creative debate over the nature and moral foundation of the interests of families and communities in research, the relationship between these interests and those of individuals, and the appropriate means by which to recognize and balance them in law and policy (Hardwig 1990; Mappes and

Zembaty 1994; Nelson and Nelson 1995; Weijer, Goldsand, and Emanuel 1999; Weijer and Emanuel 2000).

Long before that, however, select scholars in research ethics demonstrated concern for the welfare interests of patient-subjects. In particular, they were interested in the question how physicians may participate in randomized controlled trials (RCTs) in a manner consistent with their duty of care, which requires them to act in the best medical interests of patient-subjects (Fried 1974; Marquis 1983; Gifford 1986; Freedman 1987; Hellman and Hellman 1991). All of the participants in the debate accepted that the duty of care correlates to a *bona fide* entitlement enjoyed by patient-subjects. The entitlement, variably referred to as a right to 'personal' or 'competent' care, was thought to obligate physicians involved in research to take due steps to protect and promote patient-subjects' best medical interests in the design and conduct of RCTs. It was understood that the duty applies to physicians in clinical care settings, but recognition and adherence to it was deemed particularly important in research settings, given that research presents a greater risk of other (personal, social, and scientific) interests coming into intolerable conflict with those of patient-subjects (Fried 1974).

Precisely what the duty of care requires of physicians involved in RCTs has been the subject of considerable disagreement (Miller and Weijer 2003). Some argued that it effectively forbids physicians from participating in RCTs to the extent that it requires the exercise of individualized clinical judgement, and so is necessarily violated by the random assignment of treatments in RCTs (Hellman and Hellman 1991). Most commentators have, however, insisted it is possible to design and conduct RCTs in a manner consistent with the duty of care. Suffice to say that the debate has, for the most part, centred on specification of the moral condition establishing this consistency (Miller and Weijer 2003). Charles Fried, writing in the mid-1970s, suggested that a physician-researcher meets her duty of care when she is in 'equipoise', that is, when she is genuinely uncertain as to the relative therapeutic merits of the experimental and control arms of the RCT (Fried 1974). Benjamin Freedman, writing in the late 1980s, articulated a more research-friendly version of the equipoise requirement. According to Freedman, physician-researchers meet their duty to act in the best interests of patient-subjects when a state of 'clinical equipoise' obtains, that is, when there exists, at the outset of the trial, an honest, professional disagreement amongst the community of expert clinicians as to preferred treatment (Freedman 1987). In substituting the expert community for the individual physician as the referent for the equipoise requirement, Freedman recognized that standards of competent care in medicine are socially determined.

Recent work by F.G. Miller and colleagues has called for reconsideration of the norms governing the relationship between physician-researchers and patient-subjects in clinical research (Miller and Brody 2003). Contrary to a long-held view in the research ethics literature, Miller and colleagues have argued that physician-researchers do not have a duty of care requiring them to act in the best interests of patient-subjects.

Miller and Brody have attempted to articulate an alternative account of the obligations of physician-researchers to patient-subjects in RCTs. Some commentators who endorse their work have argued that the duty to obtain informed consent exhausts physician-researchers' obligations to patient-subjects (Menikoff 2003). Miller and Brody seem uncomfortable with this view. They have repeatedly argued that consent is not sufficient for the ethical conduct of research (Miller and Shorr 2002; Miller 2003). While not always consistent, Miller and Brody usually claim that in addition to having a duty to obtain valid informed consent from patient-subjects, physician-researchers have an obligation to refrain from unduly exploiting them. Unfortunately, they neither define exploitation nor explain plausibly how exploitation is to be avoided.

The work of Miller and colleagues is problematic because it stands as an *ad hoc* response to an important problem – that of determining what norms ought to govern the conduct of clinical research. Elsewhere we provide a comprehensive and critical examination of their position (Miller and Weijer 2007). But their work raises an important challenge for the ethics of clinical research. It raises questions about the foundation and relationship between norms commonly accepted as governing the relationship between physician-researchers and patient-subjects. Their rejection of a duty of care calls for a defence of its legitimacy that articulates its foundation. Further, their recognition that clinical research raises concerns regarding exploitation that are not obviated by informed consent calls for exploration of the nature of exploitation and the relationship between norms relating to it and to consent.

In what follows, we work deliberately to derive, define, and specify norms governing the relationship between physician-researcher and patient-subject, and to explore their interconnection. We argue that rooting the relationship between physician-researcher and patient-subject in a normative theory of trust is promising. It enables derivation, definition, and specification of norms governing the relationship and appreciation of their interconnection.

2.2 The significance of informed consent in relationships of contract and trust

In order to appreciate the limited moral and legal significance of informed consent for the relationship between physician-researchers and patient-subjects, we need to become clearer about the nature of that relationship.

It is widely accepted that informed consent requirements are based on the near universal value accorded individual freedom, understood as autonomy, or in Kantian terms as the capacity of an individual to set and pursue her own ends. By respecting the autonomy of others we treat them as equals, in the sense that we recognize that they are equally entitled to set and pursue their own ends. Consent requirements are an essential, if admittedly imperfect, means by which to secure respect for autonomy (O'Neill 2002, 2003). Requirements for consent to treatment and research secure respect for our autonomy interests in relation to control over our bodies, personal information, and so on. Consent requirements, therefore, provide important protection to our autonomy interests in physical integrity and privacy, among other things. While the basis and basic import of consent requirements are relatively well known, less well appreciated are limits to their moral and legal significance.

We think that consent is a necessary and arguably sufficient moral and legal requirement for relationships in which each party can reasonably be presumed equally capable of protecting and promoting their own interests and ends. This presumption is perhaps sound for most relationships between capable adults. It certainly seems sound for arm's-length commercial relationships (e.g., most contractual relationships). Wherever the presumption is sound, consensual involvement in a relationship centred on an activity in which there are independent interests seems to suffice to obviate concerns about exploitation. We think that exploitation is most plausibly defined in Kantian terms as the use of another as a mere means to the achievement of independent ends, be they social or personal (Ripstein 2004). Whether we like it or not, for most relationships in respect of most activities, we must each assume that others are pursuing their own interests and be ready to pursue and protect ours in making informed choices. Where our right to make an informed decision has been recognized, it would seem that we have little cause for complaint when our interests fare badly in comparison with those of others. Further, in consenting to an activity in which the independent interests of others factor, one may make pursuit of their ends one's own end. One is not exploited as a mere means to the achievement of another's end when one has freely adopted that end as one's own.

Granting the fundamental value of autonomy and the corresponding importance of informed consent, it strikes us as obvious that autonomy interests are not the only human interests worthy of recognition and protection in law and ethics. The limited importance of autonomy and consent is most evident in respect of relationships in which the parties *cannot* reasonably be presumed equally capable of protecting and promoting their own interests and ends. Relationships for which this presumption is unsound include those characterized by inequality of power and dependence.

A significant minority of relationships are characterized by inequality of power and dependence. We think that at least two significant categories of relationships of inequality of power and dependence can be identified, the first encompassing relationships that are involuntary, the second encompassing those that are voluntary. Involuntary relationships characterized by inequality of power and dependence are established where one party to the relationship is actually or legally incapable, and is, as a result, dependent on the beneficial exercise of power by the other party. These relationships are involuntary in the sense that establishment of the relationship turns on a determination (i.e., incapacity) over which one has no personal control. Involuntary relationships include most notably those between parents and children. They also include relationships between incapable adults and substitute decision-makers. By contrast, voluntary relationships characterized by inequality of power and dependence are established where a capable party to a relationship entrusts another with power over important personal (e.g., medical, legal, or economic) or common interests. These relationships are voluntary in the sense that their establishment turns on a voluntary act, that is, unilateral or reciprocal entrusting of power to another person. The act whereby power is entrusted can, but need not, be formal in nature (e.g., as with agency contracts, legal mandates, medical consent forms). Voluntary relationships include those between business partners, lawyers and clients, financial advisors and clients, and physicians and patients.

Involuntary and voluntary relationships characterized by inequality of power and dependence are frequently both colloquially referred to as relationships of trust. We prefer to call involuntary relationships status relationships, and voluntary relationships trust relationships. To be clear, then, by trust relationships we mean relationships in which a capable person has voluntarily entrusted another with power over specific personal or common interests.

There are important differences between status and trust relationships, relating we think principally to their nature respectively as involuntary or voluntary, and to related differences in the scope of power wielded by the power-holder in the relationship. These differences may reasonably be expected to be reflected in a comparative assessment of the moral and legal obligations appropriate to each. That being said, we do not intend presently to explore the differences between status and trust relationships. Presently, we are interested only in making and emphasizing three key points.

First, for both status and trust relationships, structural (as opposed to merely circumstantial) inequality of power and dependence disrupt the presumption of the equal capacity of the parties to protect and pursue their respective ends in the relationship. In status relationships, the dependent party to the relationship is, by virtue of incapacity, unable and/or unauthorized to protect and pursue their interests in the relationship. The powerful party to the relationship assumes, voluntarily or by force of law, the authority and responsibility to exercise power to protect and advance the best interests of the dependent party. In trust relationships, the dependent party to the relationship voluntarily entrusts another with power to protect and pursue their interests in the relationship. In short, he cedes some considerable measure of control over his welfare to another. Indeed, trust relationships are often established for that very purpose. As with status relations, so in trust relations, the powerful party to the relationship assumes the responsibility to exercise power to protect and advance the best interests of the dependent party.

Second, for both status and trust relationships, structural inequality of power and dependence gives rise to a higher than normal risk of exploitation borne solely by the dependent party to the relationship. For relationships in which the presumption of equality and autonomy holds, each party to the relationship can be presumed equally at risk of exploitation by the other. However, for relationships where one party is dependent on the other for beneficial exercise of power, the dependent party bears the burden of the distinctive risk that her interests will be neglected, subordinated, or harmed where power is exploited to advance the independent interests of the power-holder or others. The increased risk of exploitation inheres in relationships characterized by structural inequality of power and dependence, regardless of whether the power is voluntarily entrusted, is assumed, or is imposed, and regardless of whether it is broad (as in status relations) or specific (as in trust relations).

Third, and finally, clarification of the nature of status and trust relationships is of itself indicative of the insufficiency of informed consent as a moral and legal requirement governing the conduct of the powerful party to these relationships. For relationships in which presumption of equality and autonomy holds, the parties may not only be presumed equally at risk of exploitation, they may also be presumed equally capable of recognizing and guarding against this risk through informed decision-making.

This is not so of status and trust relationships. In status relationships, the decision-making authority of the dependent party is either non-existent, or subordinate relative to that of the power-holder. In trust relationships, the dependent party may retain some measure of decision-making authority, but reliance inheres in the relationship. The dependent party to a trust relationship relies on the power-holder in ceding power over some specific personal or common interest. The reliance inhering in the trust relationship is a clear departure from vigilant self-protection that is the presumptive rule for normal arm's-length relationships between individuals. Furthermore, trust relationships between strangers are generally entered into because effective protection and promotion of the dependent party's interests requires the exercise of expert skill and/or knowledge (e.g., medical, legal, or financial) enjoyed by the powerful party. In trust relationships of this kind, informed consent is even more problematic because the dependent party relies on the power-holder for access to, and explanation of, information material to the proper exercise of their retained decision-making authority.

We are now in a position to better appreciate the limited significance of informed consent for relationships characterized by inequality of power and dependence. For status relationships, informed consent is neither necessary nor sufficient, morally or legally. For trust relationships, it is necessary but not sufficient. Recognition that inequality of power and dependence are normatively salient characteristics of status and trust relationships provides the basis for articulating their normative structure. This, in turn, enables us better to understand and articulate the distinctive moral and legal obligations beyond those relating to consent that are appropriate to these relationships.

2.2.1 The structure of trust relationships and clinical research

As Annette Baier has pointed out, moral philosophers have largely neglected questions concerning the ethics of trust relationships (Baier 1986, 1994). They have generally restricted their attention to relationships for which a presumption of equality and autonomy remain sound. Indeed, according to Baier, most have seemed utterly unaware that the presumption is just that, and as such is unsound for a wide range of relationships. She notes that on the rare occasion that a moral philosopher has recognized the significance of trust, it almost always is in consideration of relationships for which the presumption of equality and autonomy is sound, and unnoticed as such, for example, work on the role of trust in contractual relationships.

Baier recognized well that 'we need a morality to guide us in our dealings with those who either cannot or should not achieve equality of power with those with whom they have unavoidable and often intimate relationships' (Baier 1986, 249) She also suggested that trust would be the centrepiece of that morality. But while Baier did a great deal to improve our understanding of trust, she left unanswered important questions concerning the range of trust relationships, their normative structure, and the obligations appropriate to them. Scepticism seems to have prevented Baier from developing answers to these questions. Her scepticism is rooted in her suspicion of male preoccupation with moral theory as systematizing exercise oriented to the development of an exhaustive account of moral obligation (Baier 1994, 1–17).

However, despite her scepticism, Baier recognized the importance of theory and obligation. She opined that a focus on trust would be key to bridging feminists' interest in relationships characterized by inequality of power and dependence with male moral philosophers' historical fascination with the development of systematic theories of moral obligation (Baier 1994, 10).

We affirm Baier's criticism of the neglect of trust in moral philosophy and agree that it is the key to the development a moral theory inclusive of relationships characterized by inequality of power and dependence. We certainly do not make pretence to providing such a theory presently, even in outline. However, we do aim to provide some substantial starting points for such a theory, building on her work and on a resource untapped by moral theorists to date – the experience of courts and academicians in theorizing trust relationships and trust-based obligations in fiduciary law (Miller and Weijer 2006a).

Trust relationships may be set into different categories. In one category of trust relationship, relationships are established where one party entrusts another with power over specific personal (e.g., medical, legal, economic, familial, spiritual) interests. We call these personal trust relationships. In personal trust relationships, the power-holder may be entrusted with power on the grounds of personal familiarity, or on the basis of social expectations generated by her professional calling, or other social role. A wide range of relationships come within this category, including those between doctor and patient, psychologist and patient, parent and childcare provider, priest and confessor, and service provider and customer. This category of trust relationship is narrower than but significantly parallel to the legal category of fiduciary relationship.

The core normative structural feature of all trust relationships is the inequality and dependence generated by the voluntary act of entrusting power to another. This feature founds an obligation common to all trust relationships, namely, that requiring the entrusted party to exercise entrusted power to serve (e.g., protect or advance) the ends or interests for which the power was entrusted.

Status relationships are also characterized by structural inequality of power and dependence. This structural characteristic also generates a core obligation on the power-holder to exercise power to serve the ends or interests of the dependent party (e.g., it is well known that parents and substitute decision-makers have an obligation to exercise their decision-making powers in the best interests of those under their care). Importantly, however, in trust relationships the inequality of power and dependence are generated by a voluntary act establishing the relationship. Furthermore, because the relationship is voluntarily entered into largely for the protection or advancement of a specific interest, the inequality of power and dependence characteristic of trust relationships is circumscribed (i.e., it is not broad or total, as in status relationships). This difference in the normative structure of trust and status relationships shapes our understanding of the obligations appropriately imposed on the powerful party to them. For instance, the powerful party to a trust relationship has a duty of disclosure designed to protect the decision-making authority retained by the dependent party. No similar obligation can sensibly be imposed on the powerful party to a status relationship given their involuntary nature. Further, the power held by the powerful party to a trust relationship is specific in nature, and this specificity is reflected in the core duty to act in the best interests of the dependent party, that is, the duty is to act in the specific, for example, medical, interests of the dependent person.

Having identified the normative structure of trust relationships we are now positioned to consider the nature of the relationship between physician-researcher and patient-subject. In our view, it falls squarely within the personal category of trust relationship. We have already noted that doctor – patient relationships fall within this category of trust relationship. Why should we think that the relationship between physician-researcher and patient-subject likewise falls within it? The reasons for thinking that it does are straightforward (Miller and Weijer 2006b). The physician-researcher enjoys many, if not all, of the powers enjoyed by the physician. That is, the patient-subject entrusts the physician-researcher with the power to administer often invasive and potentially harmful medical and diagnostic procedures in an environment of close physical proximity. Physician-researchers are clearly entrusted with substantial powers over important welfare interests of patient-subjects, namely, their physical and psychological interests in health and wellbeing.

Furthermore, physician-researchers exercise their powers on grounds substantially the same as those supporting physicians' exercise of their powers. Physicians' involvement in clinical research does not change the fundamental character of their social or professional role, nor the expectations that attach to their relationship with patients as a result. Physician-researchers are, at root, physicians conducting scientific research with patients as their subjects. They are not merely scientists. Exercise of many of their powers in the context of research is conditioned on their medical training and exclusive socially sanctioned professional licence to diagnose and treat illness. As a result, we think that patient-subjects reasonably entrust physician-researchers with their powers on the understanding that they will employ them to protect and promote their medical interests.

In voluntarily entering into the relationship, the patient-subject must, of course, entrust the physician-researcher with the power to administer some non-therapeutic procedures, understanding that access to experimental treatment is conditioned on participation in research. He must also accept that the administration of therapeutic procedures will reflect the requirements of study design. But this does nothing to lessen the moral obligation occasioned by the trust placed in the physician-researcher. If anything, it strengthens it, for the level of trust must be greater. As a result of the informed consent process, the patient-subject should know that the safety and efficacy of the experimental treatment are not proven, that research participation brings incremental increased risks associated with the administration of non-therapeutic procedures, and that the experimental treatment will not be administered in an individualized manner. He nonetheless trusts that the physician-researcher will exercise her powers as physician and scientist to design and run the trial in such a way as to minimize the risk of harm, and maximize the potential medical benefit to him. This placement of trust establishes a moral obligation upon the physician-researcher to act accordingly.

2.3 **Moral obligations and trust relationships**

Our account of moral obligations generated by trust relationships is largely based on the range of fiduciary obligations identified by legal scholars, and it rests on our recognition that fiduciary relationships and this category of trust relationship share an identical normative structure (Miller and Weijer 2006a, 2006b). In short, both are relationships in which one party enjoys power over the personal interests of another. Both inherently give rise to inequality of power, dependence, and vulnerability to exploitation on the part of the dependent party as a result of the establishment of the relationship. As such, we think it reasonable to expect that the obligations applicable to these relationships will be roughly parallel.

We think that the obligations governing the conduct of a person entrusted with power over personal interests are best understood as falling into two categories. The first category, of core obligations, includes obligations the content of which reflect and correspond to the morally salient features of the normative structure of the trust relationship. They include duties of discretion, care and loyalty in relation to entrusted power. The second category, of peripheral obligations, includes obligations the content of which reflect morally salient aspects of the circumstances in which trust relationships of this kind are usually established. Peripheral obligations are fundamentally supportive in nature. They include duties of disclosure and confidence, and their function is to protect and enable the formation and maintenance of trust relationships. In light of limitations of space, we shall confine our attention to the core obligations.

We have said that the core obligations reflect morally salient aspects of the normative structure of trust relationships. We argued above that the core normative structural feature of all trust relationships is the inequality and dependence generated by the voluntary act of entrusting power to another. We have suggested that the dependence generated by entrusting power over one's interests to another founds a moral obligation on the entrusted party to act to protect or advance those interests. We have, it then seems, already articulated the core obligation applicable to the conduct of powerful parties to trust relationships. That is, in all trust relationships, the person entrusted with power is morally obligated to exercise that power to protect and advance the specified interests over which power was entrusted. We have, however, indicated that we think that there is a *category* of core obligations for trust relationships. We say this, because we think that an effort at specifying the *prima facie* core obligation reveals two distinct obligations, and that further reflection on the normative structure of trust relationships reveals a third.

The first core obligation is the duty to exercise the power with which one has been entrusted (duty of discretion, for short). The second is the duty to show reasonable care, diligence, and skill in exercising the power (duty of care, for short). The distinction between these duties is perhaps best appreciated in thinking about the ways in which a person may be said to be wronged by a person entrusted with power. Violation of trust encompasses at least two core wrongs. First, one can be wronged where the entrusted person fails entirely to exercise the power she has been entrusted with. She simply fails to make a decision or judgement, to act or render advice.

In essence, she violates our trust by doing nothing at all to advance or protect our interests. The wrong she commits is one of neglect. Second, one can be wronged where the entrusted person exercises the entrusted power, but fails to show reasonable care, diligence or skill in doing so. As noted above, we usually entrust strangers with power over personal interests because of the special (often professional) skills or expertise they have enabling them to more effectively advance or protect certain interests of ours. For example, we trust lawyers with power over our legal interests in recognition of their specialized knowledge of law and procedure, and their skills in negotiation and advocacy. We likewise trust doctors with power over our health in recognition of their knowledge of disease and treatment, and their skills in diagnosing and treating injury and illness. In entrusting such people with power, we reasonably expect that they will show reasonable levels of expertise and skill in their exercise of power. We also reasonably expect that these powers will be exercised in a reasonably diligent manner and with reasonable care.

This brings us to the third and final core obligation. We noted above that trust relationships, like status relationships, carry a distinctive risk of exploitation borne by the dependent party by virtue of structural inequality of power and dependence in the relationship. Again, in relationships where one party is dependent on the other for beneficial exercise of power, the dependent party bears the burden of the distinctive risk that her interests will be neglected, subordinated, or harmed where the power is exploited to advance the independent interests of the power-holder or others. We are, therefore, of the view that violation of trust encompasses a third core wrong, namely, exploitation or abuse of trust.

As its name suggests, the duty of loyalty requires the powerful party to a trust relationship to demonstrate loyalty to the person subject to the entrusted power. It is met by the powerful party avoiding or properly managing conflicts of interest, in faithful pursuit of the best interests of the dependent party. The duty of loyalty can be breached in at least two ways. First, and most obviously, it is breached where the person entrusted with power uses her position of power to further some personal interest of her own. For example, the duty is breached where the entrusted person uses her position of trust to gain for herself economic profits or opportunities, sexual gratification, or honorific advantages. Second, and equally importantly, the duty is breached where the entrusted person takes on duties to act for the benefit of others whose interests clearly and necessarily conflict with those of the person subject to the entrusted power. For example, the duty is breached where a lawyer agrees to act on behalf of a client who intends to sue a current or former client.

We pause to recognize that it might be thought that the duty of loyalty effectively prevents physicians from participating in clinical research. It might be thought to do so to the extent that independent and potentially conflicting interests of others parties (e.g., the physician-researcher, institution, sponsor, society) inevitably must factor and be reflected in the design and conduct of RCTs. If the duty of loyalty were to require physicians and others entrusted with power to avoid any activity in which the interests of others factor, it would be impossibly demanding. Fortunately, we think that properly interpreted it is not this demanding.

As we have defined it above, the duty of loyalty requires the person entrusted with power to exercise it faithfully in protecting and promoting the best interests of the dependent party to the trust relationship. We have argued that it is met by avoiding or properly managing conflicts of interest. It goes without saying that the conduct of clinical research does present risks of conflicts of interest which, if left unaddressed, could result in exploitation in violation of the duty of loyalty. However, the same is true of trust relationships in other contexts. Physicians must on an everyday basis balance interests potentially conflicting with those of their patients, including their own personal interests in remuneration and rest, social interests in the fair allocation of limited health care resources, and, in the United States at least, their employers' financial interests in health care provision. Lawyers, in turn, must balance their client's legal interests with their personal interests in rest and remuneration, social interests reflected in the standards imposed upon them as officers of the court, and their employers' financial interests in the provision of legal services. In clinical research, as in legal and clinical practice, the risks of exploitation associated with potential conflicts of interest can be appropriately managed. The duty of loyalty cannot be taken to require that *only* the interests of beneficiaries of entrusted power be pursued in any given trust relationship. Rather, in our view, it requires that the person entrusted with power grant clear and overriding priority to the interests of the dependent party to the trust relationship. They do this by working to ensure that possible or actual conflicts of interest are identified and communicated, avoided where possible, and otherwise transparently justified and managed so as to pose minimal interference with the best interests of the dependent party.

2.4 **Conclusion**

Having clarified the distinctive nature of the risk of exploitation in trust relationships, and having identified and explained the obligation that serves to mitigate it, we can now bring our argument full circle. Recall that we promised that clarification of the nature of the relationship between patient-subjects and physician-researchers would help us better to understand the link between a risk of exploitation unmitigated by consent and the duty of care. We are now in a position to understand that link. In short, in our view, the duty of care and the duty of non-exploitation, treated in a disconnected way by Miller and Brody, must be seen, together with the duty of discretion, as an analytically inseparable expression of the normative structure of trust relationships. None of the three core obligations makes sense when one attempts to sever one from the others.

Recall that trust relationships of the kind we are discussing here are established when one party entrusts another with power over their personal interests. Recall, too, that we have said that the entrusting of power gives rise to inequality of power and dependence, these being the core normative structural features of trust relationships. In consideration of the nature and normative structure of trust relationships of this kind, it makes little sense to say that the powerful party to the relationship has a duty to exercise entrusted power, but no duty of care in doing so. Likewise, it makes little sense to say that the power-holder has a duty of care in relation to the entrusted power, but no duty to exercise it. But most important in consideration of our debate with Miller and Brody, it makes no sense to say that the powerful party to a trust relationship operates under a duty of loyalty, but does not operate under a duty of care.

The distinctive risk of exploitation inhering in trust relationships arises precisely because of the inequality of power and dependence generated by entrusting one's personal interests to the care of another. A duty requiring one to *faithfully* act in the best interests of another is nonsensical in the absence of a duty requiring one simply to act in that other's best interests. This point has been made most clear by distinguished legal scholar Peter Birks. Discussing the relationship between the duty of loyalty (which he refers to as the duty of disinterestedness) and the duty of care, Birks observes that:

> The obligation of disinterestedness cannot be severed from the obligation to promote and preserve. It does not make sense without that principal obligation. An independent obligation [of disinterestedness] … is unintelligible, certainly unworkable … [the obligation] is an obligation of disinterestedness in the course of *doing* something: the trustee [here, physician-researcher] shall not pursue any interest of his own which might possibly conflict with his duty to the beneficiary, *scilicet* his duty to promote and preserve the interest of the beneficiary. (Birks 2000)

In sum then, in order to recognize the special risk of exploitation facing patients in clinical research, and to identify the obligation beyond consent that can effectively mitigate it, one must recognize that the relationship between physician-researchers and patient-subjects is one of trust. But we have discovered that core obligations of discretion, care and loyalty applicable to the powerful parties to trust relationships are inseparable as a unified expression of its normative structure. In our view, therefore, to the extent that Miller and Brody wish to recognize and effectively remedy the distinctive risk of exploitation facing patients in clinical research, they have no choice but to accept the duty of care, the rejection of which has been the singular focus of their recent work.

References

Annas, G.J. and Grodin, M.A. (eds) (1992). *The Nazi Doctors and the Nuremberg Code: Human Rights in Human Experimentation*. New York: Oxford University Press.

Baier, A.C. (1986). Trust and anti-trust. *Ethics*, **96**, 231–60.

–ibid.– (1994). *Moral Prejudices: Essays on Ethics*. Cambridge, MA: Harvard University Press.

Beauchamp, T.L. and Childress, J.F. (2001). *Principles of Biomedical Ethics* (5th edition). New York: Oxford University Press.

Birks, P. (2000). The content of the fiduciary obligation. *Israel Law Review*, **34**, 3.

Faden, R. and Beauchamp, T.L. (1986). *A History and Theory of Informed Consent*. New York: Oxford University Press.

Freedman, B. (1987). Equipoise and the ethics of clinical research. *New England Journal of Medicine*, **317**, 141–5.

Fried, C. (1974). *Medical Experimentation: Personal Integrity and Social Policy*. Amsterdam: North Holland.

Gifford, F. (1986). The conflict between randomized clinical trials and the therapeutic obligation. *Journal of Medicine and Philosophy*, **11**, 347–66.

Hardwig, J. (1990). What about the family? *Hastings Center Report*, **20**, no. 2 5–10.

Hellman, S. and Hellman, D.S. (1991). Of mice but not men: problems of the randomized controlled trial. *New England Journal of Medicine*, **324**, 1585–9.

Jonsen, A.R. (1998). *The Birth of Bioethics*. New York: Oxford University Press.

Mappes, T.A. and Zembaty, J.S. (1994). Patient choices, family interests, and physician obligations. *Kennedy Institute of Ethics Journal*, **4**, 27–46.

Marquis, D. (1983). Leaving therapy to chance. *Hastings Center Report*, **13**, no. 4, 40–7.

Menikoff, J. (2003). Equipoise: beyond rehabilitation? *Kennedy Institute of Ethics Journal*, **13**, 347–51.

Miller, F.G. (2003). Ethical issues in research with healthy volunteers. *Clinical Pharmacology and Therapeutics*, **74**, 513–15.

Miller, F.G. and Brody, H. (2003). A critique of clinical equipoise: therapeutic misconception in the ethics of clinical trials. *Hastings Center Report*, **33**, no. 3 19–28.

Miller, F.G. and Shorr, A.F. (2002). Unnecessary use of placebo controls. *Archives of Internal Medicine*, **162**, 1673–7.

Miller, P.B. and Weijer, C. (2003). Rehabilitating equipoise. *Kennedy Institute of Ethics Journal*, **13**, 93–118.

–*ibid.*– (2006a). Fiduciary obligation in clinical research. *Journal of Law, Medicine and Ethics*, **34**, 424–40.

–*ibid.*– (2006b). The trust-based obligations of the state and physician-researcher to patient-subjects. *Journal of Medical Ethics*, **32**, 542–7.

–*ibid.*– (2007). Equipoise and the duty of care in clinical research: a philosophical response to our critics. *Journal of Medicine and Philosophy*, **32**, 117–33.

Nelson, H.L. and Nelson, J.L. (1995). *The Patient in the Family: an Ethics of Medicine and Families*. New York: Routledge.

O'Neill, O. (2002). *Autonomy and Trust in Bioethics*. Cambridge: Cambridge University Press.

–*ibid.*– (2003). Some limits of informed consent. *Journal of Medical Ethics*, **29**, 4–7.

Ripstein, A. (2004). Authority and coercion. *Philosophy and Public Affairs*, **32**, 2–35.

Rothman, D.J. (1992). *Strangers at the Bedside: a History of how Law and Bioethics Transformed Medical Decision-making*. New York: Basic Books.

Weijer, C. and Emanuel, E.J. (2000). Protecting communities in biomedical research. *Science*, **289**, 1142–4.

Weijer, C., Goldsand, G., and Emanuel, E.J. (1999). Protecting communities in research: current guidelines and limits of extrapolation. *Nature Genetics*, **23**, 275–80.

Chapter 3

Consent and private liability in clinical research

Paul B. Miller and Josephine Johnston

3.1 **Introduction**

The principle that informed consent is necessary for research involving humans to be ethical was established during the second half of the 20th century. The experiments performed by Nazi scientists during World War II and by US physicians in the Tuskegee Syphilis Study are two famous examples of research that was considered unethical in part because the subjects did not provide free and informed consent (Tuskegee Syphilis Study Legacy Committee 1996).

But even if the subjects had consented, the experiments would still have been unethical because the risk of harm to research subjects was unacceptably high and disproportionate to the value of the knowledge to be gained from the research. Consent thus came to be appreciated as a necessary but not sufficient condition for research involving humans to be considered ethical.

The legal significance of informed consent for research involving humans is similar. Without informed consent, many of the acts involved in research – injecting, cutting, or otherwise touching the research subject – would amount to criminal battery and administration of an experimental drug or device would very likely amount to trespass and negligent care. But just as informed consent is not always sufficient to shield the researcher from ethical censure, so too it is also not always sufficient to shield her from liability for breach of contract, negligence, or breach of fiduciary duty (*Grimes v. Kennedy Krieger Institute* 2001).

In this chapter, we raise and explore general theoretical questions relating to consent and private liability in clinical research, focusing on the implications of consent for private law duties of care governing the relationship between physicians and patients in clinical research. Limits on the legal significance of consent are typically overlooked in the bioethics literature and the question how these limits might operate between a physician-researcher and a patient-subject has received surprisingly little consideration in legal scholarship.

We do not purport to provide a comprehensive account of private liability in clinical research, a practical guide to the establishment of liability, a detailed review of authorities, or an exploration of criminal or regulatory liability. Further, our focus will be on the relationship between physicians and patients in clinical research and not researchers and research subjects more generally because the relationship between the former is *prima facie* governed by several private law duties of care and because differences between clinical care and research raise interesting problems. These differences include the presence of interests potentially conflicting with those of the patient (e.g., of sponsors, future patients, and the general public), aspects of research design that serve scientific rather than therapeutic purposes (randomization, blinding, administration of non-therapeutic procedures), and the prevalence of therapeutic misconception whereby patients can fail to understand differences between clinical care and research (Appelbaum *et al.* 1987b).

In what follows, we discuss the significance of consent in the foundation, content, and application of duties of care in tort, contract, and fiduciary law. We identify points of variation in the significance of consent across these categories of private liability. We also trace the implications of each category of liability and the points of difference between them for the relationship between physicians and patients in clinical research. We conclude with some brief remarks on potential problems reconciling these differences in the event of concurrent liability.

3.2 The nature and meaning of informed consent

We cannot here recount the considerable literature on the nature and meaning of informed consent. Suffice to say, consent to participation in research must come from the research subject or an authorized representative and should usually be recorded in writing. It must be free (i.e., made in the absence of undue influence, duress, or coercion), and it must be informed (i.e., it must evidence understanding of the nature of the research and appreciation of the risks and benefits it poses). The latter criterion, in particular, has proved difficult to satisfy, in part because there is no objective measure of comprehension. That some research subjects are children, mentally ill, or adults with compromised capacity, coupled with evidence of a persistent therapeutic misconception among patient-subjects, further complicates the informed consent process. Nevertheless, free and informed consent remains a cornerstone of research ethics.

Because research subjects must give their informed consent to participate in research, it might be assumed that they thereby forgo rights to sue for harm suffered as a result of their participation. This assumption might seem particularly compelling where the research subject was informed of the particular risk or risks that materialized. However, as we explain below, the law generally does not consider consent to be a complete defence to private liability for conduct that results in harm where the risk of same is objectively unreasonable.

3.3 Consent and the duty of care in tort

Under tort law, a duty of care in negligence arises by operation of law wherever it is reasonably foreseeable that one's conduct poses a risk of harm to another. The duty is thus said to encompass persons and injuries that fall within the ambit of reasonably foreseeable risk generated by one's conduct. The duty was famously expounded by Lord Atkin in *Donoghue v. Stevenson* as follows:

> There must be, and is, some general conception of relations giving rise to a duty of care, of
> which the particular cases found in the books are but instances. ... The rule that you are to

love your neighbour becomes in law, you must not injure your neighbour; and the lawyer's question, Who is my neighbour? receives a restricted reply. You must take reasonable care to avoid acts or omissions which you can reasonably foresee would be likely to injure your neighbour. Who, then, in law is my neighbour? The answer seems to be – persons who are so closely and directly affected by my act that I ought reasonably to have them in contemplation as being so affected when I am directing my mind to the acts or omissions which are called in question.

(Donoghue (or McAlister) v. Stevenson 1932, 580)

While the duty of care in negligence does not presume a pre-existing relationship between those having the benefit and the burden of the protection it provides, certain relationships presumptively give rise to a duty of care because reasonable foreseeability of harm is entailed by the proximity generated by the relationship and the nature of the conduct expected to occur within it. The relationship between physicians and patients is one such relationship: 'It has long been accepted that a medical practitioner owes a duty to exercise reasonable skill and care in his treatment of a patient, even where no contract exists between them.' (Jackson and Powell 2007, 13-006).

A duty of care is an obligation to exercise reasonable watchfulness, prudence, and care towards another in the performance of an act or omission that could foreseeably harm that other. In the case of physicians and other professionals, the duty of care further requires reasonable skill to be displayed in regulated professional conduct (*ibid.*, 13-022). If this duty is breached and harm is caused, a cause of action lies in negligence. In contrast with contract, the duty of care in tort arises irrespective of consent. A physician owes an unconscious patient a duty of care in tort even though the latter has not provided consent to treatment because the duty arises from the fact of the relationship rather than from the terms of any contract or other agreement between the parties.

Similarly, the content of the duty of care – the standard of conduct to which one will be held – depends not upon consent but upon the nature of the relationship. While lay people are in their interactions with one another held to the ordinary standard of reasonable care, a physician will be held to a higher standard when acting as a physician that takes as its benchmark the level of skill and knowledge that would be reasonably expected within the medical profession. Therefore, medical negligence is an act or omission by a medical provider, often a physician, that falls below the standard of care established by the medical community and that causes injury to someone to whom the provider owes a duty of care (*Bolam v. Friern Hospital Management Committee* 1957, 586; *Sidaway v. Governors of Bethlem Royal Hospital* 1985, 881; *Crits v. Sylvester* 1956, 502). Considerable American case law exists on medical negligence.

There is an emerging body of law supporting the notion that research subjects – both patients and healthy subjects – are owed a duty of care by researchers (*Halushka v. University of Saskatchewan* 1965; *Whitlock v. Duke Univ.* 1986; *Kernke v. The Menninger Clinic* 2001; *Grimes v. Kennedy Krieger Institute, Inc.* 2001). However, the contours of liability are not yet clear. Researchers may be held to the heightened standard of care that physicians owe their patients or instead to the ordinary standard that laypeople owe one another. Alternatively, the standard may vary with the nature of the relationship and the status of the parties.

Some cases involving subjects who are patients and researchers who are physicians indicate that the duty owed will be equivalent to that owed by physicians to patients in practice (*Burton v. Brooklyn Doctors Hospital* 1982; *Kernke v. The Menninger Clinic* 2001). Thus, physicians will need to show reasonable care and skill in the selection and administration of diagnostic and therapeutic interventions to patients in clinical research. Giesen argues that discharge of the duty of care in these circumstances will require that the interests of patients in receipt of competent care be granted priority: 'The interest of the sick person in receiving therapeutic treatment, where this is most conducive to his recovery, always takes precedence over the interests of science and medical progress. Thus, treating a patient with new procedures must be regarded as malpractice where approved methods may be expected to produce the same degree of success with less risk' (Giesen 1995, 29).

Some US cases, relying on notoriously difficult to define distinctions between research and practice (*Craft v. Vanderbilt* 1998; *Payette v. Rockefeller University* 1996), suggest that principles of 'ordinary negligence' should apply in research. However, English authority suggests, to the contrary, that the application of principles of negligence liability ought to be based on reasonable expectations of competence, not context, and that there is thus no meaningful distinction to be drawn between 'therapeutic' and 'non-therapeutic' contexts (*Gold v. Haringey Health Authority* 1988, 489). To the extent that the adoption of an ordinary negligence model would erode the level of protection afforded to patients, we suggest that it is inappropriate. A patient who enrols in research involving the administration and evaluation of therapeutic interventions may reasonably expect that physicians involved in recruitment, protocol design, and conduct of the research are subject to the standard of care that applies in clinical practice. For example, a patient might reasonably expect that a physician injecting an experimental drug will do so as expertly and carefully as a physician injecting an approved treatment. Similarly, a patient might reasonably expect that a physician who observes a serious adverse reaction to an experimental treatment will intervene in circumstances where competent care would ordinarily require intervention in practice.

One might be accustomed to thinking that negligence law is applicable to physicians primarily with respect to the degree of care and competence shown in the selection and administration of medical or scientific interventions. The adequacy of informed consent to treatment or research, for its part, has traditionally been understood as a matter for the law of battery (*Canterbury v. Spence* 1972). Intuitively, the wrong committed by a physician who acts without valid consent seems to be one of acting without true authority and thus in violation of the patient's right to dictate what should be done with or to her body. In short, the wrong is one of battery. However, in Canada and elsewhere the law has witnessed a revolution whereby deficiencies of consent may give rise to a claim in negligence (*Reibl v. Hughes* 1980; *Sidaway v. Governors of Bethlem Royal Hospital* 1985). This is so particularly where it is claimed that a physician has failed to explain material risks of an intervention or the comparative merits of alternative interventions. In these circumstances, the physician is said to have breached her duty of care in respect of disclosure of information to the patient.

The application of principles of negligence liability to informed consent is philosophically and doctrinally inelegant. Though there may, in some circumstances, be an element of negligence underlying the failure to obtain adequate consent, this element seems inessential to establishing the wrong. Nevertheless, it is clear that physicians in research as well as practice may be liable in negligence for failing to obtain proper informed consent. It therefore merits notice that physicians have been deemed subject to a higher standard of care in obtaining consent to research than applies in practice (*Halushka v. University of Saskatchewan* 1965; *Weiss v. Solomon* 1989). This higher standard may be warranted given that research entails greater uncertainty for the patient and the presence of interests potentially diverging from those of the patient.

Consent thus can be the object of an action in negligence. But can it obviate one? The authorities suggest that consent – or voluntary assumption of risk (volenti) – will rarely preclude liability for negligence.[1] Proof of voluntary assumption of risk requires establishment of consent to the highest standard. The party seeking to avoid liability must prove that the person injured by his negligence was fully aware of the risk of harm and 'bargained away' the right to sue.[2] Proof to this standard, while not impossible, is rarely made out. We would think that proof would be especially difficult for physicians in a research context given the prevalence of therapeutic misconception and patients' generalized vulnerability to and dependence upon medical professionals. Further, there is some authority for the proposition that consent cannot absolve physicians of liability for negligence to patients on public policy grounds.[3] This seems reasonable given that the medical profession publicly presents itself as committed to competent care of patients and given the high levels of public trust its members attract on that footing.

---

[1] Estey J.: 'while volenti is in principle available ... the defence will only be made out in unusual circumstances' (*Dube v. Labar* 1986, 658). 'In almost every negligence action of modern times where the defence of volens has been raised it has failed' (Williams 1951, 307–8).

[2] Estey J: 'volenti will arise only where the circumstances are such that it is clear that the plaintiff, knowing of the virtually certain risk of harm, in essence bargained away his right to sue for injuries incurred as a result of any negligence on the defendant's part. The acceptance of risk ... will arise ... only where there can truly be said to be an understanding on the part of both parties that the defendant assumed no responsibility to take due care for the plaintiff, and that the plaintiff did not expect him to' (*Dube v. Labar* 1986, 658–9).

[3] Melvin J.: 'As a matter of public policy, I seriously question whether surgeons should be allowed to contract out of liability for harm created by their negligence in the course of surgical procedures, regardless of the wording of the release form used ... the nature of the event being a surgery, and the complete reliance by a patient on a surgeon, dictates a negative answer' (*Hobbs v. Robertson* 2001, para 35).

3.4 **Consent and the duty of care in contract**

Freedom of contract – the idea that individuals should be at liberty to establish the terms upon which they interact without interference from legislatures or courts – enjoys considerable support in American law (*Lochner v. New York* 1905), where it is considered an innate right originating in the Constitution (Blum 2001, 10). In addition to being an ideological commitment, freedom of contract serves the pragmatic goal of enhancing commerce by enabling individuals to enter into enforceable transactions as they see fit. However, the values underlying freedom of contract are plainly premised on the assumption that parties to a contract are able to freely consent and that they would not consent to an improvident exchange. Over time, therefore, courts and legislatures have placed limits on freedom of contract to protect the rights and interests of weaker parties or to assert a state interest – early cases included litigation over the state's ability to require that employers pay a minimum wage (*West Coast Hotel Co. v. Parrish* 1937). Accordingly, freedom of contract is tempered under American law; not all contracts are upheld by courts, even when both parties consented to the bargain.

A patient who consents to participate in research might be considered to have thereby entered into a contract with physician-researchers and others (e.g., research sponsors). At its core, a contract is a legally binding exchange of value marked by offer and acceptance of terms supported by consideration (i.e., value paid for a promise). For example, people who agree to exchange a specified sum of money for a particular good or service will usually be considered to have entered into a contract. In the case of a patient-subject and a physician-researcher, the law might consider the consent to research participation to be a contract under which the patient-subject agrees to participate in the research in exchange for money, additional monitoring and care, access to the experimental intervention itself, or some other named benefit, such as a year's supply of the experimental drug following cessation of the research (*Dahl v. HEM Pharmaceuticals Corporation* 1993, 1401).

We say that the law *might* consider consent to participate in clinical research to be a contract because the case for equating consent with contract is not clear cut. Some of the hallmarks of contract are missing from, or otherwise ill-fitting of, the relationship between physician-researchers and patient-subjects. For instance, it is not clear that there is a market for opportunities to participate in clinical research; consent to research participation is not usually marked by negotiation or bargaining over terms; research participation may happen without consent or with the consent of a proxy who is not legally authorized to act as an agent (i.e., to bind the patient as principal through contract); consent to research participation can be valid without consideration (i.e., without the patient or the researcher, for that matter, providing something of value); and it is not clear whether the law would countenance enforcement of consent in an action for breach of contract (i.e., allow a researcher or sponsor to sue a patient for withdrawing from a trial or a patient to sue the researcher or sponsor for a trial halted early).

Surprisingly, few suits have been brought by patient-subjects against physician-researchers, research sponsors and/or research institutions and most have claimed negligence rather than breach of contract. While the philosophical appeal of the

contract model has been questioned (Hall and Schneider 2008), there is some authority for treating the relationship between physicians and patients in clinical practice as
contractual.[4] Further, the idea that a contractual relationship exists between patient-
subjects and physician-researchers received some support from the Maryland Court
of Appeals in the case of *Grimes v. Kennedy Krieger Institute*.

Grimes involved two actions brought by the parents of children who developed ele-
vated levels of lead in their blood while participating in a research study led by the
Kennedy Krieger Institute, a research institute associated with Johns Hopkins
University. The purpose of the experiment was to assess the effectiveness of different
methods of removing lead paint from residential buildings. During the experiment,
different lead abatement methods were employed and healthy children who lived in
the rental properties were tested to measure levels of lead dust in their blood. The
children's parents claimed that the research institute negligently failed to warn them
about, or otherwise protect their children from, exposure to dangerous doses of lead.
The research institute argued that it had no duty to warn the parents about the dan-
gers because it did not have a contractual or other relationship with the parents or
their children on which such a duty could be based.

Although negligence claims were the major focus in *Grimes*, the court addressed the
question whether a contractual relationship existed between the research institute and
the parents. It found that the parents' agreement that their children would participate
in research, as laid out in the informed consent document, met formal conditions for
the establishment of a valid contract (*ibid.*, 843). Further, by way of general statement,
the court held that

> [r]esearcher/subject consent in nontherapeutic research can, and in this case did, create a
> contract.

(ibid., 844)

The *Grimes* court declined to state whether the same could be said of consent to
therapeutic research (*ibid.*, note 35), the purpose of which it defined as 'to directly
help or aid a patient who is suffering from a … condition the objectives of the
research are designed to address' (*ibid.*, 811). Yet, it also gave no reason why consent to
participate in 'therapeutic research' could *not* give rise to a contract. Because consent
to treatment in clinical practice has already been deemed to found a contract between
physicians and patients, we would suggest that consent to participation in research
involving therapeutic interventions may likewise be deemed to found a contract
between physician-researchers and patient-subjects.

Under contract law, the terms of the contract include what each party has expressly
agreed to and any term the court considers to have been implied in the bargain or to

---

[4] 'It was recognized over 300 years ago that a contract existed between a doctor and patient, the
breach of which afforded the patient a cause of action. But the tort of negligence better covered most situations where a patient was given substandard medical care and very few suits
were brought for breach of contract alone' (Picard and Robertson 2007, 430). See also *Oliver v.
Brock* (1976), *Osbourne v. Frazone* (1968), *Rigelhaupt* (1980), *Quill* (1983, 228–34).

be necessary as a matter of law. In the context of consent to clinical research, express terms would thus encompass the language used in the consent form as well as any collateral oral or written representations. Implied terms are read into contracts on the basis of expectations deemed reasonably generated by the conduct of the parties or by industry custom. They might, for instance, encompass an expectation that medically relevant research results will be shared, or that patient confidentiality will be protected.

If the relationship between physician-researcher and patient-subject were deemed contractual, the latter could sue the former for breach of express or implied terms of contract. Liability for breach of contract is ordinarily strict: the breaching party is responsible for compensating the non-breaching party for the expectation of performance of the terms of the contract regardless of fault. The patient-subject could also sue for negligent performance of specific terms of a contract. Indeed, courts have traditionally considered that breach of terms bearing on the provision of professional services (e.g., administration of treatment, provision of legal, medical, or financial advice) requires fault in the form of negligence (Jackson and Powell 2007, 2-007–2-012). The idea underlying this rule is that contracts for professional services are not intended to provide a warranty for the success of services rendered; rather, they are intended to give the party paying for services the benefit of competent (i.e., non-negligent) performance (e.g., a person who contracts to have his tax return prepared can expect to have the return not just prepared but *competently* prepared) (Smith 2005, 170–1). Given the manifest complexity of consent to research participation, it may be difficult to distinguish terms bearing on the provision of professional services (attracting liability only on proof of fault) from ordinary terms (attracting strict liability). Nevertheless, one might imagine that a claim for harm suffered due to incompetent administration of a medical intervention will require proof of negligence while a claim that promised benefits were not provided (e.g., payment, access to treatment) will have the benefit of strict liability.

Unlike the duty of care in tort, contractual duties of care are generated by the terms of a contract and bear on the performance of those terms. Accordingly, a contract will not protect a patient from negligence at large by a physician. This follows from the truism that, generally speaking, the scope of contractual liability is determined by the terms agreed upon by the parties. Of particular significance for patient-subjects, a valid contract will provide no protection against harm caused by a physician-researcher's negligent failure to provide competent care if that care was not included in the consent (contract). Consent is thus clearly crucial to the establishment of liability in contract. Without consent, there is no valid contract, and without consensual adoption of a particular term, there can be no liability in contract for negligent failure to confer a benefit that may be contemplated by such a term (unless the term in question is deemed to be implied in the contract).

However, just because parties to a contract have consented to a term does not mean it will be enforced. Courts have a long history of refusing to enforce contracts and contract terms that are deemed contrary to public policy. They have been especially wary of clauses purporting to waive or exclude liability where the relationship between the parties is not an ordinary arm's-length commercial relationship but is rather one of confidence and trust (*George Mitchell Ltd v. Finney Lock Seeds Ltd* 1983;

Hunter Engineering Co. v. Syncrude 1989). Relationships of the latter sort raise the inference that the waiver was not the product of ordinary bargaining but was the product of undue influence. In the absence of special consideration paid for the waiver, it has all the appearance of an improvident transaction. In these circumstances, courts will refuse to give effect to the waiver on the basis that it would be unconscionable to do so.

Unsurprisingly, courts have considered relationships between physicians and patients to be amongst those warranting special scrutiny when determining whether to give effect to a purported waiver (*Hobbs v. Robertson* 2001) Thus, there is authority for the proposition that researchers cannot, through consent forms or otherwise, 'contract away' duties of care they would otherwise owe research subjects. The case of *Vodopest v. MacGregor* is instructive. In this case, the plaintiff claimed to have suffered brain injuries caused by the defendant's negligence whilst participating in a study of breathing techniques to combat altitude sickness during a trek in the Himalayas. In her defence, the defendant argued that the plaintiff had voluntarily waived her right to sue when she signed an agreement releasing the plaintiff 'from all liability, claims and causes of action arising out of or in any way connected with my participation in this trek' (*Vodopest v. MacGregor* 1996, 845).

The Supreme Court of Washington refused to recognize the defence, holding that the 'pre-injury release' was unenforceable as contrary to public policy. In reaching this conclusion, the court was influenced by the fact that medical research is of great importance to society and that medical researchers generally have significant control over the safety of human research subjects. Although careful to note that releases may be effective in other circumstances, it concluded 'Medical research using human subjects is one of those settings where public policy reasons for preserving an obligation of care owed by the researchers to the subject outweighs our traditional regard for freedom of contract'(*ibid.*, 856).

The *Vodopest* court was influenced by federal regulations on human subjects research. These regulations, which apply to research funded by the US public health service, include a provision to the effect that informed consent cannot serve to waive a research subject's legal rights or release researchers (or institutions and sponsors) from liability for negligence (45 C.F.R 46 1994 S. 46. 116). Although the regulations do not apply to all human subjects' research, the *Vodopest* court cited with approval several academic authorities for the general point that exculpatory clauses waiving the rights of research subjects to recover for negligence are of doubtful enforceability.[5] We are inclined to agree.

3.5 Consent and the duty of care in fiduciary law

The implications of fiduciary law for relationships between physicians and patients in clinical practice and research are not well understood. Few cases have been litigated at

---

[5] Citing Bowker W (1982), Hershey and Miller (1976), Annas *et al.* (1977), Appelbaum *et al.* (1987a), Maloney (1984).

the appellate level in commonwealth jurisdictions or in the United States. In Canada, the Supreme Court of Canada has granted the physician–patient relationship recognition as a category of relationship that enjoys fiduciary status in cases that arose in a clinical context (*Norberg v. Wynrib* 1992; *McInerney v. MacDonald* 1992). Canadian commentators have suggested that the fiduciary characterization extends to all relationships between medical professionals and patients (Ellis 1995). However, appellate courts in other jurisdictions have declined to recognize physician–patient relationships as having presumptive fiduciary status (*Sidaway v. Governors of Bethlem Royal Hospital* 1985; *Breen v. Williams* 1996). It is thus impossible to say with certainty or generality whether all relationships between physicians and patients are to be considered fiduciary and if not under what circumstances they might be.

Uncertainty generated by the absence of authority is exacerbated by uncertainty arising from a broad failure of consensus on several fundamental doctrinal matters in fiduciary law. Courts around the world disagree over how fiduciary relationships are established, how they ought to be recognized, what obligations they attract, whether and under what circumstances those obligations may be modified or waived, and what remedies ought to be available for breach of fiduciary duty. Uncertainty on such basic points of principle renders it difficult to say whether and when relationships between physicians and patients ought to be considered fiduciary.

Elsewhere, one of us (P.B.M.) has argued that in spite of this it is possible to define the fiduciary relationship, to identify duties arising from it, and to articulate the connection between the relationship and these duties. On this footing, it was argued that the relationship between physicians and patients in clinical research ought to be recognized as fiduciary (Miller and Weijer 2006). A review of the basis for that claim is beyond the scope of this work. Its cogency is to be assumed for the sake of argument. Here we shall focus upon the significance of consent for the establishment and possible modification or waiver of fiduciary liability in relationships between physicians and patients in clinical research.

While there is no consensus in the authorities on the nature of the fiduciary relationship, it is generally understood that fiduciary liability is premised upon its establishment. In other words, fiduciary duties are occasioned by the fiduciary relationship. They do not otherwise arise. One might thus reasonably suppose that fiduciary duties respond to certain distinctive features enjoyed by all fiduciary relationships. Building upon that supposition, and having mind to characteristics most typically attributed to it, the fiduciary relationship may be defined as follows:

> A fiduciary relationship is one in which one person – the fiduciary – enjoys discretionary power to set or pursue the practical interests of another – the beneficiary.

(Miller 2008, 146)

The relationship between physicians and patients in clinical research may be considered fiduciary under this definition to the extent that physicians are authorized to perform interventions that require the exercise of discretion relative to the medical interests of patients. While the scope of fiduciary obligation is the subject of dispute, fiduciaries are widely deemed subject to two principal duties: the duty of care and the duty of loyalty. The duty of care requires the fiduciary to show reasonable care, diligence, and skill in exercising discretion over the practical interests of the beneficiary. The duty of loyalty requires the fiduciary to exercise that discretion faithfully in the interests of the beneficiary. Hence she must avoid or properly manage conflicts of interest and duty. The duties of care and loyalty presuppose a distinct anterior duty. This duty – the duty of discretion – requires the fiduciary to exercise the discretion attached to her authority to act. These duties may usefully be understood as arising in response to structural properties of the fiduciary relationship (in particular, to specific ways in which beneficiaries are rendered vulnerable to fiduciaries by virtue of the discretionary power wielded by the latter over the practical interests of the former).

Taken in sum, fiduciary duties require physicians to act reasonably in exercising clinical judgement for the benefit of patients in clinical research and in doing so, to privilege the interests of patients over their own interests or those of others (e.g., research sponsors, future patients) in the design and conduct of research.

The essence of the fiduciary relationship is that the fiduciary enjoys authority to act in a discretionary manner in setting or pursuing specific practical interests of the beneficiary. Recognized categories of fiduciary relationship suggest three modes of authorization: agreement, undertaking, and constructive authorization (i.e., authorization by law). Fiduciary relationships established by agreement are those in which each party consents to the exercise of authority by the fiduciary: the beneficiary by voluntarily entrusting the fiduciary with it and the fiduciary by voluntarily undertaking it. Agreement is a legitimate mode of authorization only where the consent underlying it is valid. Fiduciary relationships established by undertaking arise solely upon the consent of the fiduciary in the form of a voluntary undertaking of authority. Undertaking is a legitimate mode of authorization only where the beneficiary is incapable of providing consent, preservation of his or her practical interests demands action, and there is no authorized substitute decision-maker. Fiduciary relationships established by constructive authorization are deemed to exist as of right irrespective of the consent of either party. They are exceedingly rare, the only known example being that between birth parents and their children. It is apparent, then, that consent plays a significant but inessential role in the establishment of fiduciary relationships. Fiduciary relationships can, in limited circumstances, be established without the consent of the beneficiary or indeed either party. Fiduciary law to this extent tracks the common understanding of the role of consent in authorizing medical and scientific interventions upon patients. Typically, the consent of a patient or a substitute decision-maker will authorize certain interventions and will specify those who undertake to perform them. But in cases of emergency, interventions may be carried out in the absence of consent by or on behalf of the patient (McRae and Weijer 2002). Here, the physician who undertakes to intervene upon the patient assumes the authority to do so.

Fiduciary duties – including the duty of care – may thus arise in the absence of mutual consent. They therefore differ from contractual duties of care, which arise solely as a result of the mutual consent that lies at the foundation of contract. They also differ from the tort duty of care, which is imposed by law whenever one person lies within the ambit of risk of the other's conduct such that harm to that person is reasonably foreseeable. The means by which fiduciary duties arise encompass but extend beyond the means by which tort and contractual duties arise. Like the duty of care in tort, the fiduciary duty may in very rare circumstances arise by sheer operation of law. Like the duty of care in contract, it may arise by mutual consent. But it may also arise by unilateral undertaking. In that respect, and in respect of the varied means by which they may arise, fiduciary duties are unique.

The significance of consent in the establishment of fiduciary liability is also unique. Consent has no direct role in the establishment of tort liability in negligence. But it does have well-known significance for tort liability in battery, where consent usually negates liability that would otherwise attach to physical interference. Consent has a different function in contract. In contract, mutual consent is reflected in the offer and acceptance of terms governing an exchange of value. By giving their consent, parties to a contract signal that these terms are to be binding on pain of a remedial duty to pay compensation for the expectation of performance. In fiduciary law, where consent is operative in the establishment of a fiduciary relationship, it serves to authorize one person to exercise discretion relative to the practical interests of another and/or to signal the acceptance of an authority conferred or undertaken. In either case, it founds fiduciary liability by effecting authorization to which fiduciary duties are attached.

There are also important differences in the significance of consent for the modification and waiver of liability across tort, contract and fiduciary law. In tort, consent may in rare cases exclude liability for negligence to the extent that it may be seen as constituting a voluntary assumption of risk. Voluntary assumption of risk usually constitutes only a partial defence to liability (where it is analysed under the guise of contributory negligence) and it will be recognized only where consistent with public policy. In contract, by contrast, consensual modification and waiver of default rules of contract (i.e., terms supplied by law rather than agreement) is generally permitted. Consistent with freedom of contract, parties to a contractual relationship are accorded largely unfettered freedom to set the terms of their interaction by agreement. Thus, clauses purporting to waive or modify liability for breach of contract (including breach of implied terms such as non-negligent performance) will usually be respected. Fiduciary liability is far less susceptible to modification or exclusion by consent. Absolute waivers of liability have been deemed unenforceable even when executed *ex ante* (Frankel 1983, 821). Furthermore, to the extent that modifications or partial waivers favour the fiduciary, they may be deemed presumptively unenforceable when executed *ex post* because fiduciary relationships generate a presumption of undue influence. Even where a beneficiary has provided valid *ex ante* consent to conduct by a fiduciary that would otherwise entail breach of fiduciary duty, the fiduciary remains obliged to ensure that the beneficiary is treated fairly, and that his interests are protected by an independent fiduciary (Jackson and Powell 2007, 2-139–2-141). The fiduciary is thus not permitted to treat consent as excusing conduct that is exploitative, abusive, or otherwise unreasonable in the circumstances.

The implications of these differences are profound. To the extent that the relationship between physicians and patients in clinical research is properly considered fiduciary, the obligations attendant upon it privilege the interests of the patient and accord little room for that privilege to be eroded or compromised by consent. Fiduciary law reveals sufficient flexibility to allow physicians and patients to interact in circumstances (e.g., clinical research) in which the interests of physicians and others are engaged and pursued along with those of patients. But patients remain entitled to responsible and reasonable exercise of clinical judgement through which their medical interests may be protected, promoted, or otherwise advanced.

3.6 **Concurrent liability**

Legal categorization of the nature of the relationship between physicians and patients in clinical research and the kinds of wrong that may be realized within it is not an either/or proposition. In any given case, the circumstances of the relationship and the conduct that forms the basis of a complaint could found concurrent claims in tort, contract, and fiduciary law. Indeed, to the extent that a duty of care is imposed by each category of private liability, a complaint by a patient that a physician has failed to exercise due care or skill in the selection or administration of interventions may found an action for negligence, breach of contract, and breach of fiduciary duty.

The prospect of concurrent liability raises the challenge of reconciling differences in the content, scope, and purpose of the various duties of care as well as the significance of consent to their establishment and continuing applicability. As for the establishment of the duty, it is clear that the duty of care may arise in tort irrespective of consent, in fiduciary law it will typically but not invariably be consequent upon mutual or unilateral consent, while in contract, mutual consent is essential. This suggests that a cause of action in contract will not lie if the relationship between the physician-researcher and patient-subject is not founded in a consent that can be construed as a binding agreement (e.g., where a proxy is not authorized to act as agent) or if the consent is invalid from the perspective of contract law (e.g., due to mistake).

The content of the duty of care is generally consistent across tort, contract, and fiduciary law, with the exception that tort and fiduciary law place greater emphasis upon skill and knowledge than is evident in contract. But the purpose of the duty varies considerably between the various categories of obligation. In tort, the duty of care reflects a universally held right to be free from the imposition of unreasonable risk of harm by others. In contract, the duty protects the expectation of competent performance of services that are the object of a binding exchange of value. In fiduciary law, the duty protects the expectation of competent, diligent, and skilful exercise of discretionary power by one over the practical interests of another.

The varying purposes served by the duty of care in tort, contract, and fiduciary law are reflected in differences in the scope of potential liability the duty generates. In tort, the duty is quite broad, encompassing all reasonably foreseeable risks of harm generated by one's conduct. In fiduciary law, the duty is narrower, attached as it is to the exercise of discretionary power by the fiduciary. In contract, the duty is narrower still, securing only the competent performance of specific contractual terms.

Differences in the significance of consent for the modification or waiver of liability in tort, contract, and fiduciary law also reflect differences of purpose and different assumptions concerning the interests and capacities of the parties. Consent will only rarely exclude liability for negligence in tort, reflecting the assumption that it will seldom be the case that one has truly contemplated and accepted that another is to be under no obligation to exercise due care in one's interactions with that person. Consent will generally not exclude liability for breach of fiduciary duty; and where it does, the effects are diminished by the imposition of additional duties. This is consistent with the presumption that the fiduciary relationship makes beneficiaries particularly dependent upon and vulnerable to fiduciaries. By contrast, consent will typically exclude liability for want of due care in the performance of a contract, provided that the relationship between the parties is an ordinary commercial one of arm's length.

Clearly consent is not straightforwardly decisive of liability in tort, contract, or fiduciary law. But its significance is undeniably greater in contract than in tort or fiduciary law. The challenge presented by the prospect of concurrent liability lies in what to make of these differences in attempting to discern eventual liability. It may be put concretely in contemplation of the relationship between physician-researchers and patient-subjects. Assuming that liability is triggered in tort, contract, and fiduciary law, is the scope of the duty of care to be fixed by the scope of the fiduciary relationship (i.e., with reference to the interests of the beneficiary and authority vested in the fiduciary), the scope of the contract (i.e., with reference to specific express or implied terms of contract), or reasonable foreseeability of harm? Is liability presumptively subject to exclusion or modification by consent (as in contract) or not (as in tort and fiduciary law)? If founded in contract, the duty of care may require only that a physician-researcher exercise reasonable care and skill in the performance of interventions contemplated by the protocol for which consent was obtained, and liability for negligent performance may – if the court is unwilling to disrupt the presumption of arm's-length dealing – be excluded by express language in the consent form. If founded in fiduciary law, the duty of care would require a physician-researcher to exercise reasonable care, diligence, and skill in exercising clinical judgement with respect to the selection and administration of interventions to patient-subjects and liability will typically not be subject to exclusion by consent. If founded in tort, the duty of care establishes a blanket obligation to act with reasonable care, which has been interpreted as requiring physicians to meet professional standards of competent care. Again, liability is typically not subject to exclusion by consent.

These differences are such that a court may be unable to reconcile the various claims and instead be required to determine whether the wrong should be construed as lying in contract, tort, or fiduciary law. Contract and fiduciary law regulate relationships. Tort regulates conduct at large. Given that interactions between physicians and patients in practice and research take place within the context of identifiable relationships, the merits of proceeding under contract or fiduciary law seem to us to be the obvious starting point for discussion. Setting aside the question of the merits of proceeding under tort, which may be the default starting point as a matter of practice, attention ought to be paid to the comparative merits of contract and fiduciary law as a matter of principle.

Ardent advocates of freedom of contract and *laissez faire* economics tend to assert that contract 'trumps' other categories of private law, with the implication that non-contractual liability is, or should be, defeasible by contract (Easterbrook and Fischel 1993). But such assertions are grounded in ideology, not argument or authority. In fact, the various categories of private liability make no claims upon each other. Private law doctrine is articulated within, not across, categories. There is nothing in contract doctrine itself to support the idea that contract 'trumps' fiduciary law or tort (Waddams 2003). Similarly, there is nothing in tort or fiduciary doctrine to support the idea that principles of tort or fiduciary liability 'trump' principles of liability in contract (*ibid.*). Rather, the accommodation of various categories of private liability is resolved on a case-by-case basis with the focus lying upon the facts giving rise to concurrent liability. There is thus nothing to be said in the abstract as to whether contract or fiduciary law should be preferred in cases where their respective principles of liability are conflicting.

Nevertheless, relationships between physicians and patients ordinarily have certain characteristics that suggest that fiduciary law should be afforded priority over contract. We have already noted that recognized indicia of contract are missing from many relationships between physician-researchers and patient-subjects (e.g., mutual consent, bargaining over terms, consideration, and a reasonable prospect of mutual enforcement). But it should also be noted that presumptions concerning the positioning of the parties to a contract will also frequently be untenable as applied to relationships between physician-researchers and patient-subjects. Chief amongst these are presumptions attached to ordinary arm's-length commercial dealings, the most important being that the parties are acting independently in mutual self-interest. These presumptions are untenable in light of the fact that patients in clinical research continue to be highly dependent upon and vulnerable to physicians. Evidence of therapeutic misconception beyond indicating flaws in consent processes further suggests that patients trust and expect physicians in research to act with their interests in mind. These circumstantial features of the relationship between physician-researchers and patient-subjects supplement and reinforce the formal character of fiduciary relationship. To the extent that the relationship between physician-researchers and patient-subjects satisfies a reasonable definition of the fiduciary relationship, conflicts generated by concurrent liability should be resolved in favour of the application of fiduciary principles.

This conclusion is well supported (Mehlman 1990). Mark Hall and Carl Schneider, for example, argue that fiduciary principles constrain the application of contract principles in the 'medical marketplace':

> [T]he very disabilities that make people patients make them poor consumers. The relationships among patients, doctors and hospitals make ordinary commercial relations uneasy and undesirable. And providers can compel patients to sign blank checks which providers can complete in dismaying ways ... The law responds to patients' exceptional vulnerability by altering several assumptions about commercial relationships. For example, the law spurns caveat emptor and the presumption that parties contract at arm's length and instead makes the doctor a fiduciary.

(Hall and Schneider 2008, 667)

Hall and Schneider explain well the perils of applying ordinary contract principles to relationships between physicians and patients:

> The standard 'freedom of contract' view works dreadfully in the medical context. Patients are not conventional consumers. They are strangers in a strange land, vulnerable because they are sick and because the market for health care is incomprehensible and dangerous. In their need, patients build relationships of dependence and trust with the people who care for them.

(ibid., 688)

These arguments are equally compelling as applied to relationships between physicians and patients in research. The patient is no less ill or vulnerable and the physician is no less capable of beneficial exercise of power that meets standards of competent care in research as in practice. The rhetoric and ideology of freedom of contract is not permitted to erode the protection that principles of private liability afford patients in clinical practice. There is no justification for greater laxity in clinical research.

3.7 **Conclusion**

Relationships between physicians and patients in clinical research are established in different ways. It is uncontroversial that physicians are required to act with reasonable care in these relationships. But the character of this duty depends on its legal foundation. The legal footing upon which people interact depends in turn upon the nature of their relationship and/or qualities of their interaction. We have argued that relationships between physicians and patients in clinical research are such that they may found a duty of care in tort, contract, or fiduciary law. We have also explained that the significance of consent varies across these categories of private liability. The variation is such that the prospect of concurrent liability may generate conflict between principles of liability and as such require one category to be granted priority over another. Resolution of the conflict will ultimately turn on the facts of particular relationships. However, in our opinion, the circumstances of relationships between physicians and patients in clinical research will typically be such as to require that priority be afforded to principles of fiduciary liability. Established on a fiduciary footing, the duty of care may arise in the absence of mutual consent, extend beyond terms established by consent, and survive purported exclusion by consent. Even where established in tort or contract, our analysis reveals that consent does not invariably enjoy the primacy of place it is often thought to have in the bioethics literature. Rather, appropriately enough, the significance of consent in private law is complex and contested, depending on the factual and legal character of relationships and the needs, interests, and expectations of the parties to them.

References

Annas, G.J., Glantz, L.H., and Katz, B.F. (1977). *Informed Consent to Human Experimentation: The Subject's Dilemma*. Cambridge, MA: Ballinger.

Applebaum, P.S., Lidz, C.W., and Meisel, A. (1987a). *Informed Consent, Legal Theory and Clinical Practice*. New York: Oxford University Press.

Applebaum, P.S., Roth, L.H., Lidz, C.W., Benson, P., and Winslade W. (1987b). False hopes and best data: consent to research and the therapeutic misconception. *Hastings Center Report* **17**, no.2, 20–4.

Atiyah, P.S and Smith, S. (2005). *Atiyah's Introduction to the Law of Contract* (6th edition). Oxford: Clarendon Press.

Blum, B.A. (2001). *Contracts: Examples and Explanations* (2nd edition). Gaithersburg, NY: Aspen Law and Business.

Bolam v. Friern Hospital Management Committee (1957). 1 W.L.R. 582 at 586.

Bowker, W.F. (1982). Exculpatory language in consent forms. *IRB: A Review of Human Subjects Research*, **4**(3):9.

Breen v. Williams (1996). 70 A.L.J.R. 772.

Burton v. Brooklyn Doctors Hospital 1982, 45 N.Y.S. 2d 875.

Canterbury v. Spence 464 F. 2d 772 (D.C. Cir. (1972).

Crits v. Sylvester (1956). 1 D. L.R. (2d) 502 (Ont. C.A.).

Title 45, Code of Federal Regulations, Part 46, S. 46. 116.

Craft v. Vanderbilt 1998, 18 F. Supp. 2d 786.

Dahl v. HEM Pharmaceuticals Corporation 7 F.3d 1399 (9th Cir. 1993).

Donoghue (or McAlister) v. Stevenson (1932). AC 562.

Dube v. Labar (1986). 1 S.C.R. 649.

Easterbrook, F.H. and Fischel, D.R. (1993). Contract and fiduciary duty. *Journal of Law and Economics*, **36**(1), 425–51.

Ellis, M. (1995). *Professional Fiduciary Duties*. Toronto: Carswell.

Frankel, T. (1983). Fiduciary law. *California Law Review*, **71**: 795–836.

George Mitchell Ltd v. Finney Lock Seeds Ltd (1983). Q.B. 284 (C.A.), aff'd [1983] 2 A.C. 803 (H.L).

Giesen, D. (1995). Civil liability of physicians for new methods of treatment and experimentation: a comparative examination. *Medical Law Review*, **3**, 22–52.

Gold v. Haringey Health Authority (1988). Q.B. 481 at 489.

Grimes v. Kennedy Krieger Institute, Inc. 782 A2d 807 (Md. (2001).

Hall, M.A. and Schneider, C.E. (2008). Patients as consumers: courts, contracts, and the new medical marketplace. *Michigan Law Review*, **106**, 643–89.

Halushka v. University of Saskatchewan (1965). 52 W.W.R. 608 (Sask. C.A.).

Hershey, N. and Miller, R.D. (1976). *Human Experimentation and the Law*. Aspen systems crop, Germantou MD.

Hobbs v. Robertson (2001). B.C.J. No. 190 (S.C.).

Hunter Engineering Co. v. Syncrude (1989). 1 S.C.R. 426 (S.C.C.).

Powell, J.L. and Stewart R. (2007). *Jackson and Powell on Professional Liability* (6th edition). London: Sweet and Maxwell.

Kernke v. The Menninger Clinic 172 F. Supp. 2d 1347 (D. Kan. (2001).

Lochner v. New York, 1905 198 U.S. 45. U.S.S.C.

Oliver v. Brock (1976). (Ala) 342 So 2d 1,

Osbourne v Frazone (1968) 58 Tenn App 15.

McInerney v. MacDonald (1992). 2 SCR 138 S.C.C.

McRae, A. and Weijer, C. (2002). Lessons from everyday lives: a moral justification for acute care research. *Critical Care Medicine*, **30**, no. 5, 1146–51.

Maloney, D.M. (1984). *Protection of Human Research Subjects: A Practical Guide to Federal Laws and Regulations*. New York: Plenum Press.

Mehlman, M.J. (1990). Fiduciary contracting: limitations on bargaining between patients and health care providers. *University of Pittsburgh Law Review*, **51**, 365–418.

Miller, P.B. (2008). *Essays Toward a Theory of Fiduciary Law*. Ph.D. Thesis, University of Toronto.

Miller, P.B. and Weijer, C. (2006). Fiduciary obligation in clinical research. *Journal of Law, Medicine and Ethics*, **34** no. 2, 424–40.

Norberg v. Wynrib (1992). 92 D.L.R. (4th) 229.

Payette v. Rockefeller University, 1996, 643 N.Y.S.2d 79.

Picard, E.I. and Robertson, G.B. (2007). *Legal Liability of Doctors and Hospitals in Canada* (4th edition). Toronto: Thomson Carswell.

Quill, T. (1983). Partnerships in patient care: a contractual approach. *Annals of Internal Medicine*, **98**(2), 28–34.

Reibl v. Hughes (1980). 114 D.L.R. (3d) 1 (S.C.C.).

Rigelhaupt, *What Constitutes Physician–Patient Relationship for Malpractice Purposes*, (1982) **17** ALR 4th, 132–160.

Sidaway v. Governors of Bethlem Royal Hospital (1985). A.C. 871 (H.L.).

Tuskegee Syphilis Study Legacy Committee (1996). *Final Report of the Tuskegee Syphilis Study Legacy Committee*. Virginia: University of Virginia Health Sciences Library.

Vodopest v. MacGregor (1996). 128 Wn.2d 840 (Wash.).

Waddams, S.M. (2003). *Dimensions of Private Law: Categories and Concepts in Anglo-American Legal Reasoning*. Cambridge: Cambridge University Press.

Weiss v. Solomon (1989). 48 C.C. L.T., 280 (Que. S.C.).

West Coast Hotel Co. v. Parrish (1937). 300 U.S. 379 (U.S.S.C).

Whitlock v. Duke Univ. (1986). 637 F. Supp. 1463 (M.D.N.C.).

Williams, G.L. (1951). *Joint Torts and Contributory Negligence: A Study of Concurrent Fault in Great Britain, Ireland and the common-law dominions*. London: Stevens.

Chapter 4

The decision to decline to enrol in a clinical trial: a blind spot in the literature on decision-making for research participation

Claire Snowdon, Diana Elbourne, and Jo Garcia

4.1 Introduction

The decisions that people make about clinical trial participation have been the focus of a great deal of empirical study. The available literature is, however, an eclectic and somewhat heterogeneous body of information. Data on actual decisions made by individuals (as opposed to hypothetical decisions, a common focus of research) have been placed in the public domain by authors from several different epistemological backgrounds; by trialists, clinicians, and researchers from academic fields such as medical ethics, psychology, sociology, philosophy, and medical anthropology. There are great methodological variations in the data, which range from correlations between clinical and demographics variables and acceptance or refusal rates (van Bergen *et al.* 1995), simple records of reasons for decisions (Spiro *et al.* 2000) through surveys, and questionnaire-based studies (Jenkins and Fallowfield 2000; Madsen *et al.* 2002), to in-depth analysis of qualitative interview-based data (Snowdon *et al.* 1997, 2006; Featherstone and Donovan 1998; Cox 1999, 2000; Gammelgaard *et al.* 2004; Costenbader *et al.* 2007).

Whilst the body of evidence is substantial and is derived from many sources, if considered as a collective it can be seen to be subject to particular limitations. It is circumscribed by research aims which are themselves bounded by specific areas of interest and concern. Much of the research in this area is driven, but also limited, by two dominant driving forces; the need to increase and sustain accrual rates for clinical trials, and the ethical imperative to protect individuals by improving standards of consent for trial enrolment. Whilst the importance attached to effective and ethical research management has fostered these two intersecting fields of inquiry, it is our contention that the dominance of these particular perspectives on decision-making has also resulted in a significant blind spot. In this blind spot, there are important issues relating to the decision to decline participation in a clinical trial which have been left under-researched and outside of theoretical consideration.

4.2 **The need to increase and sustain accrual rates for clinical trials**

In spite of our contention that declining enrolment in a clinical trial is under-researched, many accrual-related studies have produced data on the subject. Research relating to accrual has flourished as trialists and their funders are, quite rightly, concerned that their trials should recruit an adequate number of participants. Inadequate recruitment is a perennial problem. It has serious consequences, not only in terms of the success or failure of individual trials, but also in relation to the wider use of unevaluated interventions and impediments to medical progress (Gotay 1991; Gates *et al.* 2004).

In accrual-related research, both acceptance and the decision to decline are of interest as potentially crucial determinants of the success or failure of individual trials. The earlier studies focused very much on generating simple lists of why those who were eligible for trial participation said they had accepted or declined. Some such studies were to an extent self-limiting, given the commonly used technique of assessing lists of factors as if each was a discrete element in decision-making, unmediated, and uncomplicated. More recently research which seeks to understand decision-making in this context has grown in sophistication. There is now recognition that the decision-making process is subject to many influences, and there has been exploration of the contributory effects of a range of factors such as information leaflets (Wragg *et al.* 2000), perceptions of the views of recruiters (Grant *et al.* 2000), recruitment style (Donovan *et al.* 2002), and aspects of research design (Hutton *et al.* 1990; Plaisier *et al.* 1994; van der Windt *et al.* 2000).

Although methodological approaches have changed, the decision about participation itself can still, however, be viewed in somewhat simplistic and rather partisan terms, and often from a single vantage point. The dominant terminology which frames decision-making is highly revealing in this respect. Declining to enrol in a trial is commonly termed 'refusal' and the factors which are thought to promote and underlie acceptance are known as 'facilitators' while those associated with 'refusal' are commonly and uncritically described as 'barriers', 'obstacles', and 'hurdles'. Gaining an appreciation of these barriers is frequently presented as the key to encouraging greater participation in subsequent trials. Here declining participation is not seen as a multi-faceted phenomenon, nor is it viewed as being of potential consequence in the lives of individuals. Instead it is largely a methodological problem to be overcome. This model of research as a means to understand behaviour in order to change it is predicated on the assumption that it is appropriate to do so. The perception of consent as the right decision and 'refusal' as correctable, is fundamental to accrual-related research.

4.3 **The ethical imperative to protect individuals and to improve standards of consent for enrolment into clinical trials**

Whilst researchers in one field explicitly work to reduce the numbers of decliners and promote higher consent rates, researchers working in other fields often consider decision-making for trial enrolment with different aims in mind. A very clear imperative exists to protect individuals and improve the standards of communication and decision-making around enrolment to clinical trials. The principle of informed consent, 'the bedrock ... of protection of human research subjects' (Kraybill, 2004), holds that the decisions of those who agree to participate in biomedical research should be free, informed, autonomous, and voluntary (Beauchamp and Childress 1994). The principle of informed consent was enshrined in the Declaration of Helsinki, which was most recently refined in Tokyo in 2004 (see http://www.wma.net/e/policy/b3.htm). In accordance with this ethically driven approach to clinical research, many aspects of the decision to consent to research participation have been subject to close scrutiny in a variety of settings.

Typically, the decisions made by trial participants are measured against ideals of non-coercive and informed consent. It has been demonstrated very clearly that the decision to enter a trial very often falls short of ideal (Appelbaum et al. 1982; Benson et al. 1985; Appelbaum et al. 1987; Snowdon et al. 1997; Featherstone and Donovan 1998; Lidz et al. 2004). Much empirical effort has been made to understand the underlying difficulties that exist. How respondents understand and interpret trial participation is often examined in relation to the specific medical and research-related setting in which the decision-making process takes place. Oncology patients, for instance, make their decisions in the context of potentially life-threatening illness (Featherstone and Donovan 2002); myocardial infarction patients (Williams et al. 2003; Gammelgaard et al. 2004) and those with subarachnoid haemorrhages (Yuval et al. 2000) are asked to consider trial participation in an emergency setting, some in pain, and with varying levels of consciousness.

Studies to assess competency to consent have been carried out with patient groups whose decision-making capacity is particularly likely to be impaired, such as emergency patients (Smithline et al. 1999) and older patients with debilitating physical and mental illness (Dunn and Jeste 2003; Stroup et al. 2005). The views of adults who have been asked to make proxy decisions for incapacitated relatives have been explored (Elad et al. 2000; Sugarman et al. 2001), and a rapidly increasing number of studies have involved parents making decisions in diverse settings. Parents can be asked to make enrolment-related decisions on behalf of their children for trials involving behavioural interventions (Glogowska et al. 2001), surgical interventions (Tait et al. 2003), treatments related to chronic illness (van Stuijvenberg et al. 1998), serious illness (Wiley et al. 1999; Kupst et al. 2003; Greenley et al. 2006), and intensive care (Snowdon et al. 1997, 2006; Allmark and Mason 2006). At the most extreme end of the spectrum are the decisions made by patients with terminal conditions and no further treatment options to enter phase I toxicity trials. This has generated a subfield of enquiry driven by what Nurgat and colleagues (2005) refer to as 'genuine concern for the welfare of individual patients' (e.g., Daugherty et al. 1995; Hutchison 1998; Schutta and Burnett 2000; Cox 2002, 2003; Weinfurt et al. 2003). The studies which have explored these many different situations have indicated how at the point of weighing information and making decisions, potential trial participants can be calm or they can be confused and anxious, well or sick and in pain, and their decisions can be made with or without time for reflection or consultation. Their decisions can reflect different impulses and have different meanings for individuals. For some the act of entering a trial is a positive proactive step as shown in the accounts of some men participating in HIV/AIDs trials (Ross *et al*. 1994). In contrast, some phase I trial participants have accepted a research protocol because of the lack of other options and have been described as 'desperate volunteers' (Minogue *et al*. 1995).

Decisions have also been assessed as part of a larger complex process, as potential participants interact with recruiting clinicians, treating clinicians, and family members. Much of the research in this area has focused on the views of these actors as discrete groups, but attempts have been made to understand patterns of interaction, especially family involvement in decision-making (Snethen *et al*. 2006). There has been a growth in research comparing the views and concerns of the parties involved (Daugherty *et al*. 1995; Joffe *et al*. 2001; Meropol *et al*. 2003) and in observational research in which the dynamics of the consent process are assessed (Kodish *et al*. 2004; Miller *et al*. 2005).

Researchers have increasingly turned their attention to the post-consent period, to gain insights into perceptions of the burdens and benefits of trial participation (Kinmonth *et al*. 1983; Henzlova *et al*. 1994). They have also explored changing expectations of participation during the course of a trial (Stone *et al*. 2005) and subsequent levels of satisfaction with, or decisional regret over, the decision to consent (Pope *et al*. 2003; Stryker *et al*. 2006). Such issues are of particular importance for long-term trials which require a high level of commitment over many years from those who consent to participate. One very careful study of the experience of long-term involvement in a diabetes trial focused on the impact of trial closure, discussing how best to address 'trial bereavement' for participants making the transition back to routine care (Lawton *et al*. 2003). The possible effects of informing patients of their allocation at trial closure (Di Blasi *et al*. 2005) and of feedback of trial results have also been considered (Snowdon *et al*. 1998; Dixon-Woods *et al*. 2006). The experience of trial participation has been seen as conferring a form of expertise (Snowdon *et al*. 1999) and recommendations of previous participants have been sought in order to improve consent processes in subsequent trials (Eder *et al*. 2007).

4.4 **A blind spot**

Even this brief overview of some of the available research ethics-related literature indicates that consent to participate in a trial is now seen as a complex phenomenon. The literature considers this decision and subsequent participation in a broad socio-cultural context, exploring immediate and longer term sequelae for individuals, and suggests a level of concern for the wellbeing of those involved. Data on the quality and the personal consequences of the decision elucidate the impact of association with research upon trial participants, as well as being indicators of ethical standards in research. By comparison, the decision to decline has been considered far less frequently, and is often viewed in a much more limited fashion.

With a small number of exceptions (e.g., Mohanna and Tunna 1999; Stevens and Ahmedzai 2004), decliners' conceptions of a trial, their experiences and their wellbeing have rarely been the explicit and main focus of research. They do not appear to have been widely consulted as lay experts on how to improve or manage trial procedures. Quite notably, despite concerns surrounding phase I clinical trials, we have found no research on the reasons for declining such trials, the impact of this decision, or the possibility of decisional regret. Some first-person accounts, and a small number of studies in which decliners have been included, do provide some helpful data on the decision to decline (Madsen *et al.* 2002; Gammelgaard *et al.* 2004; Patel *et al.* 2004; Canvin and Jacoby 2006; Costenbader *et al.* 2007; Madsen *et al.* 2007) but often response rates for this group are very low and they can constitute a minority of the sample. Nonetheless, these sources suggest that declining trial participation is in fact an area particularly worthy of further study.

The accounts given by Thornton (1992), a breast cancer patient, and Blewitt (1994), a mother of a critically ill baby, both demonstrate in different ways how individuals can and do carefully assess the personal implications of participating in research. For some, this may include evaluations of the research itself, as authors of two recent publications have argued; decliners in their studies saw different implications in the trials that they were offered than those who consented, focusing on possible risks rather than possible advantages in novel treatments and research regimes (Costenbader *et al.* 2007; Madsen *et al.* 2007). Similarly, pregnant women who declined a trial aimed at preventing preterm labour were shown to view the possibility of risk of any medication for their unborn baby as their foremost consideration, even when the likelihood and risks of preterm delivery were high (Mohanna and Tunna 1999). There is some evidence that in comparison to those who accept, those who decline are less convinced that their clinicians are being wholly honest about the background level of evidence about treatment (Mills *et al.* 2003). They have been found to be less supportive of research, and less familiar with details of the research that they have rejected than those who have accepted participation (Tait *et al.* 2003; Williams *et al.* 2003; Sharp *et al.* 2006).

One study suggested that the small number of decliners who were included ($n = 4$) were reluctant to pass over control of their care to a random process (Canvin and Jacoby 2006), a finding which has also been reported in the accrual-related literature (Ross *et al.* 1999). In a rare interview study assessing views and experiences subsequent to rejecting participation in a breast cancer trial, Stevens and Ahmedzai (2004) reported that some women felt guilt about their decision. They also suggested that over time, as their fear of cancer returning increased, some women wished that they had chosen to enrol and some asked to reverse their decision and to join the trial in question. These studies tantalizingly suggest that decliners may be different from, or may even become different from, those who enter research, but they constitute a relatively small body of evidence.

It is likely that potential difficulties associated with research with those who decline contribute to the disparity of empirical data on the views and experiences of consenters and decliners. Access to decliners can be very difficult, with both research ethics committees and clinicians acting as gatekeepers (Williams *et al.* 2007), and individuals possibly being reluctant or disinclined to discuss research that they have already rejected. It is also possible that declining trial participation is of minimal interest outside of the accrual-related literature; non-participants are not subject to trial

interventions, and their decision clearly indicates that their right to decline to participate has been upheld. The Declaration of Helsinki requires only that potential participants are 'informed of the right to abstain from participation' (paragraph 22) and that
'the refusal of a patient to participate in a study must never interfere with the patient–
physician relationship' (paragraph 31) http://www.wma.net/e/policy/b3.htm).

The potential needs of decliners and the possibility that researchers might have
responsibilities towards them which extend beyond non-coercion and reassurance,
appear not to have been sufficiently considered. Whether the experience and personal
implications of declining trial participation might, like those associated with consent,
be related to context-specific factors or relate to clinical settings, types of trials, and
types of interventions, has not been explored.

Where decliners have been included in research, it would seem that their choice has
largely been considered from one of two somewhat contradictory perspectives; the
decision is seen in one literature as problematic, and in the other a demonstration
that ethical standards of non-coercion have been met. Whether or not such decisions
are informed has rarely been considered in either body of literature. It is important
that declining to take part in research is considered not just as an impediment to
progress, or in relation to the management process of clinical trials, but as an individual and a social experience with personal implications. A small amount of relevant
data which shed light on some potential aspects of declining participation are
available from the Study of Participants' Views of Perinatal Trials.

4.5 Study of participants' views of perinatal trials

This qualitative study was designed to consider views and experiences of randomized
controlled trials (RCTs) from multiple perspectives. It involved interviews with clinicians
and parents who were associated with one or more of four clinical trials: two antenatal
(TEAMS, ORACLE) and two neonatal (INNOVO, CANDA). Research ethics committee
(REC) approval for the study was given by North Thames Multi-centre REC and by all
relevant local RECs.

A specific aim of this study was to include the views of parents who declined to take
part in these trials. Access proved to be very difficult and, as in other studies, they constitute a minority of the interviews. The study included 78 parents in total but only 12 parents, from 8 interviews, had declined to participate in a trial; three interviews were with
parents who had declined TEAMS, one with parents who had declined ORACLE, and
four with those who declined the CANDA Trial. Their views, and further details of the
four trials, have been represented within reports of the larger study (Snowdon 2005;
Snowdon *et al.* 2006) but not as a group of parents who declined participation. Each trial
created different circumstances and was subject to very different rates of refusal. With
such unexpected small numbers from each trial, the parents could not be taken as representative of the decliners for a given trial, and collectively their circumstances, attitudes,
and experiences were so diverse that it was also difficult to conduct a comparative analysis.
There were, however, three interviews involving five parents which showed such striking
similarities that they became the focus of the more detailed analysis reported here. In each
case the parents had declined to participate in the CANDA Trial (Ainsworth *et al.* 2000).

As with all of the parental interviews in this study, the three interviews were carried out in the parental home. In two cases both parents were present, and one was a lone interview. With parental consent they were tape recorded, and the recordings were fully transcribed. The interviews were semi-structured and the interview was broadly ordered around the story of the events leading up to and following their decision about trial participation. This started with pregnancy and the difficulties that arose, moving through to delivery and care of their preterm baby, and on to the subsequent post-discharge period. Within this structure the interviews explored respondents' accounts of the CANDA Trial and their decision-making process. Discussions were flexible and covered other areas of interest to the participants, but the main focus analysis was the parents' accounts of the trial itself, the reasons for their decisions, and the significance they attached to these decisions. The thematic analysis was aided by the textual analysis computer package, Atlas-ti.

Whilst a number of important themes were identified which cut across these accounts, only three of the themes are presented here. Each is presented in detail through a single interview. Each account draws heavily on the participants' own words, to highlight their own voices, and their own reconstruction of events, as far as possible. Pseudonyms have been used in each case.

These accounts are put forward to suggest the value of a potential line of inquiry and to provide material for further debate. They are not proposed as being representative of those who decline, but as testimonies which might act as a catalyst for reflection and to highlight the possible value of further research.

4.5.1 The CANDA Trial

The parents whose accounts are explored here were asked to consider enrolling their baby into the CANDA Trial. This trial compared two types of surfactants given shortly after birth to preterm babies born between 25 and 30 weeks' gestation. Surfactant prevents the lung walls from sticking together but its manufacture is limited at this gestation. With inadequate levels of surfactant breathing can be very difficult for preterm babies and its routine administration on delivery undoubtedly confers a major benefit for compromised babies. Surfactant in different forms has been the subject of many RCTs and has been referred to as 'one of the most effective and safest interventions in neonatology' (Halliday 2006).

The CANDA Trial aimed to identify small potential differences between two commonly used forms of surfactant. Curosurf is derived from the lungs of pigs; ALEC (Artificial Lung Expanding Compound) is a synthetic form of surfactant. It was hypothesized that differences between these two forms, even if small, might affect length of hospital stay and so costs associated with care. The CANDA Trial clinicians who were also interviewed for the qualitative study generally viewed the trial as low risk as each arm involved a well-researched and widely used form of surfactant, and because babies whose parents declined to participate in the trial would still receive the locally preferred form of surfactant on delivery (Snowdon 2005).

Recruitment to the trial took place between May 1998 and December 1999. When the trial team were advised of the likelihood of a preterm delivery, parents were approached, either on the antenatal ward or in varying stages of labour, and asked to consider allowing their baby to be enrolled into the CANDA Trial. Parents of 199 babies agreed and parents of 37 were known to have declined (84% consent rate).

4.5.2 Three accounts of declining to enrol a baby in the CANDA Trial

Analysis of the three case studies suggested a number of different possible dimensions to declining to participate in a clinical trial. Each account is presented to highlight one of three themes which appeared to be particularly important; 'distortion', 'alienation', and 'threat'. The themes are presented through a detailed reporting of very personal stories, and this detail allows the decision to decline to be seen in the context of extraordinarily difficult events. It makes clear the significance of apparently distinct elements of the parental experiences, and helps to track how their choice related to circumstances, a sense of parenthood and to relationships with medicine.

4.5.2.1 Distortion – Gillian and Kelvin

Gillian developed pre-eclampsia at 27 weeks of pregnancy. At this gestation pre-eclampsia can develop into a serious threat to maternal health, and after two weeks as an inpatient in her local hospital, she was transferred to another hospital for delivery. She was very young at the time and described herself as fearful and emotional, sure that her baby would be stillborn. Induced labour failed to progress and an emergency caesarean was performed with a general anaesthetic. Gillian was approached and asked to consider enrolment in a trial before surgery.

> Someone come in and asked if they could do medical research on him, and I said yeah because they wouldn't know what they do today if they hadn't done nothing like that.

(Gillian)

This was unexpected as Gillian was being interviewed for the Study of Participants' Views of Perinatal Trials because she was listed in the trial records as having declined participation. Her partner, Kelvin, arrived and joined the interview part way through. His different, albeit patchy, recollection of events completely changed the direction and content of the discussion. His presence removed Gillian's certainty that she had agreed to a trial during labour, and introduced a dynamic element to the interview as the couple tried between them to recreate past conversations and to work out what had happened.

Gillian and Kelvin's account was convoluted and somewhat difficult to understand during the interview. They created a story with temporal and factual inconsistencies which did not make obvious sense. It was, however, evident that they had moved from some initial confusion to a point where their jointly constructed model worked and made sense for them and where they felt that they had given an account of their experiences and views. The key events and the emotions that they provoked were vividly recalled and these details gave their account substance and resonance. This account appeared to satisfy Gillian and Kelvin but the basis of their shared model was not fully disentangled for the research team until a later stage.

It became clear that Gillian and Kelvin had been asked to consider enrolling their baby in two different neonatal trials at two different time points. As the CANDA Trial involved an intervention to be given during the first minutes of life, decisions were made prior to delivery and Gillian had fleetingly remembered being approached during labour (as quoted previously).

The couple went on to describe how they had taken several days to make their decision about whether or not to give their consent. The longer decision-making process that they came to focus on appears to relate to a second trial which compared long and short lines for delivering nutrition, which they were asked to consider at a later point in neonatal intensive care. As Gillian and Kelvin did not hold these two trials as distinct entities, it was only possible to make sense of this account because C.S. became aware that a second trial was open to recruitment when the subject was raised by another couple in their interview. Gillian and Kelvin's confusion over the timing of events was seen in a number of other interviews in the Study of Participants' Views of Perinatal Trials. Here, however, events had not only been reordered; key features of the two trials that were suggested to them were combined to produce a composite version of a trial, surrounding events and the emotions that were provoked.

They described a single trial which involved two distinct elements. They were aware of two types of medical equipment being used in the trial, a long line and a short line which they knew would deliver a product to their baby. They were not concerned about the use of either of the two lines and accepted these. What they were not happy about was what they felt one of the lines would deliver. The following extract illustrates the shuffling of key features of the trials and is crucial to understanding their emerging amalgamated account of their decision-making process.

> Kelvin: I know there was something mentioned about a long line and a short line, and I think it was the long line one that they wanted to try more, because they were only used to using the short line, or it might have been the other way round. And there was two, there was ALEC and there was another one where they used artificial blood in the other one. Is that right, artificial blood?
> Gillian: Yeah. I can't remember.
> Kelvin: And I think we didn't feel comfortable with using the artificial blood.
> Gillian: That one, yeah, they were going to use pigs' blood or something?
> Kelvin: They were going to use pigs' blood, so we didn't um …
> C.S.: And were you asked about that at the same time, or was it a different doctor?
> Kelvin: It was the same time, everything was asked at the same time.

Notably here one of the lines is given the name of one of the forms of surfactant, ALEC, and the reference to it carrying artificial blood most likely derives from its full title, Artificial Lung Expanding Compound. Curosurf, the second surfactant, is a porcine product and this accounts for the reference to pigs, but not for the reference to blood. It is not clear whether they felt that an artificial blood was being compared to pigs' blood, or whether the artificial blood was derived from pigs' blood. Whatever the model, they presented the trial as constituting a long-term threat to their baby's health, as Kelvin explained:

> If they'd have said we're going to use normal human blood, and possibly put vitamins into the blood, or something like that, then that wouldn't have been a problem, not with humans' blood, but the fact that it was going to be pigs' blood, it don't matter how many times you filter it, no matter how many times you do whatever to it, there's always going to be a chance that something could go wrong, with animals' blood. … I always remember

thinking 'oh he's going to get mad cow's disease or mad pig's disease or summat.' … If [they] hadn't have mentioned pigs' blood it would have been a big possibility that we would have went ahead with it, but obviously they had an obligation to tell us everything.

(Kelvin)

Kelvin described the decision that they had to make as 'massive'. As very new and very young parents they were being asked to make a choice which was not simply about the acceptability of research participation, but was about parental responsibility for the choices made for one's children, and their duty to protect them. In describing their decision-making, Kelvin drew upon recollections of the intensity of the emotions that had been provoked. He felt burdened by the degree of responsibility he felt for making a potentially influential choice for a preterm baby in such a vulnerable condition.

At the time our baby was nearly dying. … It was one of the … hardest decisions we'll have to make in our lives. … [I]f we had made that decision to let them go ahead, and anything did happen, I would have possibly blamed myself, yeah, because the method that they used was tried and tested, but this method that they wanted to use was relatively new, so if anything did have happened, I'd have been, like, we should have stuck with the tried and tested method.

(Kelvin)

Although they felt that they had been offered something which was unacceptable to them, they were very positive about the doctors involved in their care. Kelvin felt that they were tolerant of his own suspicion and irritability.

I think the doctors put it the best way they could, because … I was very ratty at the time … because what I'd got into my head was they were using him as a guinea pig. … I made it clear that I wasn't happy with it, and the doctors just sat down and had a word with us and said 'Look, there's no way in the world we would put him at risk, it's just something being tested at other hospitals and we are just wanting to test it here.'

(Kelvin)

Although there was much confusion in this interview, Gillian and Kelvin had described their experiences in terms which suggested that they felt that they had weighed important factors in a difficult decision and had acted in their baby's best interest. They were not averse to research itself, but would not countenance participation in research which they felt may be to the detriment of their baby. In rejecting research, they felt that they had acted responsibly and the confusion that was evident in their shuffling of key features in the interview was not associated with any self-doubt or requests for further clarification from the interviewer, common features in the interviews with parents who had accepted trial participation. They were, however, left with the impression that the doctors caring for their baby, whatever their statements about risk, were prepared to carry out strange and, to them, unacceptable research, on vulnerable neonates.

4.5.2.2 Alienation – Shelley and Evan

Shelley went into early labour at 26 weeks of pregnancy and was transferred from her local hospital by ambulance to a larger hospital with appropriate neonatal facilities. Her labour stopped and she felt very positive.

I was fine. The pains had stopped and the contractions were slowing down, so we were like 'Okay, this is obviously going to work.' Because they'd started to slow down … [we were] quite cheerful. … [W]e were quite mellow, [feeling] 'I think we might stop this, and you know, we'll go home and [be] quite happy'.

(Shelley)

At this point, they were approached by a neonatologist. When there is a strong likelihood that a baby will be delivered early, it is common practice to try to introduce parents to aspects of neonatal intensive care before the event. The neonatologist described some of the problems that their baby might face if delivered. Shelley and Evan repeatedly referred to this conversation throughout the interview, both saying that they were told that their baby 'only had a ten per cent chance of survival' and that there was a possibility of brain damage. The suggestion that labour might continue was an unexpected and devastating blow given their earlier confidence. It seemed to represent a turning point in their experience.

That was when it all sort of like dawned. Once you knew, deep down that there is the risk of having a baby that early, and all the possibilities of them dying – until they actually said it, we hadn't really, you know, considered it. As far as I was concerned, you know, it was stopping and she was going to be fine.

(Shelley)

The neonatologist then went on to describe the CANDA Trial and ask whether they would consider enrolling their baby, if delivered. Shelley felt that this was insensitive.

I think he chose the wrong time to ask us, because he was telling us the worst case scenario and what could happen to her, and then in the next sort of breath he was telling us 'Can we use this new drug?'

(Shelley)

They instantly and unanimously declined to participate in the trial. In the interview they were unclear about what the trial involved, talking only about 'a new thing' and a 'new procedure'. As they were unaware of the animal origin of Curosurf, this was not an element in their concern. The risks that they perceived were unspecific but did include the idea of testing drugs. They focused very simply on the experimental nature of research. They saw involving a vulnerable new baby in such research as wholly unacceptable. Evan said:

I thought, a young baby that wasn't going to have much chance of survival, and they want to use an experimental type procedure! Well, the first thing we thought was 'No, no way!'

(Evan)

They stated that they did not feel under pressure to consent, and that the neonatologist was 'fine' about their refusal. They felt that he was 'a very good doctor' (Evan) but was 'very uncomfortable' (Evan), and 'very nervous' (Shelley) in his approach to them. Shelley sympathized with his position, feeling that it must have been very difficult for him. Her comment, 'I wouldn't like to be put in *that* situation. I wouldn't like to have to go up and ask people *that*!' indicates that she saw the neonatologists as having been obliged to make a very difficult request.

Why they saw the request as being so difficult for the neonatologist, and why it seemed so utterly insensitive and unacceptable, hinged not on the details of the research itself, but on connections that they made between different parts of the conversation about the threat to their baby from early delivery and discussions of the trial. Evan explained why they were being asked to allow their baby to participate in research:

> [She] didn't have much chance of survival, and they wanted to try this new procedure out on her! Well just because she didn't have much chance of survival, why would they try this new procedure out!

> (Evan)

They both felt that it was precisely because of the likelihood that their baby would die that they were being asked to agree to allow a novel treatment to be tested on her. Unlike other parents, there was no weighing of possible risks and benefits and, in contrast to Gillian and Kelvin, there was no consideration of possible effects in the long term; in this account there was no long term, precisely the reason for the approach to consider research in the first place. Evan said: 'we were just adamant that it wasn't going to happen!'

4.5.2.3 Threat – Janine

Janine was admitted to hospital at 29 weeks of pregnancy in early labour. She continued to move in and out of labour over four days. In a similar situation to Shelley and Evan, she described herself as 'shocked' and her husband as 'terrified' by a discussion with a consultant of their baby's chances of survival if delivered at that stage. At a later point, when Janine was in established labour, they were approached by a neonatologist and asked to consider enrolling their baby in the CANDA Trial.

Her accounts of the discussion during her labour were very negative and she was clearly still angry about her experience. It was evident in the interview that her emotions were gaining momentum and she became increasingly disparaging. In her initial account of her encounter with the neonatologist who had approached her during labour, she said that she was given a very brief explanation of the research which she described as seeming innocuous at the time. She offered reassurance that she was not making accusations of duplicity.

> I don't want you to think that it was someone who was trying to be false because he wasn't. ... It wasn't forceful it just ... seemed so insignificant. That's probably why I was going to do it. Because it seemed so like, well, this is what you need to do. That was why I was going to do it, because it didn't seem important. ... [But] it was *so* important!

This last comment is indicative of how she came to view the research. As she described the events involved, she became increasingly negative. She explained that she did not give much thought to the trial at first and said that she was about to consent, essentially to get the doctor to leave her to get on with her labour.

> I nearly just sort of went 'well yeah, give it here' because you're not thinking. You are just like – 'go away!' you know.

Janine explained that the midwifery staff intervened as the neonatologist had not brought an information sheet and requested some written details that they could go over with her. Janine discussed the trial with the midwifery staff and subsequently declined to participate in the CANDA Trial. She felt that she had narrowly avoided being 'railroaded' into the trial. A crucial aspect in her account was her description of a gradually increasing sense of the research being much more significant and threatening than it had originally seemed.

Janine's account of the trial, and of why it seemed to be so threatening, appears to be a fusion of information about the CANDA Trial itself with details of treatments that she and her baby are very likely to have received in preparation for a premature birth. Women in preterm labour are routinely given injections of antenatal steroids in labour to help to mature the baby's lungs and so aid breathing on delivery, and this appeared to be interwoven with the trial-related administration of surfactant on delivery, also to aid breathing. Janine felt that the trial was comparing a steroid, which she identified specifically as dexamethasone, to another substance which she described as a 'pig derivative'. She saw the trial as posing a direct and serious threat to her baby, involving risk on two levels. She felt that it had already been decided that if she consented to the trial her baby would receive the 'pig derivative'. Participation would, therefore, have meant exposure to the unknown risks of what was to her a deeply unsettling intervention, but would also have resulted in severing access to the known benefits of dexamethasone. As she came to view the trial in this way, she felt shocked that she had almost placed her baby at risk and denied him an effective treatment, by an unconsidered acceptance of the trial. She characterized the effects of her consent had she given it as 'my tiny tiny delicate baby having pig shoved in him!'

Her concern over the denial of an effective treatment arose again later in the interview in her account of seeing other babies on the neonatal intensive care unit.

> As soon as he was born and I saw that every other baby in the [neonatal] unit was on dexamethasone, it's what made me think I had no doubts whatsoever that I'd done the right thing.

Like Gillian and Kelvin, Janine pulled together different important elements in her experience and used them to make an apparently linear narrative. It was in fact an account which appeared to be a product of much temporal re-evaluation of events, a gradual piecing together of disparate pieces of evidence until the story made sense. This story was very heavily and very obviously embedded into difficult emotions and these emotions are probably the most instructive data of all. Like Shelley and Evan, she was left with a sense that she and her baby were a means to an end, despite the difficulty of their circumstances. Janine felt that somehow her baby was under threat from the proposed research and that she had only just managed to give him the protection that he needed.

4.6 **Discussion**

The views of those who decline to participate in research have largely been considered in terms of their possible or actual role in the failure of clinical trials. Choosing not to participate as a product of particular events and experiences, and indeed as an event and experience in itself, has largely been ignored. The extent of the disparity between the interest in the wellbeing of participants and of non-participants is staggering.

The three accounts presented here do little to redress that balance, and, being so small in number, reveal little about the potentially complex and variable nature of refusal. They are, however, sufficient to indicate the necessity of a wider, less partisan, exploration of this phenomenon. The three themes which were picked out for consideration, distortion, alienation, and a sense of threat, are powerful indicators of this need to gain an understanding of what declining participation means for individuals as well as for research.

There are hints of these thematic concerns in the broader literature. It is already very well known that those who enter research can often do so with an incomplete understanding of the nature of the research to which they have given their consent. The notion that therapeutic misconceptions often underpin consent is widely acknowledged and has been shown to operate in large mixed samples of trial participants (Lidz 2006). A small number of studies have also shown that those who decline to participate can be less knowledgeable about key features of research than those who consent (Tait et al. 2003; Williams et al. 2003; Sharp et al. 2006), and a recent study of those who opted out of a cross-sectional survey on activities in retirement reported that widespread misconceptions of the aims of the research underpinned the decision to decline (Williams et al. 2007). Without more detailed research, it is not clear whether shortfalls in knowledge and misconceptions for those who decline participation are similar or different from those who consent.

Certainly, these parental accounts do show an incomplete understanding of the research but this is not simply a knowledge deficit, an absence of key facts. They involve the distortion of available information into something far more problematic with ramifications for the individuals concerned. In contrast to the 'therapeutic misconception' (Appelbaum et al. 1982; Lidz and Appelbaum 2002; Lidz et al. 2004) which derives from a positive model of research in which the offer of trial entry is thought to be driven by concern for patient wellbeing and acceptance grounded in trust in clinicians, these three accounts derive from a negative model of research. Here patient wellbeing is not discussed and the offer is entirely separate from notions of care. These models appear to involve far more unsettling notions than those which have been reported in relation to the therapeutic misconception.

The sense of alienation that is expressed by these parents suggests that they felt the researchers were setting their baby's needs aside in favour of the needs of research. They were perplexed at the offer of an experimental treatment when acceptable alternatives, such as 'normal blood transfusions' (Gillian) and routinely used effective drugs (Janine) were available. This may have been tapped by other research. A generalized concern about 'being a guinea pig' has been said to underlie the reasons for non-participation for some patients (Patel et al. 2004; Quinn et al. 2007; Sullivan et al. 2007), but those described by these parents are very specific and relate to what they felt had been suggested and why. It is possible that this sense of alienation and suspicion may also be relevant to the decisions of those who declined to participate in a trial of management strategies for localized prostate cancer. This group of men were said to understand the concept of equipoise between treatment strategies, but were reported as being unconvinced that it really existed; the authors commented that 'belief in clinical equipoise was key to participants' consent to randomization'

(Mills *et al.* 2003). Similarly, authors of a qualitative study which included women with breast cancer who had declined participation in a clinical trial suggested that for some their decision was based upon disbelief in equipoise and some mistrust of the 'internal control of doctors' (Madsen *et al.* 2007).

If individuals do not feel that they are being given accurate or complete information, or feel that they are being used as a means to an end, it is not surprising that some may articulate a sense of threat. These parents all saw the CANDA Trial as involving something new and experimental and felt that they had had to protect their baby from the unacceptable and unnecessary risks involved. For Shelley, Evan, and Janine, the proposed research was seen as irresponsible and unethical, involving opportunistic experimentation on the dying, and deliberate and irresponsible withholding of a beneficial drug from a sick baby. The level of risk to which the parents felt the trialists were willing to expose their babies was such that in each case they attributed survival to their choice not to consent.

Although the parents all gave different accounts of what the CANDA Trial involved, the common ground between them suggests that theirs are not simply idiosyncratic interpretations of research. Their commonality highlights the value of further reflection on how or why views such as these may arise. They may, for instance, originate if the circumstances in which individuals are approached are particularly difficult. Trials of drugs and interventions involving women in labour are known to involve particular difficulties (Mohanna and Tunna 1999; Ferguson 2000; Kenyon *et al.* 2006) and this may in part account for some of the confusion. This degree of distortion and concern was not, however, present in the accounts of the other parents who consented to the CANDA Trial, most of whom were also approached in active labour.

Problems may arise from the style and content of actual recruitment processes, and it is possible that these processes are different for those who go on to refuse. Shelley stated that they had made it clear that they did not want to listen to the neonatologist once they became upset, and agreed that it was very likely that as a result they had only been given limited and truncated information about the research. This would suggest that difficulties might in some ways be a result of the inclination and subsequent decision to decline participation itself. When research is discussed, those who are inclined to refuse may be less interested in specific details, and subsequently less likely to retain irrelevant information. It is important that future observational research should include follow-up of those who decline to participate in trials to explore this possibility. Unlike those who consent, non-participants do not receive subsequent reminders of the nature of a research project through administration of research procedures or further contact with research staff. Whatever the causes, there are undoubtedly consequences of the perceptions of research which are reported here. There is confusion in the short and long term and it seems that anxiety, distress, and suspicion were still operating for some of these parents. These accounts suggest the need for more empirical work on declining trial participation as a topic of interest in its own right.

There is also further theoretical work to be done. The accounts clearly fall short of what we might hope for after a substantive and informed refusal, but this concept, although subject to debate elsewhere in medicine, especially in relation to rejection of blood products (Dixon and Smalley 1981; Bodnaruk *et al.* 2004), surgery (Bramstedt and Nash 2005) and emergency care (Derse 2005; Moskop 2006), is infrequently invoked as a concept of relevance to decisions around trial participation. Whilst it seems intellectually appropriate to aim for informed refusal, in practice, it may well be difficult to achieve. It may even be an unreasonable expectation. It is, however, important to consider whether refusal should (ideally) be made with the same (ideal) level of understanding of research as consent, or whether different standards might apply where individuals indicate that they are disinterested in research or disinclined to participate. Persistent information-giving may improve knowledge and understanding, but like consent processes in certain circumstances, could also be charged with being 'needlessly cruel' (Tobias and Souhami 1993) if not coercive. It is likely that some of the theoretical ground that has already been covered in relation to consent will need to be revisited in reflections on refusal.

It is also important that very practical issues involved with the management of discussions around refusal are considered. Should, for instance, potential participants be told, as suggested by Williams and colleagues (2007), that there is a potential negative impact of non-participation on the success of a trial, so that they may incorporate this information into their decision-making process? Would this help them to make more sophisticated decisions about trial participation, or would it firmly delineate this choice as a socially undesirable action? This example alone is indicative of the thin and problematic line that might exist between information-giving and coercion.

Much effort has been made to further our understanding of the decision to participate in a trial, of the multifarious factors which affect this decision, and of the different ways in which it is or is not of consequence for those involved. Similar attention and effort is required to bring declining research participation into view. Until the offer of a trial is seen as an intervention in the lives of those involved, irrespective of the direction of the decision that they make, it will not receive the sensitive consideration that it requires.

References

Ainsworth, S.B., Beresford, M.W., Milligan, D.W., *et al.* (2000). Pumactant and poractant alfa for treatment of respiratory distress syndrome in neonates born at 25–29 weeks' gestation: a randomized trial. *Lancet*, **355**, 1387–92.

Allmark, P. and Mason, S. (2006). Improving the quality of consent to randomized controlled trials by using continuous consent and clinician training in the consent process. *Journal of Medical Ethics*, **32**, 439–43.

Appelbaum, P.S., Roth, L.H., and Lidz, C. (1982). The therapeutic misconception: informed consent in psychiatric research. *International Journal of Law and Psychiatry*, **5**, 319–29.

Appelbaum, P.S., Roth, L.H., Lidz, C.W., Benson, P., and Winslade, W. (1987). False hopes and best data: consent to research and the therapeutic misconception. *Hastings Center Report*, **17**, 20–4.

Beauchamp, T.L. and Childress, J.F. (eds) (1994). *Principles of Biomedical Ethics* (4th edition). New York: Oxford University Press.

Benson, P.R., Roth, L.H., and Winslade, W. (1985). Informed consent in psychiatric research: preliminary findings from an ongoing investigation. *Social Science and Medicine*, **20**, 1331–41.

Blewitt, A. (1994). The hardest decision. *Midwives Chronicle*, **107**, 317–18.

Bodnaruk, Z.M., Wong, C.J., and Thomas, M.J. (2004). Meeting the clinical challenge of care for Jehovah's Witnesses. *Transfusion Medicine Reviews*, **18**, 105–16.

Bramstedt, K.A. and Nash, P.J. (2005). When death is the outcome of informed refusal: dilemma of rejecting ventricular assist device therapy. *Journal of Heart and Lung Transplantation*, **24**, 229–30.

Canvin, K. and Jacoby, A. (2006). Duty, desire or indifference? A qualitative study of patient decisions about recruitment to an epilepsy treatment trial. *Trials*, **7**, 32.

Costenbader, K.H., Brome, D., Blanch, D., Gall, V., Karlson, E., and Liang M.H. (2007). Factors determining participation in prevention trials among systemic lupus erythematosus patients: a qualitative study. *Arthritis and Rheumatism*, **57**, 49–55.

Cox, K. (1999). Researching research: patients' experiences of participation in phase I and II anti-cancer drug trials. *European Journal of Oncology Nursing*, **3**, 143–52.

–ibid.– (2000). Enhancing cancer clinical trial management: recommendations from a qualitative study of trial participants' experiences. *Psychooncology*, **9**, 314–22.

–ibid.– (2000). Assessing the quality of life of patients in phase I and II anti-cancer drug trials: interviews versus questionnaires. Soc Sci Med 2003 Mar; 56(5):921–34

–ibid.– (2000). Informed consent and decision-making: patients experiences of the process of recruitment to phases I and II anti-cancer drug trials Patient Educ Souns. 2002 Jan: 46(1): 31–8

Daugherty, C., Ratain, M.J., Grochowski, E., *et al.* (1995). Perceptions of cancer patients and their physicians involved in phase I trials. *Journal of Clinical Oncology*, **13**, 1062–72.

Declaration of Helsinki – http://www.wma.net/e/policy/b3.htm

Derse, A.R. (2005). What part of 'no' don't you understand? Patient refusal of recommended treatment in the emergency department. *Mt Sinai Journal of Medicine*, **72**, 221–7.

Di Blasi, Z., Crawford, F., Bradley, C., and Kleijnen, J. (2005). Reactions to treatment debriefing among the participants of a placebo controlled trial. *BMC Health Services Research*, **5**, 30.

Dixon, J.L. and Smalley, M.G. (1981). Jehovah's Witnesses. The surgical/ethical challenge. *Journal of the American Medical Association*, **246**, 2471–2.

Dixon-Woods, M., Jackson, C., Windridge, K.C., and Kenyon, S. (2006). Receiving a summary of the results of a trial: qualitative study of participants' views. *British Medical Journal*, **332**, 206–10.

Donovan, J., Mills, N., Smith, M., *et al.* (2002). Quality improvement report: improving design and conduct of randomized trials by embedding them in qualitative research: Protect (prostate testing for cancer and treatment) study. Commentary: presenting unbiased information to patients can be difficult. *British Medical Journal*, **325**, 766–70.

Dunn, L.B. and Jeste, D.V. (2003). Problem areas in the understanding of informed consent for research: study of middle-aged and older patients with psychotic disorders. *Psychopharmacology (Berl)*, **171**, 81–5.

Eder, M.L., Yamokoski, A.D., Wittmann, P.W., and Kodish, E.D. (2007). Improving informed consent: suggestions from parents of children with leukemia. *Pediatrics*, **119**, e849–59.

Elad, P., Treves, T.A., Drory, M., *et al.* (2000). Demented patients' participation in a clinical trial: factors affecting the caregivers' decision. *International Journal of Geriatric Psychiatry*, **15**, 325–30.

Featherstone, K. and Donovan, J.L. (1998). Random allocation or allocation at random? Patients' perspectives of participation in a randomized controlled trial. *British Medical Journal*, **317**, 1177–80.

–ibid.– (2002). 'Why don't they just tell me straight, why allocate it?' The struggle to make sense of participating in a randomized controlled trial. *Social Science and Medicine*, **55**, 709–19.

Ferguson, P. (2000). Testing a drug during labour: the experiences of women who participated in a clinical trial. *Journal of Reproductive and Infant Psychology*, **18**, 117–31.

Gammelgaard, A., Mortensen, O.S., and Rossel, P. (2004). Patients' perceptions of informed consent in acute myocardial infarction research: a questionnaire based survey of the consent process in the DANAMI-2 trial. *Heart*, **90**, 1124–8.

Gates, S., Brocklehurst, P., Campbell, M., and Elbourne, D. (2004). Recruitment to multicentre trials. *British Journal of Obstetrics and Gynaecology*, **111**, 3–5.

Glogowska, M., Roulstone, S., Enderby, P., Peters, T., and Campbell, R. (2001). Who's afraid of the randomized controlled trial? Parents' views of an SLT research study. *International Journal of Language and Communication Disorders*, **36**, Suppl: 499–504.

Gotay, C.C. (1991). Accrual to cancer clinical trials: directions from the research literature. *Social Science and Medicine*, **33**, 569–77.

Grant, C.H. 3rd, Cissna, K.N., and Rosenfeld, L.B. (2000). Patients' perceptions of physicians' communication and outcomes of the accrual to trial process. *Health Communication*, **12**, 23–39.

Greenley, R.N., Drotar, D., Zyzanski, S.J., and Kodish, E. (2006). Stability of parental understanding of random assignment in childhood leukemia trials: an empirical examination of informed consent. *Journal of Clinical Oncology*, **24**, 891–7.

Halliday, H.L. (2006). Recent clinical trials of surfactant treatment for neonates. *Biology of the Neonate*, **89**, 323–9.

Henzlova, M.J., Blackburn, G.H., Bradley, E.J., and Rogers, W.J. (1994). Patient perception of a long-term clinical trial: experience using a close-out questionnaire in the Studies of Left Ventricular Dysfunction (SOLVD) Trial. SOLVD Close-out Working Group. *Controlled Clinical Trials*, **15**, 284–93.

Hutchison, C. (1998). Phase I trials in cancer patients: participants' perceptions. *European Journal of Cancer Care (Engl)*, **7**, 15–22.

Hutton, J.D., Wilkinson, A.M., and Neale, J. (1990). Poor participation of nulliparous women in a low dose aspirin study to prevent preeclampsia. *New Zealand Medical Journal*, **103**, 511–12.

Jenkins,V. and Fallowfield, L. (2000). Reasons for accepting or declining to participate in randomized clinical trials for cancer therapy. *British Journal of Cancer*, **82**, 1783–8.

Joffe, S., Cook, E.F., Cleary, P.D., Clark, J.W., and Weeks, J.C. (2001). Quality of informed consent in cancer clinical trials: a cross-sectional survey. *Lancet*, **358**, 1772–7.

Kenyon, S., Dixon-Woods, M., Jackson, C.J., Windridge, K., and Pitchforth, E. (2006). Participating in a trial in a critical situation: a qualitative study in pregnancy. *Quality and Safety in Health Care*, **15**, 98–101.

Kinmonth, A.L., Lindsay, M.K., and Baum, J.D. (1983). Social and emotional complications in a clinical trial among adolescents with diabetes mellitus. *British Medical Journal (Clin Res Ed)*, **286**, 952–4.

Kodish, E., Eder, M., Noll, R.B., *et al.* (2004). Communication of randomization in childhood leukemia trials. *Journal of the American Medical Association*, **291**, 470–5.

Kraybill, E.N. (2004). The challenge of informed consent in neonatal research. *Journal of Perinatology*, **24**, 407–8.

Kupst, M.J., Patenaude, A.F., Walco, G.A., and Sterling, C. (2003). Clinical trials in pediatric cancer: parental perspectives on informed consent. *Journal of Pediatric Hematology/Oncology*, **25**, 787–90.

Lawton, J., Fox, A., Fox, C., and Kinmonth, A.L. (2003). Participating in the United Kingdom Prospective Diabetes Study (UKPDS): a qualitative study of patients' experiences. *British Journal of General Practice*, **53**, 394–8.

Lidz, C.W. (2006). The therapeutic misconception and our models of competency and informed consent. *Behavioural Sciences and the Law*, **24**, 535–46.

Lidz, C.W. and Applebaum, P.S. (2002). The therapeutic misconception: problems and solutions. *Medical Care*, **40**(9 Suppl), V55–63.

Lidz, C.W., Appelbaum, P.S., Grisso, T., and Renaud, M. (2004). Therapeutic misconception and the appreciation of risks in clinical trials. *Social Science and Medicine*, **58**, 1689–97.

Madsen, S.M., Mirza, M.R., Holm, S., Hilsted, K.L., Kampmann, K., and Riis, P. (2002). Attitudes towards clinical research amongst participants and nonparticipants. *Journal of Internal Medicine*, **251**, 156–68.

Madsen, S.M., Holm, S., and Riis, P. (2007). Attitudes towards clinical research among cancer trial participants and non-participants: an interview study using a Grounded Theory approach. *Journal of Medical Ethics*, **33**, 234–40.

Meropol, N.J., Weinfurt, K.P., Burnett, C.B., *et al.* (2003). Perceptions of patients and physicians regarding phase I cancer clinical trials: implications for physician–patient communication. *Journal of Clinical Oncology*, **21**, 2589–96.

Miller, V.A., Drotar, D., Burant, C., and Kodish, E. (2005). Clinician–parent communication during informed consent for pediatric leukaemia trials. *Journal of Pediatric Psychology*, **30**, 219–29.

Mills, N., Donovan, J.L., Smith, M., Jacoby, A., Neal, D.E., and Hamdy, F.C. (2003). Perceptions of equipoise are crucial to trial participation: a qualitative study of men in the Protect study. *Controlled Clinical Trials*, **24**, 272–82.

Minogue, B.P., Palmer-Fernandez, G., Udell, L., and Waller, B.N. (1995). Individual autonomy and the double-blind controlled experiment: the case of desperate volunteers. *Journal of Medicine and Philosophy*, **20**, 43–55.

Mohanna, K. and Tunna, K. (1999). Withholding consent to participate in clinical trials: decisions of pregnant women. *British Journal of Obstetrics and Gynaecology*, **106**, 892–7.

Moskop, J.C. (2006). Informed consent and refusal of treatment: challenges for emergency physicians. *Emergency Medicine Clinics of North America*, **24**, 605–18.

Nurgat, Z.A., Craig, W., Campbell, N.C., Bissett, J.D., Cassidy, J., and Nicolson, M.C. (2005). Patient motivations surrounding participation in phase I and phase II clinical trials of cancer chemotherapy. *British Journal of Cancer*, **92**, 1001–5.

Patel, A., Wilke, H.J. 2nd, Mingay, D., and Ellis, J.E. (2004). Patient attitudes toward granting consent to participate in perioperative randomized clinical trials. *Journal of Clinical Anesthesia*, **16**, 426–34.

Plaisier, P.W., Berger, M.Y., van der Hul, R.L., *et al.* (1994). Unexpected difficulties in randomizing patients in a surgical trial: a prospective study comparing extracorporeal shock wave lithotripsy with open cholecystectomy. *World Journal of Surgery*, 1994 Sep-Oct; 18(5): 769–72.

Pope, J.E., Tingey, D.P., Arnold, J.M., Hong, P., Ouimet, J.M., and Krizova, A. (2003). Are subjects satisfied with the informed consent process? A survey of research participants. *Journal of Rheumatology*, **30**, 815–24.

Quinn, G.P., Bell, B.A., Bell, M.Y., *et al.* (2007). The guinea pig syndrome: improving clinical trial participation among thoracic patients. *Journal of Thoracic Oncology*, **2**, 191–6.

Ross, M.W., Jeffords, K., and Gold, J. (1994). Reasons for entry into and understanding of HIV/AIDS clinical trials: a preliminary study. *AIDS Care*, **6**, 77–82.

Ross, S., Grant, A., Counsell, C., Gillespie, W., Russell, I., and Prescott, R. (1999). Barriers to participation in randomized controlled trials: a systematic review. *Journal of Clinical Epidemiology*, **52**, 1143–56.

Schutta, K.M. and Burnett, C.B. (2000). Factors that influence a patient's decision to participate in a phase I cancer clinical trial. *Oncology Nursing Forum*, **27**, 1435–8.

Sharp, L., Cotton, S.C., Alexander, L., Williams, E., Gray, N.M., and Reid, J.M. (2006). Reasons for participation and non-participation in a randomized controlled trial: postal questionnaire surveys of women eligible for TOMBOLA (Trial Of Management of Borderline and Other Low-grade Abnormal smears). *Clinical Trials*, **3**, 431–42.

Smithline, H.A., Mader, T.J., and Crenshaw, B.J. (1999). Do patients with acute medical conditions have the capacity to give informed consent for emergency medicine research? *Academic Emergency Medicine*, **6**, 776–80.

Snethen, J.A., Broome, M.E., Knafl, K., Deatrick, J.A., and Angst, D.B. (2006). Family patterns of decision-making in pediatric clinical trials. *Research in Nursing and Health*, **29**, 223–32.

Snowdon, C. (2005). Collaboration, participation and non-participation: decisions about involvement in randomized controlled trials for clinicians and parents in two neonatal trials. PhD thesis. University of London.

Snowdon, C., Elbourne, D., and Garcia, J. (1997). Making sense of randomization; responses of parents of critically ill babies to random allocation of treatment in a clinical trial. *Social Science and Medicine*, **45**, 1337–55.

–ibid.– (1998). Reactions of participants to the results of a randomized controlled trial: exploratory study. *British Medical Journal*, **317**, 21–6.

–ibid.– (1999). Zelen randomization: attitudes of parents participating in a neonatal clinical trial. *Controlled Clinical Trials*, **20**, 149–71.

–ibid.– (2006). 'It was a snap decision': parental and professional perspectives on the speed of decisions about participation in perinatal randomized controlled trials. *Social Science and Medicine*, **62**, 2279–90.

Spiro, S.G., Gower, N.H., Evans, M.T., Facchini, F.M., and Rudd, R.M. On behalf of the Big Lung Trial Steering Committee (2000). Recruitment of patients with lung cancer into a randomized clinical trial: experience at two centres. *Thorax*, **55**, 463–5.

Stevens, T. and Ahmedzai, S.H. (2004). Why do breast cancer patients decline entry into randomized trials and how do they feel about their decision later: a prospective, longitudinal, in-depth interview study. *Patient Education and Counseling*, **52**, 341–8.

Stone, D.A., Kerr, C.E., Jacobson, E., Conboy, L.A., and Kaptchuk, T.J. (2005). Patient expectations in placebo-controlled randomized clinical trials. *Journal of Evaluation in Clinical Practice*, **11**, 7–84.

Stroup, S., Appelbaum, P., Swartz, M. *et al.* (2005). Decision-making capacity for research participation among individuals in the CATIE schizophrenia trial. *Schizophrenia Research*, **80**, 1–8.

Stryker, J.E., Wray, R.J., Emmons, K.M., Winer, E., and Demetri, G. (2006). Understanding the decisions of cancer clinical trial participants to enter research studies: factors associated with informed consent, patient satisfaction, and decisional regret. *Patient Education and Counseling*, **63**, 104–9.

Sugarman, J., Cain, C., Wallace, R., and Welsh-Bohmer, K.A. (2001). How proxies make decisions about research for patients with Alzheimer's disease. *Journal of the American Geriatrics Society*, **49**, 1110–19.

Sullivan, P.S., McNaghten, A.D., Begley, E., Hutchinson, A., and Cargill, V.A. (2007). Enrollment of racial/ethnic minorities and women with HIV in clinical research studies of HIV medicines. *Journal of the National Medical Association*, **99**, 242–50.

Tait, A.R., Voepel-Lewis, T., and Malviya, S. (2003). Do they understand? (part I): parental consent for children participating in clinical anesthesia and surgery research. *Anesthesiology*, **98**, 603–8.

Thornton, H.M. (1992). Breast cancer trials: a patient's viewpoint. *Lancet*, **339**, 44–5.

Tobias, J.S. and Souhami, R.L. (1993). Fully informed consent can be needlessly cruel. *British Medical Journal*, **307**, 1199–201.

van Bergen, P.F., Jonker, J.J., Molhoek, G.P., *et al.* (1995). Characteristics and prognosis of non-participants of a multi-centre trial of long-term anticoagulant treatment after myocardial infarction. *International Journal of Cardiology*, **49**, 135–41.

van der Windt, D.A., Koes, B.W., van Aarst, M., Heemskerk, M.A., and Bouter, L.M. (2000). Practical aspects of conducting a pragmatic randomized trial in primary care: patient recruitment and outcome assessment. *British Journal of General Practice*, **50**, 371–4.

van Stuijvenberg, M., Suur, M.H., de Vos, S., *et al.* (1998). Informed consent, parental awareness, and reasons for participating in a randomized controlled study. *Archives of Disease in Childhood*, **79**, 120–5.

Weinfurt, K.P., Sulmasy, D.P., Schulman, K.A., and Meropol, N.J. (2003). Patient expectations of benefit from phase I clinical trials: linguistic considerations in diagnosing a therapeutic misconception. *Theoretical Medicine and Bioethics*, **24**, 329–44.

Wiley, F.M., Ruccione, K., Moore, I.M., *et al.* (1999). Parents' perceptions of randomization in pediatric clinical trials. Children Cancer Group. *Cancer Practice*, **7**, 248–56.

Williams, B., Irvine, L., McGinnis, A.R., McMurdo, M.E., and Crombie, I.K. (2007). When no might not quite mean no; the importance of informed and meaningful non-consent: results from a survey of individuals refusing participation in a health-related research project. *BMC Health Services Research*, **7**, 59.

Williams, B.F., French, J.K., and White, H.D. (2003). Informed consent during the clinical emergency of acute myocardial infarction (HERO-2 consent substudy): a prospective observational study. *Lancet*, **361**, 918–22.

Wragg J.A., Robinson, E.J., and Lilford, R.J. (2000). Information presentation and decisions to enter clinical trials: a hypothetical trial of hormone replacement therapy. *Social Science and Medicine*, **51**, 453–62.

Yuval, R., Halon, D.A., Merdler, A., Khader, N., Karkabi, B., Uziel, K., and Lewis, B.S. (2000). Patient comprehension and reaction to participating in a double-blind randomized clinical trial (ISIS-4) in acute myocardial infarction. *Archives of Internal Medicine*, **160**, 1142–6.

Chapter 5

Beyond a rebarbative commitment to consent

Kathleen Liddell

5.1 **Introduction**

In medical law, a strange and fascinating tension surrounds the issue of consent.[1] On the one hand, judicial decisions and parliamentary regulation evince a powerful belief that the autonomy of patients is protected by seeking their consent. Yet at the same time there is a palpable reluctance to specify what constitutes valid consent or legitimate exceptions to the rule. To this day, there is in England no single or clear doctrine of consent at common law (Young 1986) or in statute.[2]

What could explain this polarity? It is, I believe, a reflection of wider confusion in society. Consent is exalted as a mechanism to protect the individual's freedom, their dignity and identity. It promotes trust, gives grip to rights, and ensures that someone somewhere (i.e., the individual themselves) is responsible for overseeing what is done to people and their property. A person with the power to agree or (more importantly) to object to the propositions of others is an *individual* with freedom, rights, and a separate existence from the mêlée that is the rest of society. This is the advantage of consent: it is a bulwark against the mistakes and excesses of society. To set limits on consent is to open up the possibility that individuals will on some occasions be subsumed by amorphous, irresponsible, incompetent, unpredictable society, and its so-called expert advisors. In the healthcare context, this is seen as a grave danger, particularly in the context of human experimentation. Prominent historical examples serve as reminders of what society will do or let happen if permitted.

Given time, the law has done what is bid of it. It has tuned into the perils of hard paternalism and elitism. The ambiguity in *Sidaway v. Board of Governors of the Bethlem Royal Hospital*[3] about the reasonableness of professional judgement has given way to a much more definite emphasis on the rights of patients to control decisions

---

[1] This chapter is concerned with the law that applies in England.

[2] The most complete statutory definition is to be found in the Medicines for Human Use (Clinical Trials) Regulations 2004 Sch 1, paragraph 3.

[3] [1985] AC 871; *Bolam v. Friern Hospital Management Committee* [1957] 1 WLR 582.

about their health care. The decision in *Chester v. Afshar* is a key example.[4] In the statutory context, a bevy of new legislation also sets consent as the fundamental principle of legitimacy. For instance, consent is the opening gambit in the Human Tissue Act 2004 (UK), and was equally prominent in the Minister's Second Reading Speech and government discussion papers. The Medicines for Human Use (Clinical Trials) Regulations 2004 (UK) also stress the importance of consent.[5] Freely given informed consent must be obtained from every competent adult prior to participation in a clinical trial. The idea of consent even penetrates the governance of clinical trials involving adults and children *unable* to give their consent. In these circumstances, a representative must give 'consent' to stand in place of the individual's agreement. Similarly, the Data Protection Act 1998 (UK) and the common law of confidentiality are perceived to require consent prior to the use or sharing of health records for research save in the most exceptional cases. The importance of consent is emphasized so strongly that researchers are not even permitted to contact patients *to ask* whether they consent to participate in research. The approach must be made by the health service provider rather than the researcher. This is because, or so the reasoning goes, in the absence of specific consent a clinician is not permitted to pass on contact details to a researcher. Ironically, it is accepted that the patient may be contacted by an unfamiliar secretary, nurse or contractor who is engaged by the GP or hospital.

Informed consent, as this demonstrates, is heralded not just as an ethical panacea (Corrigan 2003) but also as a legal cure-all.

But is this thesis truly accurate? And was the bald assertion above justified in saying that the law's preoccupation with a strong and indefinite concept of consent is powered by confusion? The purpose of this chapter is to examine more closely the extent to which the law governing medical research is mesmerized by a narrow paradigm of consent. From a legal perspective, what is there beyond consent?

5.2 **The Human Tissue Act 2004**

Given the constraints of a single chapter, I will confine my analysis to a single area of law – the Human Tissue Act 2004 (**'the Act'**).[6] The Act is (to date) the high-water mark of the ideological shift from stern gatekeeping by the profession to consent tollbooths. More than any of the other recent reforms, it makes informed consent the

---

[4] 2005] 1 A.C. 134 (HL). A physician who performed an operation failed to warn the patient that it carried a small risk of paralysis, which eventually came to pass. He was held liable in negligence when she was paralysed even though he had performed the operation competently and the patient conceded that had she been warned, she would have agreed to the operation at a later date after pausing to consider the risk. While the surgeon's action had not *caused* the paralysis in strict terms, the court felt a finding of liability was necessary or the duty to inform would be a hollow one.

[5] Although interestingly consent does not dominate all other considerations. The Regulations give as much prominence to risk/benefit assessment, scientific soundness and ethics committee review. This is consistent with the argument run in the remainder of this chapter.

[6] All statutory references are to the Act unless otherwise specified.

supreme touchstone of legitimacy in dealings with the human body. As such it serves as a good case study.

5.2.1 The emphasis on consent

As with any piece of legislation there were several motivations for the Act. But first and foremost, it was a response to the public outrage and parents' grief on finding that their children's organs and tissues had been retained at Bristol and Alder Hey hospitals. This sad and distressing turn of events began with an inquiry about paediatric cardiac services at the Bristol Royal Infirmary. Doctors' evidence highlighted a side issue of which the general public was relatively unaware. Thousands of congenitally malformed hearts had been retained from the deceased infants, stillborn children and fetuses without the positive consent of their parents not only at Bristol, but at many other hospitals. A Royal Commission was directed at the largest collection thought to be at the Alder Hey Children's Hospital ('Alder Hey Report'). It found that an extraordinary retention of organs had taken place between 1988 and 1995 under the guidance of Dr Van Velzen (Alder Hey Report 2001). Professor Van Velzen instructed his staff to remove and retain every organ in fetal and infant post mortems (Alder Hey Report 2001, [10.3]). The public inquiry went on to conclude that in Van Velzen's case 'research purposes were the main, if not only motivation', which led the media and public to perceive researchers as untrustworthy and self serving (Alder Hey Report 2001, [14.2]).[7] Body parts from deceased adults were also retained at other hospitals (Department of Health 2003). On final analysis, it was estimated that throughout the UK 54 000 organs, body parts, stillborn children, and fetuses had been retained between 1970 and 2001.

The question most asked was 'how could this have been allowed to happen?' and the answer most often given was 'because the Human Tissue Act 1961 (the old Act) did not insist that organs taken at post mortem be stored and used only with prior consent'.[8] The government swiftly promised that it would enact new legislation. The initial proposal was to introduce a simple, two-clause Bill (Department of Health *et al.* 2001, 38; Price 2003; Liddell and Hall 2005). This was soon passed over in favour

---

[7] Professor Van Velzen was expected to run a clinical pathology service for the hospital and develop an international research program on cot death for the University and its sponsors. Faced with a chronic shortage of resources for his tasks, his idea was to develop a stock of organs from his growing clinical workload (with which he could not cope) for subsequent research examination. The hypothesis he intended to research was that SIDS babies were vulnerable as a result of the effect of intrauterine growth retardation which affected the development of their organs. Depending on the timing of the growth retardation, different organs might be affected and in different ways. The University had expertise in the three-dimensional measurement ('stereology') that would assist with this study (Alder Hey Report 2001, [4.2], [4.4]).

[8] The 1961 Act provided that a person lawfully in possession of the body of a deceased person may authorize the removal of tissue and organs for medical education or research if 'having made such reasonable enquiry as may be practicable, he has no reason to believe' that the deceased person had previously objected or that any surviving relative objects.

of a broadbrush review. The new law would emphasize the importance of seeking consent not only from families at a post mortem, but also from all living persons whenever human material (organ, tissue, or cells)[9] was used or stored. In addition, the new legislation would establish a criminal offence – the first of its kind – for holding DNA with an intention to analyse it for an impermissible purpose without consent. These aspects of the legislation went well beyond the problems experienced at Alder Hey and Bristol. They reflected an abiding concern with consent and the rights of individuals to control absolutely the tissue excised from their body. Many amendments were proposed, but time and time again the Minister retorted:

> Without wanting to use language that is too emotive, I should say that the amendment, though sincerely meant, would drive a stake through the heart of the Bill because it goes against its basic principle; namely, that people should be able to decide what happens to their bodily material. ...
>
> It is one of the fundamental tenets of the Bill that consent is needed for the use of tissue in research. The removal, retention and use of tissue from the deceased is a matter of the greatest sensitivity.[10]

The emphasis on consent was peculiar in many respects. For example, in the initial drafting the Bill required consent whether or not the tissue was anonymized. This would have criminalized the use of anonymized tissue banks as it would have been impossible to contact the relevant individuals; a perverse discouragement for research methodologies sensitive to privacy.[11] The Act also failed to provide for the fact that many adults lack the capacity to give consent.[12] Another issue was that consent was required under the Act for the *use* or *storage* of bodily material from a living person, but not for its *removal*. Further, the consent requirement applied to the use and storage of human material for specific, wide-ranging purposes but these purposes did not include clinical treatment.[13] Accordingly, nothing in the Act required a clinician (or any other person) to seek consent before taking tissue, however large the sample, from a living person. These matters were left to the common law. Of further note, the organs and tissues of the deceased could not under any circumstance be used for public health, transplantation, research, or to diagnose relatives without consent from themselves, their nominee, or the person most closely related to them. The great irony was that according to the Minister's vision, stricter rules of consent would apply to the use of *excised* pieces of tissue than the persons from whence they came, and the bodies of the deceased would be more stringently protected than the living.

---

[9] Excluding gametes, *in vitro* embryos, and hair and nail from living persons.

[10] Baroness Andrews (government) addressing the Grand Committee of the House of Lords on 16 September 2004 col. GC 474, 480.

[11] This aspect of the Bill was ultimately amended, as described below.

[12] This element of the Bill was also amended, as described below.

[13] Save where scientific or medical information relevant to any other person (including a future person) is obtained.

Most odd, the Act made a big play for the importance of 'appropriate consent' but provided minimal definition. It described the people who were eligible to provide consent and situations when consent must be evidenced in writing. But the specificity of information to be disclosed when seeking consent, and the type of response expected of individuals (i.e., explicit or implied) was left to be determined by the courts[14] and such guidance that the Human Tissue Authority develops.[15] Speeches recorded in Hansard hinted at the approach that might be taken in relation to medical research. On the issue of the information which must be disclosed prior to a request for consent, the Minister for Health insisted in the early stages of the Bill's passage that, in the case of research, disclosure should be specific.[16] However, this position softened after considerable pressure from the research community. On the issue of explicitness of response, the Minister rejected the concept of implied consent.

5.2.2 Criticisms

These elements are clear evidence that the Act was steeped in the narrowest paradigm of consent. In the eyes of many, this went unnoticed. The Act insisted on consent and that was all that mattered. But in other circles, it was roundly criticized. It was said to use a sledgehammer to crack a nut (Pincock 2004) or, as others more mockingly put it, the legislation 'is a sledgehammer that misses the nut'.[17] Most problematic it would function to 'criminalize activity that is part of normal and proper clinical, pathological and research practice that may as a result create a climate of excessive caution' which would 'harm patients ... through hindering and even preventing vital research' (Academy of Medical Sciences 2004a, 2004b).

Such comments referred in particular to the Act's impact on medical research. The standard practice of pathologists was to retain tissue blocks and slides where those samples were, or might prove, helpful in the development of generalized knowledge (the majority of blood samples are disposed of within days). Pathologists rarely have direct contact with patients. They receive the tissue from the referring doctor. The tissue may be accompanied by a consent form, but in one study this was true of less than half the samples and of those 40% of the forms were incompletely filled in (Furness and Sullivan 2004). Subsequently seeking consent

---

[14] The common law position is not well-established. Most judicial decisions on information disclosure for valid consent have concerned advice about surgical intervention where the risks include serious physical injury or psychiatric harm. In the instant scenario, where excised tissue (obtained with consent) is used or stored, the 'risk' is less significant. It is more likely to be limited to emotional distress or feelings that one's autonomy has been diminished. Rather than look to the law of negligence, the more appropriate field of precedent might be consent and waiver in an action for breach of confidence.

[15] See http://www.hta.gov.uk/guidance/codes_of_practice.cfm (last accessed 17 April 2008).

[16] Rosie Winterton, Minister of State, House of Commons, Hansard (Committee), 27 January 2004, col. 15.

[17] Correspondence between pathologists and other scientists (June 2004); Baroness O'Neill, *Lords*, Hansard (second reading), 22 July 2004, col. 396.

for research is a difficult and costly process (*ibid.*). Another study found that after 12 months' effort to contact 495 patients for permission to use surplus tissue from renal biopsy for research, the opinions of 26% could not be ascertained (Furness and Nicholson 2004). Whilst potential donors widely believe they should be notified or given a choice about the uses to which their tissue is put, studies have found that once contacted the majority of individuals willingly support the use of tissue removed during surgery for medical education and research. This casts further doubt on the allocation of extensive resources to the consent process (Start *et al.* 1996; Furness 2003; Jack and Womack 2003; Richards *et al.* 2003).

In her book, *Autonomy and Trust in Bioethics*, O'Neill presents further reasons for questioning a rebarbative commitment to mere sheer choice. A principle of consent that fails to distinguish sadistic, selfish, hostile, and competitive desires, implements a false concept of autonomy (O'Neill 2002, 33–7).

> 'Autonomous choices are distinguished from mere choices by the fact that they follow from and reflect a greater degree of self-knowledge, or of self-control, or of capacities to review, revise and endorse other desires' (*ibid.*, 33). … 'By insisting on informed consent we *make* it *possible* for individuals to choose autonomously, however that is to be construed. But we in no way guarantee that they do so' (*ibid.*, 37).

The message is that individuals sometimes (some say generally!) choose unwisely, though not in every instance. The traditional concept of informed consent gives weight to any choice so reflects a strong ideal of self-determination but an impoverished ideal of self-control or autonomy.

The genetics community was also concerned by the Act's commitment to mere sheer choice. When the Human Genetics Commission recommended an offence for non-consensual analysis of DNA it added a caveat: the offence should not inhibit 'the use of genetic testing in medical and research settings' (Human Genetics Commission 2002, [3.60]). The fact that a particular person has tested positive for a mutation may be personal information; but the fact that a particular mutation is in the family is an essentially different kind of information which should not be regulated solely with regard for the proband's preferences (Clark 2003, 80). Despite this, the government drafted a provision giving the person from whom DNA is obtained the absolute power to veto its analysis for the benefit of another family member. The emphasis in section 45 on the individual's consent disregarded these significant family interests (see Chapter Eleven).

5.3 **An alternative perspective**

Despite the problems consent presented in the Act for collective interests and reflective reasoning, the government pressed on with its fanfare about consent being the Act's 'golden thread'.[18] But intriguingly, despite the government's attitude, there is much in the Act that extends beyond consent.

---

[18] Dr Stephen Ladyman, *House of Commons*, Hansard (Committee), 27 January 2004, col. 66.

5.3.1 **Assistant and surrogate decision-makers**

The Act establishes for the first time a Human Tissue Authority whose functions include issuing licences for the storage of tissue and publishing guidance, and codes on (*inter alia*) the definition of death, existing holdings, disposal of human tissue, and communication with bereaved relatives. The members of the inaugural Authority, appointed in line with Nolan principles,[19] have diverse backgrounds from archaeology, anatomy, finance and philosophy, and viewed from one perspective we might see them as having been appointed to make some of the decisions which a process of consent is too feeble to ensure. They are, metaphorically, assistant decision-makers whose work relieves individuals of burdensome negotiations. Once a doctor approaches a bereaved family to ask whether their child's organs might be kept for research, it is too late for the family to negotiate acceptable communication standards. A patient whose tumour is removed during life-threatening surgery is unlikely to have the forethought or energy to negotiate the terms of its disposal. The Authority can attend to these matters, in advance, by preparing Codes. The Authority is also the individual's eyes and ears. Once tissue is taken, an individual is in a very weak position to monitor how it is used, stored, or disposed. The Authority is given the resources and powers to do this more effectively.

What is it though that makes the Authority a wise assistant decision-maker? Its decisions have a certain legitimacy by virtue of the power granted to it under the Act, but can its decisions be trusted to be fair? Criticisms of democratic defecit are often levelled at expert bodies. It is said to be unfair for a few unelected experts to make decisions for the rest of us.

But as John Stuart Mill is reputed to have said:

> Every one has a right to feel insulted by being made a nobody, and stamped as of no account at all. [But] [n]o one but a fool … feels offended by the acknowledgement that there are others whose opinion, and even whose wish, is entitled to a greater amount of consideration than his.

> (Mill 1865, 335)

The legitimacy and fairness of expert bodies lies in their deliberativeness and ability to see beyond the personal interests of the persons who make up the group. While not being moral oracles, in the right circumstances they develop expertise in deliberation. Ideally, they seek to understand the reasonable disagreement that divides individuals and to transcend it through a consensus (of sorts) that is politically dispositive. If the group is genuinely pluralist and broad, the consensus will not be a comprehensive consensus. Rather it will be an overlapping consensus based on propositions for fair terms of cooperation which the members believe citizens (despite their moral differences) could reasonably accept bearing in mind the

---

[19] The Nolan principles refer to the 'Ethical Standards in Public Life and the Commissioner for Public Appointments United Kingdom' (Nolan Committee 1995) which emphasize openness, accountability and integrity.

burdens of moral judgement (Rawls 1996; Liddell 2003). Their decisions are thus a variation on the idea of consent: it is consent at another level brought about through rational reflection and a motivation to cooperate.

In theory, then, decision-making by a (well functioning) deliberative body enables the citizenry to find fair compromises for collective goals without the constant need to request/grant consent. It could operate as a surrogate for individual consent where seeking consent is highly impractical or disproportionate. However, the Act does not see it this way. The Authority has few powers to substitute its judgement for an individual's consent.[20] In general, it is intended to *supplement*, rather than replace, the requirement for an individual's consent with additional regulatory standards and define the conditions of valid consent.

Research ethics committees (RECs) have the potential to play a similar role. They too are a touchstone of legitimacy within the Act, but in a slightly different way. As earlier noted, the first version of the Bill required individual consent even where tissue had been anonymized. After much pressure from the research community, the Bill was amended[21] to allow anonymized tissue from living persons to be used in research provided the research is endorsed by a REC. There are two points of interest here. First, the individual is taken out of the equation. Once the individual's identity is concealed, the decision-making function is transferred to an ethics committee. Anonymity is taken to cancel out, or substitute for, the individual's autonomy interest. This is controversial, but justifiable.[22] It can also be rationalized in another way. Rather than nullify the autonomy interest, anonymization can be seen as a means to help the individual protect their privacy. The REC is simultaneously set up as a 'surrogate' decision-maker since an individual whose identity is anonymized cannot be contacted for their decisions. A second point of interest is that the ethics committee is given more than the power to determine the acceptability of research. A failure to follow the committee's decision or to seek their approval is a criminal offence. Such a severe consequence has not previously applied. It is also a criminal offence to breach a licence condition stipulated by the Human Tissue Authority.

Surrogate decision-making is more overt in other sections of the Act, but not in relation to research. The clinical genetics community successfully pointed out that a lack of consent sometimes stems from tracing difficulties or respondent apathy rather

---

[20] An example is discussed below. See also s. 43.

[21] s. 1(7), (8), (9), (10).

[22] Some argue it is unacceptable because tissue and data retains moral significance for the individual after anonymization. The counter argument is that an individual's integrity is neither implicated nor impugned by the sheer fact that information once upon a time related to him. Individuals may not like the type of research that is done, but it does not affect them or sully their moral integrity. An analogy could be made with the use of public taxes to fund such research. Individuals might argue that taxes should not be spent on such research because the research is unethical or low priority. However, it is unconvincing to suggest that research funding would tarnish the tax payer's character or affect their life by virtue of the fact that their labour, inheritance, or intellect created the money.

than in-principle objections. The government, supported by Parliament, accordingly agreed a special exception. Consent is not required where the Authority is satisfied that the researcher has made reasonable efforts to contact the individual without receiving a response nor in situations where it is not reasonably possible to trace him.[23] In effect, the Authority is given power to substitute its decision for the individual's consent. The exception applies only where the tissue or DNA is used to assist another person. In these provisions, Parliament called on its authority as a representative, (loosely) majoritarian body to make decisions on behalf of individuals. Surprisingly, though, the exception does not apply if the effort to secure the other person's interests involves medical research. In the wake of the Alder Hey inquiry, Parliament lacked the political courage to substitute its approval for individual consent where the purpose is medical research.

The denigration of research was also plain in other areas. Part 2 of Schedule 1[24] lists purposes for which Parliament declared that the consent of an individual is not required, provided the tissue is obtained from a living person. These purposes include public health monitoring, clinical audit, health care training, performance assessment of medical products and devices, and quality assurance exercises. The characteristic shared by each of these activities is their collective nature. None can be performed without the contribution of large numbers of people, and the results improve the medical care of patients in general (the patients treated by the hospital or medical device investigated; the patients treated by the doctors trained; the epidemiological population monitored, etc.). Similarly, medical research aims to produce generalized knowledge of benefit to communities of patients rather than individuals. It is thus conspicuously missing from the Part 2 list.

5.3.2 Compliance strategies

Whilst the strategy of appointing alternative decision-makers to substitute or supplement an individual's consent – either an expert advisory group or Parliament – adds a communitarian tone, the Act in other ways tries to improve rather than replace individualism. As flagged, a problem with consent as a touchstone of legitimacy is that, in practice, the individual's power is fleeting. They have little ability to monitor whether their refusals or the terms of their consent are subsequently observed. To counteract this, the Act implements a system of deterrence and monitoring that makes compliance with consent more likely.

Deterrence is arranged through a series of criminal offences. So whilst section 1 declares certain uses of tissue to be unlawful without appropriate consent, section 5 hammers this home with a criminal offence. The Director of Public Prosecutions can

---

[23] s. 7; schedule 4, para 9.

[24] A similar division applies for DNA analysis. However, an odd quirk of the drafting is that Parliament approved a wider range of uses of DNA than tissue. For example, unlike tissue, DNA initially collected for therapeutic purposes may subsequently be analysed without consent in accordance with a court order or for the prevention or detection of crime. See s. 8.

bring criminal proceedings against a person who fails to obtain consent for the activities covered by section 1.[25] A person found guilty may be sentenced to three years' imprisonment, a fine, or both. A medical professional found guilty of a crime would also expect to face disciplinary proceedings before the General Medical Council. In fact, though, prosecutions are unlikely to be common. The primary purpose of the offence is to set consequences sufficiently dramatic to motivate people to seek and observe an individual's consent. The government was keen that the new Act should not be 'a toothless tiger imposing fuzzy rules with no provision for sanctions or redress', as was the case with the 1961 Act (Brazier 2002).[26] The Act also warns that criminal punishments may follow for non-consensual analysis of DNA, buying and selling human material beyond permitted circumstances, breaching a licence issued by the Human Tissue Authority, and removing organs from a live donor for transplant in an unrelated recipient.[27] Consent or its absence is largely irrelevant to the last three mentioned crimes.

A threat of criminal prosecution is generally perceived as more serious than liability to pay compensation. It represents condemnation by the community, rather than an individual's retribution or restitution. It takes away liberty and status, not merely financial wellbeing. But that being so, criminal penalties are normally an adjunct to civil liability. In this way, an individual has an option to seek redress for loss and damage they suffered, and the community additionally steps in to prosecute the worst breaches of law. Unusually, this is not the case in the Act. Individuals are given no power to seek compensation. So on the one hand, the government declared the most minor consent infraction to be a heinous criminal breach of an individual's fundamental rights and liberties; yet on the other, it denied individuals any right to seek compensation.[28] This is a peculiar policy, both under- and over-inclusive.

Continuous monitoring and supervision, beyond that which can be achieved by the individual, is organized through the licensing requirement. Section 16 of the Act specifies that a licence must be obtained from the Human Tissue Authority before storing human tissue, conducting anatomical and post mortem examinations, removing material from deceased persons, or displaying tissue from deceased persons in public. The Human Tissue Authority has the power to decide the fate of licence applications, including the terms on which a licence is granted. Additional powers help it administer the licensing system. The Act grants it powers of inspection, entry, search and seizure, and powers to give directions to licence holders and to revoke licences.[29]

---

[25] It is a defence for the defendant to prove he or she was reasonably mistaken about the existence or need for consent.

[26] The old Human Tissue Act 1961 specified no penalty or liability for failure to comply with its provisions.

[27] Respectively, s. 45, 32, 25, and 33. Each offence is subject to exceptions and defences.

[28] But see now the Regulatory Enforcement and Sanctions Act 2008, s. 36–38. The common law provides little assistance. In extreme circumstances, compensation may be payable for negligent malpractice: *AB v. Leeds Teaching Hospital N.H.S. Trust* [2004] E.W.H.C. 644 (QB).

[29] s. 48, 37 and Schedule 5.

In theory, then, those who use human tissue are strongly accountable to the Human Tissue Authority, which stands in for individuals who cannot practically police their interests. Each time a tissue-holder seeks a licence, the Authority will consider whether there is any evidence that they have failed to handle tissue in responsible and lawful ways. Although a licence is not required for all uses of tissue (e.g., research, audit, transplantation), the Authority could in many circumstances oversee this by virtue of its power to license tissue storage. Furthermore, while criminal proceedings will be rare, tissue users will recognize that the Human Tissue Authority may more readily use its power to refuse their licence applications or to add restrictions for poor conduct.

5.3.3 **Protecting interests other than autonomy**

In obscure ways, the Act also refers to interests beyond those that can be protected by consent. For instance it sets up a legal framework under which it is lawful to use tissue obtained from cognitively impaired persons, who lack the capacity to give or withhold consent. Embarrassingly, the government omitted such provisions in the Bill first presented to Parliament. The mistake was rectified by a general regulation-making power, meaning the details could be left to be determined the following year under the Mental Capacity Act 2005. Eventually it was decided that the tissue of incapacitated persons may be used in research provided the use is consistent with their 'best interests'. 'Best' interests differ from autonomous interests in that they are determined by other persons and are subject to legal and bureaucratic scrutiny. As the term implies, actions consistent with best interests are supposed to protect and promote the individual's health, happiness, welfare, and security. Under the Mental Capacity Act 2005 (UK), an assessment of best interests should take account of the person's past and present wishes and feelings, and the beliefs and values that would be likely to influence his decision if he had capacity.[30] The latter may include altruism and solidarity, which is the basis on which non-invasive non-therapeutic research may be permitted.[31]

Some reference to dignity interests can also be implied from provisions in the Act. Human dignity, insofar as it is a principle of constraint (Beyleveld and Brownsword 2001),[32] is an impersonal, inherent, inalienable interest (hence divorced from consent). It protects 'our humanity – that is, some essential quality that has always underpinned our sense of who we are and where we are going' (Brownsword 2004b, 209, citing Fukuyama). This interpretation accounts for the prohibitions in the Act against buying and selling human tissue for profit, public display of dead bodies, and some organ donations by live donors. In other respects, however, the Act falls dramatically short of protecting human dignity. It is silent about the lawfulness of nefarious acts such as eating human flesh, necrophilia, or making leather from human cadavers.[33]

[30] Mental Capacity Act 2005 s. 4 (see Chapter Nine).

[31] Such as observational research, research based on tissue and data, and pathophysiological research.

[32] Contrast 'dignity as empowerment', which shares strong similarities with autonomy and privacy interests.

[33] Baroness O'Neill, Lords, Hansard (second reading), 22 July 2004, col. 396.

5.4 **The justificatory power of consent**

5.4.1 **Consent as procedural justification**

The question with which we began was whether consent was indeed a legal cure-all in the Act. The sections above have shown that while policymakers present consent as an ethical panacea, the legal policy they promulgate is in fact considerably more nuanced. But there is much ambivalence in their willingness to move beyond consent (*viz.* constraints on epidemiological research, and surrogate decision-making), and reluctance to explain the importance for such moves. For more perceptive accounts, we must look to other sources. Through these, we can better understand and evaluate what is going on in the Act.

Beyleveld and Brownsword argue that consent is a procedure for avoiding a violation of rights, making an otherwise wrongful action lawful (Beyleveld and Brownsword 2007). It is an agreement to engage a private rule-set. This serves as a reason – a consensual reason – for holding a rights holder to a change of position and the power-holder to the terms of the rule-set (*ibid.*, 335–8). It signals the rights holder is willing for a power to be exercised in a particular way. Having given consent an agent is 'bound in' (*ibid.*, 338–42). Consent is thus a communicative procedure for permitting transgressions against individuals. As such, the terms of valid consent are governed by reasonable behaviour of communication. Information disclosed prior to seeking consent should seek to balance fidelity with the agent's will (to protect the agent) with reasonable transactional expectation (to protect the recipient) (*ibid.*, 343–50). It is not essential for the prior information to be as detailed as possible.

The authors go on to explain that the integrity of consent needs to be defended against two distinct kinds of threat. On the one hand, there is the familiar threat of under-valuation where consent is fictionalized. Opt-out consent regimes, implied consent, and lackadaisical form-filling are prime examples. The government's insistence that consent was the central and most important component of the Act can be understood as a reaction to this threat.

On the other hand, there is the threat of over-valuation. This threat Brownsword explains:

> is much less well-advertised. It arises where consent is viewed as the key to ethical and legal justification, where – as Onora O'Neill put it in her Gifford Lectures – communities become 'fixated' with consent (O'Neill 2002). ... [T]his less obvious threat to the integrity of consent ... [concerns] a culture of consent being overtaken by a cult of consent.
>
> (Brownsword 2004a)

This comment helps to explain why policymakers did not publicize strategies in the Act beyond consent. Cultural forces which feed, and feed off, consent fetishism pushed them along this tack. The policymakers' mistake was to advocate repeatedly that without informed consent any action is wrong, and with consent, it is most likely right. Beyleveld and Brownsword refer to these assumptions as the 'fallacy of necessity' and the 'fallacy of sufficiency' (Beyleveld and Brownsword 2007). It seems that the government did not fully adopt this stance, but repetition reinforced the fallacy in the minds of others and blocked key amendments.

A product of the fallacy of necessity is the idea that consent is its 'own free-standing justificatory standard' (Brownsword 2004). This sort of statement may be convenient shorthand for public debates. But it is important to remember, and to remind one's audience, that the shorthand presupposes that there are rights to be protected, that consent is an effective protection and that there are no alternative justifications for the action. Unfortunately, reminders of this kind are few and far between.

A further product of the assumption is to think that consent is the only justification for a wrong done to a rights-bearing agent.[34] Beyleveld and Brownsword note that legal regimes tend (rightly in their view) to recognize that procedural and substantive reasons other than consent can justify a violation of rights. This is indeed what occurs in the Act, even while the government reiterated the essential nature of consent. For example, Parliament's decision to allow tissue to be used for some purposes without consent – for example, Part 2 of Schedule 1 purposes – might be justified on this basis. Before considering this further, the fallacy of sufficiency warrants note.

The fallacy of sufficiency, Beyleveld and Brownsword explain, is to think that where a person consents to a particular act then no wrong is done. Whilst there is no *private* wrong between the person consenting and the person acting, there may be a reason for treating the act as a *public* wrong. This helps to explain the sections of the Act which protect dignity interests. Putting a monetary figure on tissue with the donor's consent may be a legitimate action as between the donor and the purchaser, but it may nevertheless constitute a wrong. The difficulty is to ascertain the circumstances where an action done with consent constitutes a breach of dignity. Typically, consent is insufficient to justify actions that harm third parties not privy to the agreement. Beyleveld and Brownsword argue that consent may also be insufficient where public interest purposes justify State intervention. They offer three sub-categories: measures taken to secure respect for the rights of other citizens; actions that protect other citizens' 'opportunity to flourish as members of a community committed to human rights and responsibilities'; and measures that give effect to prohibitions expressly authorized by members of the community (e.g., via Parliament). While the scope of the sub-categories leaves much to be debated, the general principle explains why the Act might stipulate criminal offences (i.e., public liability) rather than civil liability for trafficking organs, public display of dead bodies, and some live donor organ donations.

5.4.2 Procedural and substantive justifications other than consent

As noted, Beyleveld and Brownsword venture the view that procedural and substantive reasons other than consent can justify a violation of rights. However, they give only the broadest of examples: 'self-defence, necessity, or the like' (Beyleveld and Brownsword 2007, 335–7). Lawrence O. Gostin provides more detailed discussion in his writing on public health law.

---

[34] To forget that some actions involve no wrong and, therefore, require no consent, is another product of this fallacy.

A theme in Gostin's work is that public health and medicine are conceptually distinct. The science of medicine is familiarly oriented towards individual patients, seeks a discrete cause for the individual's disease, and concentrates on the micro-relationship between health care provider and patient. The science of public health, on the other hand, is conceptually designed to benefit the collective population, searches for root causes, and focuses on the broader relationships between the State and individuals. The public health system has come to terms with these differences. It understands, Gostin says, that people cannot and do not wish to rely on the ethics of voluntarism to defend the common welfare. The threats to public health cannot be easily reduced, and acting alone individuals cannot assure either the methods, resources, or the knowledge they need for the purpose. 'Private individuals – whether individuals, groups, or corporate entities – have incentives to engage in behaviours that are personally profitable or pleasurable but may threaten other individuals or groups [and]. … adversely affect communal health and safety' (Gostin 2000, 18–19). This echoes the concerns of O'Neill and others who worry that individuals can never be fully informed and find it difficult to reflect on interests beyond their immediate (usually stressful) circumstances.[35]

Gostin argues that to counteract these pressures citizens assert their collective power, through the law and its associated institutions, to tax, inspect, regulate, and coerce. That being so, they remain committed to the fundamental rights and liberties that they cherish in free and liberal society. Achieving a just balance between individual rights and the goals of public health poses an enduring problem, long studied by scholars and students of public health law (Gostin 2000, 20). Citizens cannot have it both ways: they must give up some privacy and forgo some collective benefits (*ibid.*, 115, 139). The law, coupled with the rule of law, is the means for tailoring this. It 'acts as both a fountain and a levee: it originates the flow of power (to preserve the public health) and curbs that power (to protect individual freedoms)' (*ibid.*, 26).[36] And it tends to forswear the possibility of bold governance in exchange for checks and balances that prevent overreaching and assure political accountability (*ibid.*, 31).

Gostin's central point is that the protection of public health is one of the few justifications, aside from consent, for violating protected human rights. Citing Tobey he notes 'the government is organized by the people, for this express purpose (among others) … and cannot divest itself of this important duty' (*ibid.*, 11). And this is how the exceptions to the consent rule in Part 2 of Schedule 1 of the Human Tissue Act can be justified. Public health monitoring, clinical audit, health care training, performance assessment, and quality assurance are the methods and basis for securing public health purposes.

The Act deviates, however, in two significant respects from Gostin's arguments. Understanding these points sharpens our understanding of the policymakers'

[35] Further theoretical support for a collective interest in health and research has been derived from the duty to assist others: see Chapter Seven.

[36] Gostin speaks in particular of constitutional law, but the principle can be generalized to other forms of law.

ambivalence and highlights where, in particular, they were misguided. First Gostin is quite clear that population-based medical research is an essential and basic element of the public health agenda, even though he notes that the trust of vulnerable communities has been strained by unethical research studies (*ibid.*, 124). In contrast, the Act draws a firm, unyielding distinction between public health and research in all circumstances. In the Act, research can be justified only by an individual's consent, never by government for the people. This rationale is driven, not by reason, but by politics in the aftermath of events at Alder Hey and Bristol. It dismisses widely accepted definitions of research. These stress that the purpose of research is not to assist particular individuals but like audit, education, and public health monitoring to conduct 'a systematic investigation ... to develop or contribute to *generalizable* knowledge' (Belmont Report 1979). It also ignores the relevance of research for evidence-based medicine.[37]

A second difference is less obvious. Gostin argues that while the government has the power and duty to protect public health, it should regard its powers as subject to restraints. Hence the secondary title of his book: *Power, Duty, Restraint.* Pared of its detail, his argument is that rather than a rigid all-or-nothing violation of rights, justification for public health requires graduated proof, and scrutiny. A complete exemption for public health monitoring, clinical audit, education and training, performance assessment, and quality assurance runs counter to this; as does a complete lack of exemption for public health research. Thus Parts 1 and 2 of Schedule 1 of the Act are both flawed.

More specifically, Gostin's systematic evaluation lists a set of principles for assessing whether a violation of fundamental rights such as privacy is justified. These principles are the tailoring Gostin speaks of when he argues that law should create *and curb* collective power. The law should require public health authorities which interfere with fundamental rights without consent to demonstrate: significant risk to members of the public or a pressing social need (based on scientific methods); the intervention's effectiveness (by showing a close fit between means and ends); the intervention is the least restrictive alternative; reasonableness of economic costs (compared with probable benefits); and a fair distribution of benefits, costs, and burdens. The level of scrutiny to be employed should be scaled to the degree of interference. In short, human tissue should only be used for the purposes of public health and research in the absence of consent where it is necessary, reasonable means are employed, the interference is proportionate, and due process is followed. An intervention that gratuitously overrides an individual's rights without seeking his or her consent is not justified.[38]

---

[37] Contrast the government's policy (which was prepared by other civil servants) in the Research Governance Framework for Health and Social Care (2005).

[38] Beyleveld and Brownsword also argue for the priority of consent: 'it is better to obtain the right-holder's consent for what would otherwise be a violation of that right than to justify wrongdoing by reference to overriding rights – if the evil is avoidable, it should be avoided rather than justified as the lesser of two evils. In this light, where legal regimes present a right-holder's consent as one of several justifying reasons, but without prioritising consent, they are defective' (Beyleveld and Brownsword 2007, 335–8).

For these ideas, Gostin draws upon US constitutional theory. However, the same sorts of principles are recognized by European human rights law and the Human Rights Act 1998 (UK). If these principles had been followed in the drafting of the Act, Part 2 of Schedule 1 would be significantly different (and improved). The list of purposes would include public health research as well as public health monitoring, clinical audit, health care training, performance assessment, and quality assurance. But none would be categorical exemptions. Tissue might be used or stored for these purposes (whether it came from deceased or living persons) if the use or storage were necessary and the violation of privacy rights it entailed (to the individual or their family) were proportionate.

5.4.3 Integrating consent and other justifications

The divide between 'governance by individual consent' and governance for public health is not as great as it first seems. First, public health regulation need not (in fact it should not) jettison a principle of consent. The principle of proportionality, which (amongst other things) insists on the least restrictive interference, supports the continuation of consent. But it encourages a more flexible account. Although the *fact* of consent is all or nothing, the requirements for valid consent are scalar and can vary according to the circumstances. Two variables are particularly significant:[39] the specificity of information disclosed when seeking consent and the overtness of the subject's response. So, where there is no pressing reason to interfere with an individual's autonomy, explicit–specific–temporally-limited consent might be required. But where there is a reason to interfere (e.g., public health research), broad–enduring consent might be sufficient. Where even this presents significant problems for community interests, implied consent, or no consent at all, would be justified provided there were other safeguards.

Second, in setting up a system of governance for public health, the Government should not impose its view of the collective good on an unwilling community. The degree to which individuals should forgo rights claims in order to achieve improved health and a higher quality of life in a given situation is an issue for political resolution within a democratic society. It, thus, calls for governance by consent at a higher order; the Parliamentary level. At this entry point, citizens have the opportunity via parliamentary representatives to consent to a rule-set for substantive and procedural justifications (e.g., public health research and monitoring), and a rule-set of surrogate decision-makers (e.g., the Human Tissue Authority (code preparation), RECs (code consideration), Secretary of State (code endorsement), Parliament (regulations and code approval), courts (best interests determinations in the event of disputes; code review)). This may seem a poor-man's version of consent, however it need not be so if the deliberativeness of the surrogates was improved.

---

[39] Other significant variables include voluntariness and the degree of subject understanding.

5.5 **Conclusion**

This chapter began by reproaching the law for supporting a narrow consent-based model of legitimate medical research. But in fact, my purpose was to interrogate this view. To what extent is the law really contributing to the blinkered and narrow paradigm of consent that has mesmerized society and many scholars? As the narrative has shown, it has not proven easy to find a discrete, generic answer, even when the focus was a single statute. But within the inevitable methodological constraints, insights emerge.

The Human Tissue Act 2004 is a good example of the ambivalent, confused, and confusing attitudes about consent that law and legal policymakers display. On the one hand, there is considerable evidence that the problems of a narrow consent model are being replayed in this recent legislation. Consent was lauded by policymakers as *the* mechanism for protecting individuals. Its importance was stressed repeatedly to the exclusion of other issues. Moreover, policymakers would not speak of its limitations or problems: not the difficulties consent presents for community and family interests, the costs of consent, nor the fact that individuals have limited information and time when making consent decisions. Nor did policymakers openly discuss the alternative mechanisms that exist for protecting autonomy, dignity, and the trust of patients. They linked the principle of consent to a concept of autonomy, without critically considering the different conceptions which abound and the implications different conceptions carry for information disclosure pre-consent. Furthermore, the principle of consent was stretched to extraordinary lengths so that any agreement (e.g., an agreement about the use of tissue from another deceased person) was discussed in the language of informed consent irrespective of whether self-determination was at stake. On the other hand, the Act is a remarkably interesting source of information about regulatory mechanisms beyond consent. These mechanisms come in two forms: 'adjuncts' and 'alternatives' to a narrow principle of consent. In the category of adjuncts, this chapter drew attention to several compliance strategies including the introduction of criminal penalties and a system of licensing overseen by the Human Tissue Authority. These mechanisms deter researchers from poor conduct and insist on regular proof of good conduct. This holds researchers to account in a way that individuals could never achieve on their own. The principle of consent is accordingly less hollow. In addition, the Act adds standards to supplement consent. This is clearest insofar as the Human Tissue Authority was given a broad remit to prepare codes. The codes will not substitute for an individual's consent. Rather they provide an additional layer of standards to be observed. These standards might have been insisted upon by an individual, were they aware of the full gamut of issues and minded to reach a fair compromise with people of opposing moral views.

'Alternatives' predominantly consist of exceptions to the consent approach which were agreed by Parliament in the passage of the Bill. The government proposed several broad exceptions, amongst other things, for public health monitoring, clinical audit, performance assessment, and existing tissue holdings. Additional exceptions were added only after concerted efforts from the medical research and genetics communities, and even then they were tightly circumscribed. For example, the DNA may be analyzed where the proband cannot be traced and the analysis of their tissue is important for another person. The government also made allowances for incapacitated persons, developing a framework based on best interests, and consultation with carers. By far the broadest amendment beyond consent was the exemption for anonymized tissue, which coupled identity protection with surrogate decision-making by RECs and criminal penalties.

Set out in this way, the government's obsequious commitment to consent looks insincere. But this would be overly critical. There was considerable political pressure from patient groups, media, and academe to implement principles of consent above all else. The government, to give it its due, was listening. The problem was that in their eagerness to achieve change, the government and interest groups lost touch with a detailed understanding of consent. Accordingly, mechanisms beyond consent were used sporadically throughout the Act and not always with consistency.

A more coherent account of consent and its justifications is required if the peculiar polarities in law are to be addressed. O'Neill, Beyleveld and Brownsword, and Gostin provide a basis for this. Their arguments demonstrate that consent does not always track autonomy, that consent can be over-valued as well as under-valued, and that actions that violate an agent's interests or rights may be justified on grounds other than consent. One such justification is public health research insofar as it constitutes a communal interest that cannot be effectively achieved by direct grants of consent by individuals. The role of government in achieving this end is critical. It cannot abdicate its responsibility to set up frameworks beyond consent which respect autonomy, privacy, dignity, and the need for trust. It must also recognize exceptions where interference without consent is necessary, reasonable means are employed, the interference is proportionate, due process is followed and compliance monitored. This involves regulating with a principle of individual (ostensibly private) consent that is procedural and scaled, and accompanied by, ostensibly public, adjuncts, and alternatives sanctioned by the community.

References

Academy of Medical Sciences (2004a). *Statement on Human Tissue Bill*. London: Academy of Medical Sciences.

Academy of Medical Sciences and the Council of Heads of Medical Schools (2004b). *Joint Letter to Ms Rosie Winterton, Minister of State*. London: Academy of Medical Sciences.

Belmont Report (1979). *Ethical Principles and Guidelines for the Protection of Human Subjects of Research*. Bethesda, MD: National Institutes of Health (Office of Human Subjects Research).

Beyleveld, D. and Brownsword, R. (2001). *Human Dignity in Bioethics and Biolaw*. Oxford: Oxford University Press.

–ibid.– (2007). *Consent in the Law*. Oxford: Hart Publishing.

Brazier, M. (2002). Organ retention and return: problems of consent. *Journal of Medical Ethics*, **29**, no. 1, 30–3.

Brownsword, R. (2004a). The cult of consent: fixation and fallacy. *Kings College Law Journal*, **15**, 223–51.

–ibid.– (2004b). What the world needs now: techno-regulation, human rights and human dignity. In *Global Governance and the Quest for Justice*, edited by R. Brownsword, N.D. Lewis and S. MacLeod, Oxford: Hart Publishing.

Clark, A. (2003). Commentary on Hallowell *et al. Journal of Medical Ethics*, **29**, 80–2.

Corrigan, O. (2003). Empty ethics: the problem with informed consent. *Sociology of Health and Illness*, **25**, no. 7, 768–92.

Department of Health (2003). *The Investigation of Events that Followed the Death of Cyril Mark Isaacs.*

Department of Health, Department for Education and Employment, and the Home Office (2001). *The Removal, Retention and Use of Human Organs and Tissue from Post Mortem Examinations: Advice from the Chief Medical Officer.* London: The Stationery Office.

Furness, P. (2003). Consent to using human tissue. Implied consent should suffice. *British Medical Journal*, **327**, no. 7418, 759–60.

Furness, P. and Nicholson, M. (2004). Obtaining explicit consent for the use of archival tissue samples: practical issues. *Journal of Medical Ethics*, **30**, no. 6, 561–4.

Furness, P. and Sullivan, R. (2004). The Human Tissue Bill. *British Medical Journal*, **328**, no. 7429, 553–4.

Gostin, L.O. (2000). *Public Health Law: Power, Duty, Restraint.* Berkeley: University of California Press.

Human Genetics Commission (2002). *Inside Information: Balancing Interests in the Use of Personal Genetic Data.*

Jack, A.L. and Womack, C. (2003). Why surgical patients do not donate tissue for commercial research: review of records. *British Medical Journal*, **327**, no. 7409, 262.

Liddell, K. (2003). *Biolaw and Deliberative Democracy: Regulating Genetic Technology in a Morally Pluralist Society.* DPhil thesis, University of Oxford.

Liddell, K. and Hall, A. (2005). Beyond Bristol and Alder Hey: the future regulation of human tissue. *Medical Law Review*, **13**, no. 2, 170–223.

Mill, J.S. (1890). *Considerations of a Representative Government.* 3rd ed., London: Longman Green.

Nolan Committee (1995). *Standards in Public Life.* Cm 2850.

O'Neill, O. (2002). *Autonomy and Trust in Bioethics.* Cambridge: Cambridge University Press.

Pincock, S. (2004). Human Tissue Bill could jeopardise research, scientists warn. *British Medical Journal*, **328**, no. 7447, 1034.

Price, D. (2003). From Cosmos and Damian to Van Velzen: the human tissue saga continues. *Medical Law Review*, **11**, no. 1, 2–47.

Rawls, J. (1996). *Political Liberalism* (2nd edition). New York: Columbia University Press.

Report of the Inquiry into the Royal Liverpool Children's Hospital (Alder Hey Report) (2001). HC 12-II.

Richards, M., Ponder, M., Pharoah, S., Everest, P. and Mackay, J. (2003). Issues of consent and feedback in a genetic epidemiological study of women with breast cancer. *Journal of Medical Ethics*, **29**, no. 2, 93–6.

Start, R.D., Brown, W., Bryant, R.J., *et al.* (1996). Ownership and uses of human tissue: does the Nuffield Bioethics Report accord with the opinion of surgical inpatients? *British Medical Journal*, **313**, no. 7088, 1366–8.

Young, P. (1986). *The Law of Consent.* North Ryde: The Law Book Company.

Chapter 6

The normative status of the requirement to gain an informed consent in clinical trials: comprehension, obligations, and empirical evidence

Angus Dawson

6.1 Introduction

Informed consent plays a preeminent role in contemporary research ethics. Given the history of medical research over the last seventy years this is understandable. However, it is not, in my view, justified. This chapter seeks to re-orientate research ethics through an exploration of the exact nature and status of the normative requirement to gain an informed consent in the context of randomized clinical trials. This chapter first focuses on this requirement in its own terms. I argue that our normative commitments need to be shaped within the framework of what is possible: where we have relevant empirical evidence that a moral requirement is impossible to attain, we are obligated to revise our moral commitments. In the second half of the chapter, I explore the status of the requirement to gain an informed consent from a different direction, through a discussion of the relationship between respect for autonomy and other moral values. I conclude that we need to situate any commitment to gaining consent to participation in research within a wider framework of plural and equal values.

6.2 Definitions and clarifications

First, I need to clarify what I mean by 'informed consent'. The exact necessary and sufficient conditions for obtaining an informed consent are subject to much debate. However, informed consent is standardly taken to involve three or four necessary elements. On this view an informed consent requires that the consenting individual:

(a) must have the required *competence* to understand the information

(b) must be subject to *no undue influence* or coercion

(c) must be in *possession* of the relevant information

and many accounts add the additional informational criterion that the consenting individual also:

(d) must *comprehend* the relevant information.

In this chapter, my focus is on the information elements contained in (c) and (d), and I will just assume in the rest of this chapter that the other two conditions will have been met. As we will see in the next section, some accounts of informed consent only require the *possession* of the relevant information, others that possession is not enough, and that the individual must also *comprehend* the information that is provided. The stronger comprehension interpretation (accepting (d) as well as (c) as necessary conditions) imposes a much greater burden on the information provider (Sreenivasan 2003). I will assume in this chapter that informed consent requires us to meet this higher threshold. This is for a number of reasons. First, the most influential and widely cited accounts of informed consent in the literature propose comprehension of the disclosed information as a necessary requirement for a genuine informed consent (Faden and Beauchamp 1986; Beauchamp and Childress 2001). Second, the comprehension interpretation seems to be a better fit with the common justification for seeking an informed consent; namely, that this is an important means of respecting an individual's autonomy. It is difficult to see how the mere *provision* of information is enough to meet this condition. Third, the alternative or weaker interpretation of the information condition makes the requirement to gain an informed consent a relatively trivial and uninteresting matter. If all that is necessary is to supply the information to the patient, why do regulations give such prominence to the idea of informed consent? Taking these issues together suggests that the most plausible accounts of informed consent must require fulfilment of all four components suggested above.

Second, this chapter is about informed consent in the context of medical research, not everyday clinical care. I focus on the case of medical research because of the force and ubiquity with which the requirement to gain informed consent is cited in this context. In this paper I assume that we are talking about competent adult participants in phase II and III trials. Such participants are assumed to be (or, in fewer cases, have actually been found to be) capable of giving an informed consent. I exclude phase I trials from this discussion, because in this chapter I focus on cases where the trial participant *may* gain some personal (medical) benefit from participation in the trial (such as when they take the form: existing treatment versus innovative treatment). I also assume that the researchers will be in equipoise, however we choose to define it (Ashcroft 1999).

I will begin in section 6.3 by presenting an argument based upon the claim that the requirement to gain informed consent (IC) cannot be met in a significant number of cases (I call this the 'unattainability argument'). I will then discuss each of the premises of this argument in turn and suggest reasons to hold them to be true. In section 6.4, I will then present a second parasitic argument (the 'revisability argument') to suggest that as a result of the 'unattainability argument', we are obligated to revise our moral beliefs in relevant circumstances (and the case of IC is one such case). In section 6.5, I outline and reject the idea that we should insist upon meeting the requirement to gain an IC because this is considered such an important moral claim (despite the existence of any empirical evidence about its impossibility). Section 6.6 explores the exact scope of the arguments that I have presented. The alternative position that I sketch in these last sections allows greater space for what I take to be the plausible claim that at least some medical research is ethical, despite the absence of informed consent.

6.3 The 'unattainability argument'

In this section, I outline and defend what I call the 'unattainability argument', so-called because it suggests that IC often cannot, in actuality, be attained. The starting point for this argument is the apparent tension between two facts. The first is that it is almost universally claimed that we must obtain a fully informed consent from competent adult participants in clinical trials. The second is that we have good empirical evidence that many (perhaps even most) competent adults cannot understand the information that is given to them to the degree necessary to hold that they have given a fully informed consent. I say that the two are in tension because if the second is true, it seems strange that the first is so widely held, expressed so forcefully, and stated in such absolute terms in research ethics guidelines and practice. The argument can be outlined as follows:

1. It is claimed that we ought to obtain IC from competent adult research participants
2. We cannot obtain IC in a significant number of cases
3. Where we cannot actually obtain IC, it makes no sense to require it.

Conclusion: It makes no sense to require IC.

I will discuss each of these premises in turn.

6.3.1 Premise 1: It is claimed that we ought to obtain IC from research participants

I will illustrate this first premise by reference to a number of different international research regulations, because of their widespread acceptance and the ubiquity of their application. One thing that is striking is that the ambiguity I noted above in relation to the information criterion for giving an IC is present in the regulations. The majority of international regulations seem to require only *possession* not *comprehension* of the information by the potential trial participant. The following quote from CIOMS is typical:

> *Before requesting* an individual's consent to participate in research, *the investigator must provide the following information,* in language or another form of communication that the individual can *understand* … for controlled trials, an explanation of features of the research design (e.g., randomization, double-blinding), and that the subject will not be told of the assigned treatment until the study has been completed and the blind has been broken.
>
> (Guideline 5) (my italics)

Here the obligation is only to *provide* information (in relation to this long list of factors) in a comprehensible form. This condition will be met if the information is written in suitably simple terms in a language that the individual understands.

There is no requirement that the participant actually understands the information provided. There are many other examples of this 'provision' interpretation of the requirement to gain an IC (EU Directive on Clinical Trials 2001; Department of Health 2004; MRC 2005; OPRR 2005).

In some guidelines, the requirement in relation to IC appears, at least on first glance, to be more demanding than the 'provision' interpretation. The best example of this is the IC requirement contained in *Guideline for Good Clinical Practice*. This document focuses on the formal recording of the consent process, and includes the stipulation that a witness is present during the act of obtaining an IC to attest to the fact that:

> the information in the consent form and any other written information was accurately explained to, and apparently understood by, the subject.

> (ICH 1996: 4.8.9) (my italics)

No actual understanding or formal evaluation of comprehension is required by these guidelines. Presumably just sitting silently and not objecting will be enough to infer that the research participant has 'apparently understood'. So in practice, this requirement is no higher than the 'provision' interpretation of IC. 'Apparent' understanding is different from actual understanding.

By contrast, other regulations seem to require the higher *comprehension* interpretation of the information criterion. The best example of this is perhaps the Helsinki Declaration, where it is stated that research participants:

> must be adequately informed of the aims, methods, sources of funding, any possible conflicts of interest, institutional affiliations of the researcher, the anticipated benefits and potential risks of the study and the discomfort it may entail. … After ensuring that the subject has understood the information, the physician should then obtain the subject's freely-given informed consent, preferably in writing.

> (Paragraph 22) (my italics)

Another example of the stronger interpretation is that given in the *Belmont Report* (NCPHSBBR 1979). This document, central to US and international research ethics since its inception, also requires comprehension as a component of the information criterion. The point is made as follows:

> Investigators are responsible for ascertaining that the subject has comprehended the information. While there is always an obligation to ascertain that the information about risk to subjects is complete and adequately comprehended, when the risks are more serious, that obligation increases. On occasion, it may be suitable to give some oral or written tests of comprehension.

> (The National Commission for the Protection of Human Subjects of Biomedical and Behavioral Research 1979. (my italics)

Helsinki and Belmont are presented in a stronger form than that of CIOMS, in their requirement that researchers ensure that participants *understand* the information. I take it that this stronger version of the information criterion is more appropriate to what is required in obtaining an IC for the reasons given above.

6.3.2 **Premise 2: We cannot obtain IC in a significant number of cases**

This second premise is far more contentious and contains the central claim in the 'unattainability' argument. I believe that this premise can be supported by appeal to a fair interpretation of the whole body of empirical work performed in relation to IC over the last 30 years. This literature, in my view, clearly and consistently demonstrates substantive problems in obtaining IC with many participants, due to lack of comprehension of the information provided (Sugarman *et al.* 1999; Corrigan 2003; Dawson 2005). However, my claim is not just that many people *do not* understand key elements of information disclosed to them, but that they *cannot* do so. If this is true, and the supporters of IC require the comprehension criterion for IC to be met, we have good grounds for holding that IC cannot be obtained in a significant number of cases. (I exclude from discussion cases of failure to comprehend due to such things as the deliberate withholding of information from participants.)

Of course, wherever we discuss empirical studies, objections can be raised over numerous potential problems. The methodology may be disputed, the sample size may be held to be too small to generalize (particularly in qualitative studies), and it might be claimed that the results are not truly representative as there may have been special reasons for the failure in a particular case. Each (or all) of these claims may well be true in relation to any particular study. However, I suggest that the body of literature in relation to apparent failures in understanding within the context of gaining an IC cannot be quickly dismissed, as the trend is remarkably consistent across patient groups, timeframes, and different methodologies. We cannot and should not ignore this evidence.

In this discussion, I will concentrate upon empirical data relating to the comprehension of the concept of 'randomization', for a number of reasons. First, and most importantly, I suggest that if a participant does not understand this key feature of the methodology governing a randomized trial, then they have clearly failed to give an informed consent. My thought is that this piece of information ('I got my treatment by chance') is so central to what it is to participate in a randomized trial, that if someone fails to comprehend this, then we have good grounds for holding that they did not give an IC. However, it should be noted that I am not suggesting that an IC is only attained if an individual comprehends *all* relevant information. Such a standard would be, arguably, too high (despite the long list of factors that Helsinki requires to be disclosed and comprehended). I will leave open what is to count as an adequate amount of information to meet the threshold for giving an IC. However, I suggest that the failure to comprehend 'randomization' is far more devastating to the claim that an individual has given an IC than a failure to understand every last minor and unlikely risk. Second, lay comprehension of this particular concept has received extensive investigation and discussion in the literature. Here, I will discuss briefly a number of key references to empirical work on participants' comprehension of randomization within trials in an attempt to justify this premise. Of course, if the reader chooses to reject these particular studies (for whatever reason) this does not defeat the general claim, as there are plenty of other studies to discuss (Sugarman *et al.* 1999; Corrigan 2003; Dawson 2005). Nor is this premise dependent upon literature relating to the comprehension of the particular concept of 'randomization', as the issues of comprehension of equipoise (Robinson *et al.* 2005) and risk (Lidz *et al.* 2004; Reynold and Nelson 2007) seem to produce very similar results.

A series of studies investigating comprehension of 'randomization' using a variety of methodologies have produced very similar results (Appelbaum *et al.* 1987; Snowdon *et al.* 1997; Featherstone and Donovan 2002; Robinson *et al.* 2004, 2005). For reasons of space, I will discuss only two of these studies here. Appelbaum and colleagues, in a large body of work, have explored what they call the 'therapeutic misconception'. This is a persistent misunderstanding by trial participants that participation in research will be of benefit to them in a similar way to therapeutic care. In their research they report that 69% of participants interviewed had 'no comprehension of the actual basis for their [own] random assignment' and only 28% were held to have 'a complete understanding of the randomization process [as a whole]' (1987, 21). One thing that is striking about the interview data that they discuss is the apparent ability of some of these participants to be able to both give a correct account of the randomization methodology in the abstract, but also hold that they did not get their own treatment by chance (even though they did). The study by Featherstone and Donovan (2002) produced very similar results, despite using a different methodology. This study involved exploring participants' (and those that had refused trial participation) understandings of interventions in relation to prostate problems with three options (a new laser treatment, a standard surgical intervention, and conservative 'wait and see' management). This study suggests that:

> Just over half of the participants (12) indicated that they had expected to receive treatment [within the research study] based on their diagnosis and an assessment of their specific needs by a clinician […] in the way that they perceived normal clinical practice to occur.

(p. 713)

That is, despite being held to have given an informed consent, they thought that their doctor would intervene in the study to ensure that they would either get the treatment option that they preferred, or, in most cases, the option that their doctor thought was in the participant's best interests. It seems as though many participants will go to elaborate lengths to explain why it was that they got the treatment that they did (where the actual reason was chance within the framework of a randomized methodology).

However, it might still be argued that at best all this evidence suggests is that many participants *do not* understand significant elements of the relevant information, not that they *cannot*. It is a very common response to the failures in understanding apparent in such studies to argue that we just need to either provide more information to participants or we need to improve the information providers' ability to communicate. In other words, it might be difficult to gain informed consent, but it is another thing to demonstrate that it is impossible. However, I do not believe this is an adequate response, and I suggest that it is reasonable to draw the inference from *do not* to *cannot* from this evidence for three reasons. The first is just the combined weight and consistency of the empirical evidence. The fact that a significant number of participants do not understand is not just a rogue result from a single study, but the persistent finding of numerous studies (Sugarman *et al.* 1999; Corrigan 2003; Robinson *et al.* 2004, 2005; Dawson 2005). The extent and variety of such problems in comprehension (covering all aspects of trials, not just randomization) requires explanation. One possibility could be that these studies illustrate a persistent failure by researchers to provide information in an accessible and comprehensive form (despite the researchers' best intentions and the oversight of research ethics committees examining the information sheets and supposedly ensuring that they are comprehensible). However, an alternative possibility could be that such empirical studies reflect an important fact about human nature. On this view, such problems in understanding are not to be seen as a failure, but rather as a discovery about the limits to human understanding.

The second reason to make the inference is again based on empirical evidence, but this time in relation to the apparent failure to dramatically 'improve' comprehension, through the many studies that attempted to do so via such things as the provision of *more* information, *different* information, the *rewording* of information, and the presentation of information using *different formats*. It might be the case that we can improve understanding through these methods by a statistically significant amount, although the current empirical evidence suggests there are strong reasons to doubt this. The differences produced through such interventions appear to be minimal at best (Flory and Emanuel 2004). There is certainly no evidence that suggests that the provision of either greater information or improved communication skills will remove the 'therapeutic misconception'. For example, some studies suggest that significantly extending the time devoted to explaining randomization has no impact on the comprehension of the concept (Kodish *et al.* 2004). This is consistent with the extensive and thorough empirical studies reported by Robinson *et al.* (2004, 2005) in a context of hypothetical trial participation. The latter research attempted to improve understanding of randomization through the use of different examples and rephrasings of information about the concept. The main effect was, apparently, not greater understanding, but a growing sense that randomization (in its use of chance allocation) was a morally problematic methodology.

Third, as I have already suggested, there is a perfectly reasonable explanation for such 'failures' in comprehension; one that does not rely upon the idea that lack of understanding results from mere miscommunication. In earlier work, I argued that we can think about failure to comprehend in two different ways. The first are what I called 'process failures'. They can be 'corrected' through the provision of information. Such failures are due to misunderstandings that are corrigible. For example, if I falsely claim that the St Lawrence is the longest river in Canada, you can correct me. The second type of failure, I called 'framing failures' (Dawson 2004). The name, of course, derives from the work of social psychologists such as Tversky and Kahneman (1981, 1984). Such 'failures' are due to the context of the individual's previous beliefs, assumptions, and experiences that 'frame' the information provided. The 'therapeutic misconception' is just one example of this general 'framing' problem in relation to IC (Dawson 2005). Participants do not fail to comprehend due to a lack of understanding of the actual information provided; it is rather that they just don't 'see' it. This does not mean that participants are intellectually inferior or deficient in any way, nor do we need to accept that they have their own alternative way of understanding the information presented (Corrigan 2003; Dixon-Woods *et al.* 2007). A focus on 'framing' allows us to accept a plausible picture of the reality of the psychological and social context for individual decision-making. On this view, as human beings we are not purely rational deliberators, able to process discrete pieces of information in a detached and logical way. Rather, our prior commitments and beliefs influence or 'frame' the information we are given to a significant extent. Some people are able to 'overcome' the influence of such factors in their understanding of some information, but many people cannot. To hold that this is a 'failure' is to miss an important fact about human nature: understanding is contextual and social.

6.3.3 Premise 3: Where we cannot actually obtain IC, it makes no sense to require it

This third premise is an application of the well known (and widely accepted) moral principle that 'ought implies can'. That is, that it is a plausible constraint upon an acceptable moral obligation that it should be possible for the relevant agent to carry out that obligation. There is more to be spelled out here than might at first appear. For example, we must be clear about the nature of the 'impossibility' we are talking about: is it conceptual, physical, or metaphysical impossibility (Howard-Snyder 2006)? I assume that we are talking about metaphysical impossibility. Some have recently contested that 'ought implies can' (Fischer 2003). I accept that it is possible to deny this principle, but consider it to be a reasonable one (although I do not think there are any finally convincing arguments in favour, despite great efforts to produce them (Streumer 2007)). I will just treat it as being true in this chapter. The supporter of IC may, then, sidestep the unattainability argument if they are willing to deny 'ought implies can'. However, given its general acceptance, I take it this will not be a popular move, and objections to my argument will have to be found elsewhere. However, it should be noted that the principle I am appealing to is a slightly different variation of 'ought implies can': namely, we cannot x, therefore, we ought not to require x. I do not believe this formulation makes any difference to the acceptability (or otherwise) of this premise.

Before concluding this section, I will respond to two possible general objections to the unattainability argument. The first is that the argument generalizes beyond the scope of the empirical evidence. This objection argues that even if we accept the evidence that I have presented, it does not suggest that in all cases all participants will fail to understand the relevant information. Therefore, it can be argued, there will be some cases where IC can be actualized. This may well be true, and my argument does not require that all participants apparently fail to comprehend the information. It is an empirical matter to be settled by further research exactly what percentage of trial participants meet the comprehension test in relation to relevant factors within a trial. However, all that is necessary for my argument is that a significant number of trial participants do, in fact, fail to comprehend, not that all participants fail to do so.

The second general objection might be that I have made the basic error of moving from an empirical to a normative claim (moving from an 'is' to an 'ought') in this argument. In a sense, I have. However, like Pigden (1991), I take Hume's claim to really be about moving from solely empirical premises to a normative conclusion (that is, it is a claim about the correct form of an ethical argument incorporating empirical premises). It should be noted that my argument has both empirical and normative premises, and that they are linked through premise 3. This means that my argument does not fall victim to Hume's objection.

In conclusion, then, despite the requirements of the international research ethics regulations and numerous writers on research ethics, I suggest we have reasonable grounds for doubting whether it makes sense to maintain that we are under a moral requirement to gain an IC in clinical trials (at least in relation to many participants).

6.4 **The 'revisability argument'**

This second or 'revisability' argument is parasitic upon the first, in the sense that it builds upon its conclusion. The thing that motivates this argument is the observation that supporters of the requirement to gain an IC in research can hardly fail to be aware of the manifold evidence in relation to the problems in gaining an informed consent, but they continue to maintain acceptance and advocacy for this requirement. What can justify such a position? Does it make any sense to remain committed to such a view? I want to argue that it does not, and that in circumstances where we have enough relevant empirical evidence about the impossibility of attaining a moral requirement (in a significant number of cases), we are required to revise our related moral beliefs.

This second argument goes as follows:

1. If relevant evidence exists that we cannot attain an apparently morally required end (in a significant number of cases), and this failure is not due to moral failing, then we ought to revise our moral beliefs about that end

2. We have good evidence that we cannot obtain IC in a significant number of cases

3. This is not due to moral failing

Conclusion: We ought to revise our relevant moral beliefs about gaining IC.

These premises should, mostly, be familiar from the previous discussion. However, I need to say something about premise 3 and what I mean by the term 'moral failing'. This premise is required so that the argument is not open to inappropriate application. For example, I don't want this argument to apply in cases where the individual is culpable in failing to perform an obligation, due to such things as laziness or weakness of will. So the mere fact that an obligation imposes significant costs upon an agent (or society) will not, in itself, count as a sufficient reason to cancel any obligation. A failure to fulfil an obligation just because it is *hard* to do so, will count as a moral failing, and so the 'revisability argument' should not be invoked in this case. We need to retain the option of holding the agent responsible for a failure to carry out the expected moral obligation. This premise attempts to limit this argument to cases where the failure to carry out the obligation is due to factors beyond the control of the agent. An example of such a case would be where the therapeutic misconception applies. Here, the failure to fulfil the requirement to gain an IC is due not to 'moral failing' on the part of the researcher, but rather to human nature or 'biases' in human reasoning (that is, factors beyond the researcher's control).

In the light of what has been outlined in this paper so far, could the advocate of IC credibly deny the 'revisability' argument? Chances are that any objection will take one of two forms. It will either focus on the evidence claim itself or the role of evidence in our moral deliberations. For example, in relation to the first claim, it might be argued that someone is just unaware of the relevant evidence. Assuming this is not disingenuous, we can just ensure that they do become aware of it (or if we are feeling more charitable, perhaps we can supply it). Alternatively, perhaps someone might argue that they are aware of the evidence, but just don't believe it. This is harder to respond to, because it will depend upon the nature of the disbelief. However, in the previous section I tried to outline what it is reasonable to believe in relation to the empirical evidence, and do not think anyone can retain the commitment to IC (in anything like its present form) if they consider the body of evidence fairly (even if they wish to dispute particular studies). The second set of objections relates to the status of empirical evidence within the context of moral deliberation itself. Perhaps someone could genuinely believe that what is actually the case does not in fact restrict our moral obligations. Such a view could contest 'ought implies can' and related principles, or appeal to the idea that some moral requirements are just so important that we must continue to uphold them, no matter what the empirical evidence suggests about our capacity to implement them in the real world. I find it hard to make sense of the latter claim, but will explore it in the next section.

6.5 Defending the moral status of IC

This section will discuss the motivation that lies behind the first premise of the 'unattainability argument'; that is, the claim that we ought to obtain IC from research participants. Although there will, of course, be other justifications for seeking an IC, perhaps the most plausible will be the idea that this is a key means of respecting a patient's autonomous decision-making. Let's assume, for now, that this is true. It might be argued that given the value we do (or should) ascribe to IC (and the need to respect any individual's autonomy), despite the empirical evidence about the problems relating to comprehension discussed earlier, we should choose to ignore them. In substance, this view claims that, given their importance as *moral* claims, IC, and autonomy considerations should always take priority in our moral deliberations, despite any concerns about the possibility of actually carrying them out. This view might, in turn, be supported by an appeal to a justification for respect for autonomy based upon an absolute duty or an account of rights containing absolute claims. If this point were to succeed, then the 'unattainability' argument will fail, and the 'revisability' argument could not be built upon it. However, I think this counter-argument will not work, because we have no grounds for giving such priority to respecting autonomy for two reasons.

First, such an argument in this context is self-defeating. How can ignoring the fact that people do not understand information be a way of respecting their autonomy?

Where evidence exists that people do not comprehend relevant information, the supporter of autonomy should be interested in this fact, because here is a potential impediment to a participant making an autonomous decision. Anyone interested in respecting autonomy should take a keen interest in, rather than ignoring, empirical evidence about lack of comprehension. This will be the case even if we are just talking about participants *not* comprehending, because then the focus ought to be on finding ways of encouraging understanding. If it turns out that many participants *cannot* comprehend the information, then the supporter of autonomy will have to come up with some strategy for dealing with such cases, perhaps arguing that this group should be held to be incompetent (and decision-making should be made on their behalf by suitable proxies: that is, individuals not party to any failures in comprehension). In either case, ignoring the evidence is not an option for the supporter of respecting autonomy.

Second, any view that claims that autonomy should always take priority is highly implausible, given the number of other possible values that will be relevant to participant decision-making. For example, it is easy to think of cases where other moral considerations such as beneficence or justice will take priority over concerns about autonomy (NCPHSBBR 1979). We can retain the idea that autonomy is an important value, as well as it being something that ought to be protected and promoted, without being committed to the idea that it must always take priority over other considerations or even that it is 'first among equals' in a range of values: that is, that it is, roughly, of equal value to other considerations, but that it should be given 'extra' priority for some reason (Gillon 2003; Dawson and Garrard 2006). If it is believed that autonomy should take priority, at the very least this needs some argumentative support. Surely only the most red-blooded libertarian would hold such a view, as almost any plausible moral theory will allow for the possibility that autonomy may be outweighed by other moral considerations (at least some of the time)? What we really need is a form of moral theory that defends an idea of a set of moral values or considerations that can be weighed against each other. Examples of such theories might include Rossian deontology, many forms of consequentialism, and at least some forms of contractarianism. I conclude that, in the absence of any good arguments, it makes no sense to prioritize autonomy over other moral considerations, or to maintain a requirement to gain IC to such an extent that we ignore relevant empirical evidence about its impossibility.

This point about the status of autonomy within a plurality of values is particularly important given the reality of individuals being, at the same time, both research participants and patients. The danger in focusing on IC is that it imposes the burden for decision-making upon the participant, and it is forgotten that they are patients as well. Participant-patients may be feeling ill and be concerned, primarily, about recovery from their ill health. For this reason, I'd suggest that even if it is held that, in general, autonomy should take priority in ethical deliberations, this looks much less plausible in phase II and III trials. In this context, the contribution of the research ethics committee (REC) is vital. Their role cannot just be to ensure that participants are fully informed about the trial in the sense that the information sheets are written in suitable language.

The REC must take a balanced approach to weighing the different factors that are relevant, and reach a defensible conclusion. This 'balanced' view is important because it means that we can question both those who explicitly want IC to play the primary role in research ethics (Edwards *et al.* 2004) as well as those who implicitly seem committed to such a view given the fact that they argue in favour of downplaying the notion of beneficence in research ethics (Miller and Brody 2003). In at least some cases, it might be appropriate not to permit research to progress, because priority ought to be given to the idea of protecting participants from potential harm (Chapter Two) (even if the participants are willing to go ahead). The more one accepts the reality of the existence of a therapeutic misconception, the more tempting a proposal for reassessing IC becomes. This is, of course, a form of paternalism, but this does not necessarily mean that it is wrong (Edwards *et al.* 2004; Garrard and Dawson 2005).

6.6 **The scope of the arguments**

In this section, I will explore more generally the scope of both the unattainability and revisability arguments presented earlier. What exactly can we conclude from them? This is important for two reasons. First, it might be argued that the correct interpretation of the requirement to gain an IC is that we only have to *genuinely attempt* to gain an informed consent, not *actually* do so. Second, even if some people fail to comprehend, we need to remember that the evidence suggests that at least some will understand, and so, it might be argued, we should focus policy on them. However, it should be noted that both points concede that there is something to the empirical evidence that I have presented, and suggest that we should not inappropriately prioritize IC.

So, first, perhaps it is enough to *attempt* to obtain IC rather than actually obtain it? The idea here is that IC is an *ideal* that we should aim towards even if we cannot actually attain it. I don't have any trouble with this restriction, except for the fact that the nature of the claims made on behalf of IC seem to go much further, and take a more absolute form, than this would suggest. If the *attempt* to gain an IC is all that is required, then I think it is worth being honest about it. (Perhaps this is why so many research ethics guidelines only require the giving of information, rather than its comprehension?) In addition, if this is indeed what is meant, we should not forget that we will still have a significant number of participants who will not understand the information about such important things as the methodology of study. Even if we choose to focus our obligation upon *genuine attempts* to gain an IC, we still need a policy that is sensitive to the fact that so many apparently fail to comprehend.

Second, even in the worst-case scenario, it is the case that not all participants will fail to understand, and it can be argued that we should, therefore, focus our guidelines on this group. On this view, we should have a presumption that people can give an IC, and so prioritize this group's concerns in our policies. This seems reasonable, although, again, the focus on an absolute requirement to gain IC looks odd from this perspective. We also need to ensure that there is enough protection, through alternative means, for those that cannot meet the comprehension standard. An excellent example of the importance of this point is supplied by Schüklenk and Ashcroft (2007) in their discussion of the therapeutic misconception in HIV vaccine trials. In such a case, failure to understand the methodology of the trial may result in increased risk of infection through behaviour change (due to participants' possibly false belief that they are protected by the vaccine). Where such failures in understanding are possible, what are we to do? We could restrict trials to those who really do understand all informational elements that are deemed essential, but we need to accept at the beginning that this will have serious implications for our research agenda (as trials will have to be smaller or take longer to recruit). The costs of such an option will, almost certainly, be too high. I think the evidence in relation to the lack of comprehension by many trial participants should motivate an attitude towards research ethics where IC plays much less of a central role: one where other ethical values such as beneficence and non-maleficence are given due prominence. On this view, whilst it is important to provide key information for those potential participants that can comprehend, this should be kept brief and should only relate to the truly vital points of the research (although other information could be available for those who really want it). In essence, whilst we have no grounds to deny that all will fail to understand the necessary information, many will do so. It seems not just unreasonable, but unethical, to continue to act as if all competent adults can give an IC (especially as we have clear evidence that they cannot).

6.7 **Conclusion**

In this chapter, I have argued that we have good reason to think that the requirement to gain an IC is impossible to achieve (at least for many competent adult research participants). If this is true, as I believe it is, then it makes no sense to continue to promote a general requirement to gain an IC. Even if this argument is not accepted, the supporters of IC need to take account of the evidence, and consider how to respond to this inconvenient truth (beyond looking the other way). In the tension between the two facts that I outlined at the start of this chapter, I have argued that it is the general requirement to gain an IC that requires revision; and that there is, indeed, a moral requirement to revise our moral beliefs (and related research guidelines) in the light of appropriate empirical evidence. The case of IC in clinical trials can serve as a paradigm case of a situation where the facts (as far as we can ascertain them) act as a constraint on what we ought to believe.

Acknowledgements

I am very grateful to audiences at the following events for their comments on earlier versions of this chapter: the symposium 'Informed consent – in whose interest?', organized by the Nordic Committee on Bioethics (13 June 2006, Sandhamn, Sweden); the 'Contemporary Ethics: Perspectives' workshop (1–2 February 2008, CREUM, University of Montreal, Canada); and the Fellows' Seminar, Centre for Ethics, University of Toronto (24 March 2008). Special thanks to John McMillan, Charles Weijer, Kathy Liddell, Oonagh Corrigan, and Danielle Bromwich for their detailed comments on previous versions. I would also like to thank the Centre for Ethics,

University of Toronto, for funding a Faculty Fellowship for the academic year 2007–8, where I completed the final version of this chapter.

References

Appelbaum, P., Roth, L., Lidz, C., Benson, P., and Winslade, W. (1987). False hopes and best data: consent to research and the therapeutic misconception. *Hastings Center Report*, **17**, 20–4.

Ashcroft, R. (1999). Equipoise, knowledge and ethics in clinical research and practice. *Bioethics*, **13**, 314–26.

Beauchamp, T.L. and Childress, J.F. (2001). *Principles of Biomedical Ethics (5th edition)*. Oxford: Oxford University Press.

CIOMS. International Ethical Guidelines for Biomedical Research Involving Human Subjects. November 2002. http://www.cioms.ch/frame_guidelines_nov_2002.htm [accessed 4/2/08].

Corrigan, O. (2003). Empty ethics: the problem with informed consent. *Sociology of Health and Illness*, **25**, 768–92.

Dawson, A. (2004). What should we do about it? Implications of the empirical evidence in relation to comprehension and acceptability of randomization. In *Engaging the World: The Use of Empirical Research in Bioethics and the Regulation of Biotechnology*, edited by S. Holm and M. Jonas. Netherlands: IOS Press.

–ibid.–(2005). Informed consent: bioethical ideal and empirical reality. In *Bioethics and Social Reality*, edited by M. Hayry, T. Takala, and P. Herissone-Kelly. Amsterdam/New York: Rodopi.

Dawson, A. and Garrard, E. (2006). In defence of moral imperialism: four equal and universal prima facie duties. *Journal of Medical Ethics*, **32**, 200–4.

Department of Health (2004). The Medicines for Human Use (Clinical Trials) Regulations (2004: Statutory Instrument (2004 No. 1031. London: Stationery Office.

Dixon-Woods, M., Ashcroft, R.E., Jackson, C.J., Tobin, M.D., Kivits, J., Burton, P.R., and Samani, N.J. (2007). Beyond 'misunderstanding': written information and decisions about taking part in a genetic epidemiology study. *Social Science and Medicine*, **65**, 2212–22.

Edwards S.L.J., Kirchin, S., and Huxtable, R. (2004). Research ethics committees and paternalism. *Journal of Medical Ethics*, **30**, 88–91.

European Union Parliament and Council (2001). Directive 2001/20/EC of 4 April 2001: http://www.eortc.be/Services/Doc/clinical-EU-directive-04-April-01.pdf [accessed 5/2/08].

Faden, R.R. and Beauchamp, T.L. (1986). *A History and Theory of Informed Consent*. Oxford: Oxford University Press.

Featherstone, K. and Donovan, J.L. (2002). 'Why don't they just tell me straight, why allocate it?' The struggle to make sense of participating in a randomized controlled trial. *Social Science and Medicine*, **55**, 709–19.

Fischer, J.M. (2003). 'Ought-implies-can', causal determinism and moral responsibility. *Analysis*, **63**, 244–50.

Flory, J. and Emanuel, E. (2004). Interventions to improve research participants' understanding in informed consent for research. *Journal of American Medical Association*, **292**, 1593–601.

Garrard, E. and Dawson, A. (2005). What is the role of the REC? Paternalism, inducements and harm in research ethics. *Journal of Medical Ethics*, **31**, 419–23.

Gillon, R. (2003). Ethics needs principles – four can encompass the rest – and respect for autonomy should be 'first among equals'. *Journal of Medical Ethics*, **29**, 307–12.

Howard-Snyder, F. (2006). 'Cannot' implies 'not ought'. *Philosophical Studies*, **130**, 233–46.

International Conference on Harmonisation (ICH) of Technical Requirements for Registration of Pharmaceuticals for Human Use (1996). *Guidelines for Good Clinical Practice*. E6 (R1). http://www.ich.org/LOB/media/MEDIA482.pdf [accessed 1/4/08].

Kodish, E., Eder, M., Noll, R.B., *et al.* (2004). Communication of randomization in childhood leukemia trials. *Journal of American Medical Association*, **291**, 470–5.

Lidz, C.W., Appelbaum P.S., Grisso, T., and Renaud, M. (2004). Therapeutic misconception and the appreciation of risks in clinical trials. *Social Science and Medicine*, **58**, 1689–897.

Medical Research Council (2005). *Medical Research Council Position Statement on Regulation and Ethics*. London: MRC.

Miller, F.G. and Brody, H. (2003). A critique of clinical equipoise: therapeutic misconception in the ethics of clinical trials. *Hastings Center Report*, **33**, no. 3, 19–28.

National Commission for the Protection of Human Subjects of Biomedical and Behavioral Research (NCPHSBBR) (1979). *The Belmont Report: Ethical Principles and Guidelines for the Protection of Human Subjects of Research*. Washington DC: GPO.

Office for Protection from Research Risk (OPRR) (2005). *Protection of Human Subjects*, 45 CFR 46 (originally 1983, revised 2005). Washington DC: GPO.

Pigden, C.R. (1991). Naturalism. In *A Companion to Ethics*, edited by P. Singer. Oxford: Blackwell.

Reynold, W.W. and Nelson, R.M. (2007). Risk perception and decision processes underlying informed consent to research participation. *Social Science and Medicine*, **65**, 2105–15.

Robinson, E.J., Kerr, C., Stevens, A., Lilford, R., Braunholtz, D., and Edwards, S. (2004). Lay conceptions of the ethical and scientific justifications for random allocation in clinical trials. *Social Science and Medicine*, **58**, 811–24.

Robinson, E.J., Kerr, C., Stevens, A., Lilford, R., Braunholtz, D., Edwards, S., Beck, S., and Rowley, M. (2005). Lay public's understanding of equipoise and randomization in randomized controlled trials. *Health Technology Assessment*, **9**, no. 8, 1–192.

Schüklenk, U. and Ashcroft, R. (2007). Editorial: HIV vaccine trials: reconsidering the therapeutic misconception and the question of what constitutes trial related injuries. *Developing World Bioethics*, **7**, no. 3, ii–iv.

Snowdon, C., Garcia, J., and Elbourne, D. (1997). Making sense of randomization; responses of parents of critically ill babies to random allocation of treatment in a clinical trial. *Social Science and Medicine*, **45**, no. 9, 1337–55.

Sreenivasan, G. (2003). Does informed consent to research require comprehension? *The Lancet*, **362**, 2016–18.

Streumer, B. (2007). Reasons and impossibility. *Philosophical Studies*, **136**, 351–84.

Sugarman, J., McCrory, D., Powell, D., Krasny, A., Ball, E., and Cassell, C. (1999). Empirical research on informed consent. *Hastings Center Report*, **29(Supp)**, S1–S42.

Tversky, A. and Kahneman, D. (1981). The framing of decisions and the psychology of choice. *Science*, **211**, 453–8.

–ibid.– (1984). Choices, values and frames. *American Psychologist*, **39**, 341–50.

World Medical Association Declaration of Helsinki (2002). Ethical Principles for Medical Research Involving Human Subjects. 52nd WMA General Assembly, Edinburgh, Scotland, October (2000, with clarification (2002. http://www.wma.net/e/policy/b3.htm [accessed 5/2/08].

Chapter 7

Is there an obligation to participate in medical research?[1]

Stephen John

7.1 Introduction

It is a commonplace of medical ethics that we ought to seek individuals' informed consent to their participation in risky forms of medical research.[2] One way in which these demands might be understood is as expressing a purely pragmatic requirement: subjects who have given their consent to participation in trials are, under normal circumstances, more likely to be cooperative than subjects who have not consented to participation in research. Therefore, research is far more likely to be successful if participants have consented to their participation. However, most debates over the relationship between consent and research make a far stronger claim: that research which involves exposing human subjects to risks of physical or psychological harm is ethically permissible *only* if research subjects have given their informed consent to their participation.[3] In turn, this claim is often supported by appeal to one (or more) of several general, ethical claims: about the obligations of physicians; about individuals' rights not to be exposed to 'excess risks'; or, most commonly, about the importance of promoting and protecting individuals' autonomy (Faden *et al.* 1986).

However, claims about the ethical limits which we ought to impose on research can seem ethically problematic to the extent that they overlook the benefit generated by research, that is, the development of new technologies which might save lives or improve health (Buchanan and Miller 2006). Of course, these kinds of worries are most pressing when it seems that adherence to strong consent procedures leads us to

---

[1] This paper has benefited greatly from the comments made by participants in the 'Beyond Consent' workshop (Hinxton, July 2005) and by this volume's editors. I have also benefited from comments by Richard Ashcroft, Michael Parker, Onora O'Neill, and Charlotte Goodburn.

[2] There is, of course, much debate over precisely to which kinds of risks we ought to consent to being exposed; for example, whether we need to consent to retention of medical information for future 'secondary research' (see Laurie (2002)). However, there seems to be widespread agreement that we need to seek consent in cases where individuals are placed at risk of physical harm; in this paper, I shall concentrate on these kinds of cases.

[3] See Faden and Beauchamp (1986) for the history of this claim. For a useful overview of recent work on consent see O'Neill (2002).

forgo useful research. However, even when it is unclear that less stringent (or simply different) consent requirements would lead to more or better research being pursued, we may still worry that an over-emphasis on questions of consent (or on a particular understanding of consent) in debates over research ethics might be morally problematic if this approach fails to recognize the moral imperative to pursue medical research.

In section 7.2 of this paper, I shall argue that proper awareness of the benefits generated by medical research leads to the conclusion that within a society such as the UK, where everyone has a guarantee of future access to state-provided medical care, each has an 'imperfect' obligation to be willing to participate in medical research.[4] In section 7.3, I claim that if we recognize the existence of this obligation, then we have good ethical reasons to change the social structures which ensure and regulate participation in research. In section 7.4, I shall then discuss the relationship between my claims and the concept of 'individual autonomy'. Finally, in section 7.5, I shall discuss the relationship between my claims and arguments about patients' rights and physicians' obligations.

7.2 A fairness-based obligation to participate in medical research?

Several writers have suggested that arguments for strong 'informed consent' conditions on medical research misrepresent the reasons why individuals might participate in research, because these arguments overlook the fact that we have obligations to participate in research. As a starting point for my arguments for the conclusion that we have a fairness-based obligation to participate in research, I shall focus on a recent article by John Harris on this theme (Harris 2005). Harris claims that accounts of the role of informed consent in research usually 'impute moral turpitude as default' by assuming that no-one would participate in medical research unless they perceived participation to be in their own self-interest (Harris 2005, 247).[5] However, Harris claims that this assumption is false, and that people are often motivated to participate in research because they believe that they have a moral obligation to do so. Furthermore, he claims, not only are people moved by the belief that they have an obligation to participate in research, but they are also right to be thus motivated: we often do have an obligation to participate in research. Of course, as Harris stresses, to say that we have an obligation to participate in research is not to say that we can

---

4 I will explain the concept of an imperfect obligation in greater detail in section 7.3 below. For now, it is important to stress merely that, unlike perfect obligations, it is normally assumed that we cannot (legitimately) be legally compelled to discharge imperfect obligations.

5 In this context, Harris is particularly concerned with arguments which combine a strong informed consent requirement on research with sociological claims about the existence of the 'therapeutic misconception' to deliver the result that placebo trials, for example, are always ethically illegitimate. However, his claims obviously have implications for a far broader range of topics related to the ethics of research.

legitimately be compelled to participate in research. However, this claim would seem to have implications for how we frame debates over the nature and limits of consent in research.

7.2.1 Harris on fairness

Harris suggests that our obligation to participate in research can be justified as falling under two broader obligations: an obligation to do no harm, and an obligation to treat others fairly. To defend Harris' argument that we harm others if we fail to participate in research would require us to deny the doing/allowing distinction. This is an extremely controversial move.[6] Therefore, I shall place to one side his claim that the principle 'do no harm' provides grounds for an obligation to participate in research. Of course, we could attempt to retrench Harris' argument by appealing, as he does, to a principle of beneficence, rather than one of non-maleficence, to support the claim that each has an obligation to participate in research. However, for the purposes of this paper, I shall concentrate on Harris' second claimed ground for an obligation to participate in research: his appeal to considerations of 'basic fairness'.

The fairness-based argument for an obligation to participate in research can be summarized thus: if we fail to take part in research, yet accept treatments or rely on medical knowledge which arose from previous research, we are 'free-riding' on the contributions of others. To 'free-ride' is to fail to treat others fairly.[7] Therefore, if we enjoy the benefits of medical treatments but refuse to take part in medical research, we breach our obligations of fairness. We all have reason to fulfil our obligations of fairness. Therefore, we all have some kind of reason to participate in research.

This kind of argument can seem intuitively plausible; there does seem to be something unfair about relying on the fruits of research, only gleaned because others have taken part in research, while failing to take part in research oneself.[8] I agree that there is a fairness-based obligation to participate in research, and that we can understand this obligation in terms of 'free-riding'. However, I also think that we must be very careful quite how we spell out this claim, for reasons I shall now elaborate.

In what follows I shall assume, as does Harris, that we each have an obligation to treat others fairly, and that we fail to treat others fairly if we are 'free-riders'. I shall adopt the following definition of free-riding: to free-ride is to receive some benefit but refuse to contribute to the maintenance of the system which generates that benefit, where widespread refusal to contribute to maintenance of the system would mean that no-one could enjoy the relevant benefit (Cullity 1995).[9] For example, if I travel

---

6 For a useful discussion of how the doing/allowing distinction (and related distinctions) might be relevant to health policy, see Pogge (2004).

7 See Klosko (1987) and Cullity (1985) for useful overviews of the nature and force of charges of 'free-riding'. Much current writing on this topic derives from Hart (1955).

8 Indeed, Martyn Evans independently made a similar claim in 2004.

9 Harris himself does not offer an explicit definition of free-riding. However, my definition seems in line with his claim that we each have a fairness-based obligation to contribute to a social system from which we have benefited and will continue to benefit. The definition above does bring

on a bus without buying a ticket then I am (literally) free-riding, because if enough people were to act as I do, then there would be no bus service at all. 'Free-riding' appears *prima facie* unfair, because it involves enjoyment of some benefit without bearing the costs that others bear (and which we too could bear) necessary for enjoyment of that benefit (Cullity 1995).

It is at this point, however, that we must be careful to make a distinction (which seems to be absent from Harris' paper) between different ways in which we might benefit from the participation of others in research. In his article, it seems that Harris understands the benefits produced by past research in terms of our enjoyment of particular medical goods or particular pieces of knowledge, or, perhaps, in terms of the more general goods, such as clean environments, that have been produced as a result of past research. However, it is not clear that my current enjoyment of the fruits of past medical research does ground on me any obligation to participate in current or future research. After all, if I receive some benefit such as treatment for an illness, but refuse to participate in research which would ensure that others enjoy an even better treatment in the future, I am not performing an action such that, were enough other people to do the same, there would be no current treatment *at all*. My refusal to bear the costs of taking part in research is not in any way unfair relative to the benefits I *currently* enjoy. If I receive the benefit of some drug but refuse to help to develop a better drug, my refusal may be morally problematic, perhaps because it displays a lack of gratitude or of solidarity. However, it would be incorrect to say that what I do in such a situation is free-riding, and thus unfair, because a charge of free-riding requires that we do something which is inconsistent with the continued enjoyment of some current benefit. Even if my enjoyment of a current benefit depends on what others did in the past, I do not free-ride if I refuse to do what would help others in the future.

These claims are not intended as a refutation of Harris' claim that we have a fairness-based obligation to participate in research. Rather, they are intended to point towards an important distinction between two ways in which we might benefit from the participation of others in research: we might now be better off than we would be otherwise either because others *have* contributed to past research, or because others continue to contribute to research. It is, I claim, only if we can show that individuals in some society currently enjoy the second of these benefits – that is, it is only if we can show that they currently benefit from the *current* participation of others in research – that we can hope to argue that they act as free-riders if they refuse to participate in research. Harris' own argument seems to me to run together these two very similar, but conceptually distinct, senses in which we might benefit from others' participation in research. However, the distinction is, for the kinds of reasons set out above, important: free-riding does not occur when we enjoy benefits which would exist whatever we do now.

out a key feature of free-riding which is not explicitly discussed by Harris (but which is, I assume, implicit in his claims): that individual acts of free-riding are (typically) compatible with the continuation of a system, although it would be impossible for everyone to free-ride simultaneously.

Furthermore, similar worries apply to a way in which we might reformulate Harris' arguments: as expressing demands of fairness more generally, rather than a demand not to free-ride in particular. Harris appeals to Nozick's formulation of the 'principle of fairness' as 'those who have submitted to ... restrictions have a right to similar acquiescence on the part of those who have benefited from their submission' (Harris 2005, 243). This principle only makes sense, I claim, if we read it in terms of a demand made by those who have *currently* submitted to some regulation can make on others who benefit from their submission. It does not make sense as a demand which those who are now long dead can now make on the living. After all, simply because my ancestors submitted to some difficult regulations which created benefits I now enjoy, there seems no reason to think *they* have a claim that *I* submit to similar regulations now. If considerations of fairness – whether framed in terms of free-riding or not – are to gain any traction in debates over consent, we need to show not only that people benefit from *past* research, but that they benefit from *current* research.

7.2.2 How to save the fairness argument

Yet, despite these difficulties there seems to be something appealing about the claim that we have an obligation of fairness to participate in research. How, then, might we argue that we have a fairness-based obligation to participate in research? To answer this question, it is necessary to move away from a focus on individuals' receipt of particular treatments, to think more generally about how people are benefited by the fact that they enjoy entitlements to medical care.[10] Consider the National Health Service (NHS) in the UK. This system seeks to ensure that medical treatment is distributed to individuals, insofar as possible, on the basis of medical need.[11] It seems reasonable to say that even if I do not *currently* make use of any of my entitlements to medical treatment (and, indeed, even if I end up never using my entitlements), I am better off than I would be otherwise in virtue of the fact that I possess such entitlements. We could explain the nature of this benefit in a number of different ways.[12] However, the basic claim that I am better off if I enjoy some kind of 'health security' than I am if I do not enjoy 'health security' seems fairly uncontroversial.[13]

From this perspective, we can also understand how we are benefited by systems of medical research. The benefits we enjoy because of the existence of the NHS depend in part on which kinds of medical research are currently pursued and how these forms of medical research are likely to be brought to bear on future provision of medical treatment. Consider, for example, someone who is a citizen of the UK and suffers a genetic disorder which makes it highly likely that, at some point in the future,

---

[10] At some points, Harris seems to argue along these lines himself. However, as I noted above, his overall strategy is (to this reader at least) slightly obscure. Therefore, I shall place exegetical issues to one side from now to concentrate on developing my own, positive argument.

[11] Newdick (2005) sets out the current legal situation in the NHS very clearly.

[12] I investigate these questions in my PhD thesis.

[13] Pogge suggested a similar point in 2006, but does not develop it. See also Wolff and de Shalit (2007), for some suggestions as to the importance of 'security'.

she will suffer from an incapacitating condition. Furthermore, imagine that there is a medical research programme, in which other members of her community willingly participate, designing treatments for the disorder from which she suffers. Presumably, if this research project will successfully generate a treatment for her condition, and if this treatment is to become available on the NHS, then this individual enjoys a higher level of 'health security' than she would do otherwise.

Taking these claims seriously makes it easier to make sense of our intuitive feeling that someone who refuses to participate in research might be breaching her obligations of fairness. I shall assume, for the sake of argument, that we are each members of a society with a system like the NHS, which benefits us by providing us with entitlements to medical care. Furthermore, I shall assume that the value of our entitlements to medical care – the contribution they make to our level of health security – depends to a large extent on the fact that medical research is pursued in our society, and that other members of our society participate in this research. If we think about the relationship between research and treatment in this manner, then we can better understand the claim that it is unfair – an act of free-riding – to refuse to participate in medical research. If an individual adopted a policy of refusing to participate in any form of medical research, then this *would* constitute free-riding, because were enough other people to adopt the same policy, then it would be the case that the *system* of research and treatment which currently benefits her by ensuring that she enjoys health security would not continue to function at all.

My suggestion, then, is that we should shift our attention away from cases where someone receives a *particular* treatment, already developed by the past contributions of others, but refuses to take part in a *particular* act of research, and concentrate instead on cases where someone enjoys the benefits that follow from a *system* where she possesses entitlements to future treatment, the value of which relies on others' participation in research, but adopts a policy of never participating in medical research herself. To adopt such a policy is to free-ride on the willingness of others to participate in research. Therefore, to adopt such a policy is to show no regard to the fact that each has an obligation of fairness to be willing to participate in (at least some forms of) medical research. I phrase this as an obligation 'to be willing to' participate in research, rather than an obligation to participate in research because it is, of course, possible that an individual benefited by a system of entitlements to medical care will never be able to participate in research: for example, because no research is being done into any conditions from which she suffers, or the condition from which she suffers is already fully researched, or her health is so poor that she would not be able to take part in research. Furthermore, as I shall explain below, even when we can participate in some kind of research, we do not necessarily act unfairly if we do not take part in that particular piece of research, insofar as so doing may be incompatible with our other obligations.

The argument that we have a fairness-based obligation to be willing to participate in research assumes a situation where each has clearly defined entitlements to future medical care, and that there is a relationship between current research projects carried out in our society and the value of these entitlements. If, for example, it were the case that all research which benefits individuals were carried out elsewhere – and would continue to be carried out whatever the benefited individuals did – it would not, I suppose, be the case that those benefited have a fairness-based obligation to be willing to participate in research, because their policy of refusing to participate in research would have no effect on the benefits they enjoy. Furthermore, my arguments do not establish a fairness-based obligation on individuals to be willing to participate in medical research which would help distant others with whom they do not share a common system of medical treatment. These are important caveats, and there are interesting questions of whether we have obligations other than those of fairness to be willing to participate in medical research, and how these are relevant to the pursuit of research in the global arena (Pogge 2006; Macklin 2004). However, I shall not discuss these issues further in this chapter.

To claim that we have a fairness-based obligation to be willing to participate in research, two conditions must be met: first, that there is some important link between research projects in which we could participate and a system of medical treatment which benefits us; second, that this research is carried out with the aid of contributions from others who can also expect to benefit from the system of health care from which we benefit. Both of these conditions are often met, I suggest, in a country such as the UK. Most of us are in a situation where we benefit from the existence of a system of health care, and much of the research which determines the value of our entitlement relationships to future medical care is carried out in our community with the participation of other members of our polity.[14] It is thus reasonable to suggest that most citizens of the UK have a fairness-based obligation to be willing to participate in medical research, because of the structure of systems of research and treatment within the UK. Of course, it will not be the case that each citizen of the UK has an unconditional fairness-based obligation to be willing to participate in *all* forms of medical research, because some kinds of research cannot be expected to have any beneficial impact on the services offered by the NHS.[15] Furthermore, it is presumably the case that we cannot have a fairness-based obligation to participate in research which would expose us to levels of risk far higher than the benefits of reduced risk we enjoy through the existence of the NHS.

Although limited in scope, these arguments provide us with a way in which to understand the intuition that those who refuse to participate in research are, somehow, free-riding on the contributions of others. I have argued that we can best

---

[14] Indeed, much of the research could only be carried out in our society, as the research is often specifically geared to improvements of current local practice.

[15] It is important to stress here that the condition that research should improve NHS services does not necessarily imply that we have no obligation to participate in research which is privately funded or which physicians are paid by private companies to pursue. What matters is the expected effect of the research, and not the intentions of those who carry out the research. Of course, having noted this philosophical point, it is important also to stress that the greater the possible conflicts of interest involved in a research project, the more careful we ought to be about claims that the research will benefit those who enjoy the benefits of the NHS.

understand our intuitions if we realize that someone who benefits from living in the kind of environment where she enjoys entitlements to medical care, but who adopts a position of refusing to participate in any kind of medical research, is acting in such a way that, were others to adopt the same policy, she would not continue to enjoy the benefits she currently enjoys.

7.3 Fairness and the role of informed consent

What are the implications for research ethics of the claim that those of us who enjoy lower levels of risk than we would otherwise, because of our possession of entitlements to future medical care, have an obligation of fairness to be willing to participate in (at least some forms of) medical research? To answer this question, I shall assume that, if only for practical reasons, most trials require that patients have consented to their participation in the trial. Imagine that we ask Jane, who benefits from her possession of entitlements to medical care, to participate in a medical trial and she refuses to take part. It does not follow from the claim that Jane has an obligation to be willing to participate in research that she does anything wrong if she refuses to take part in a particular piece of research. Jane's refusal to participate in a particular act of research might involve her breaching her fairness-based obligations, but it also might not. If, for example, Jane refuses to take part in research on the grounds that she does not wish to help others, then, clearly, she acts unfairly if she continues to enjoy the benefits of entitlement relationships underpinned by others' participation in research. If, however, Jane cannot reasonably take part in this particular research project, since doing so would lead her to lose her job, but she would be willing to participate in an alternative project, then her refusal to participate in research is not necessarily unfair.

We can sum up these claims by saying that an obligation to participate in research generates only an 'imperfect obligation' because there are often multiple ways in which we could participate.[16] One feature of imperfect obligations is that they are not normally thought to be legally enforceable, because there is no way in which to settle in advance when a particular failure to perform a particular act counts as a breach of our more general obligation.[17] Does this mean that my argument that each has a fairness-based obligation to be willing to participate in research is irrelevant to policy-making? I suggest not. Rather, the argument challenges the normal understanding of how we ought to act when someone refuses to agree to participate in research.

Let us imagine a research trial which we have reason to believe will benefit many members of the population. We ask various individuals to participate in the trial, but give them the option to refuse to participate in research; some of the people we

---

[16] See O'Neill (1996) and Rainbolt (2000) for discussion of imperfect obligations. Harris is aware that a similar point applies to his conclusions (Harris 2005, 243).

[17] Of course, the distinction between perfect and imperfect obligations will not always necessarily map completely on to the distinction between (legitimately) legally enforceable and non-legally enforceable obligations. However, these complexities are not relevant to the main argument of this chapter.

contact refuse to take part in the trial. According to the standard model of the relationship between informed consent and ethically permissible research, we ought to treat this refusal to participate in research as 'final', in the sense that we do not require any further explanation of why the individual refuses to participate, and we do not impose any kind of sanction on her for not taking part. If her choice is based on relevant information – it is informed – then it ought to be treated as final, because it reflects her autonomous decision.

However, given the arguments of section 7.2, there is an obvious problem with this way of understanding the relationship between consent and ethically permissible research. In effect, it seems to condone individuals' acting contrary to their imperfect obligations to participate in research, by treating a policy of refusing to participate in research as permissible. Indeed, we could even say that a system where we treat the subject's 'no' as 'final' might encourage people to act contrary to their obligations of fairness: the system allows people to reap the benefits of a system of research and treatment without ever paying one of the costs necessary for maintenance of that system. Taking individuals' failure to consent to research as 'final' creates a system where fairness-based reasons for individuals to participate in research are given no weight whatsoever. This, I suggest, is a serious problem. After all, even if we think that it would be wrong (or perhaps merely imprudent) to coerce someone to meet her imperfect obligations of fairness – in this sense, refusal *is* 'final' – it would seem strange to think that a social system ought to allow, or even create incentives for, free-riding.

Therefore, I suggest an alternative way in which we might structure the pursuit of medical research, and, perhaps, its relationship to treatment. I suggest that when someone is unwilling to participate in a medical trial (for which they might be a suitable research subject), rather than taking their refusal as 'final', we ought instead to try to find alternative research trials in which they would be willing to participate. An advantage of this kind of system is that it would allow us to distinguish cases where individuals are willing to fulfil their imperfect obligations of fairness but feel unable to do so in particular circumstances, from cases of genuine 'free-riding', where individuals are willing to enjoy the benefits of a system of medical care, but are unwilling to make the contributions necessary to sustain that system.

Of course, although it captures the fact that we have an imperfect obligation to participate in research and, therefore, that participation cannot be mandatory, the claim that we ought to ask those who refuse to consent in some particular piece of research whether they would be willing to participate in alternative research may seem impractical. After all, it is rarely the case that any particular researcher will have knowledge about which current research projects exist for which the individual is suitable. Therefore, for the suggestion above to be implemented would require the construction of systems which allow for ways of tracking who has participated in research, their answer, and the availability of alternative research projects. I do not pretend that it would be easy or straightforward to construct such a system.

However, it is important to stress that my primary aim in this chapter is not to outline a completely different way in which we might structure the pursuit of research here and now. Rather, it is to suggest that there is some kind of default ethical requirement on citizens of a society such as the UK to participate in research, and to suggest some ways in which this kind of default requirement *might* be practicable. One way in which to understand these arguments would be by appeal to the example of jury service.[18] The current legal system in the UK assumes that citizens have a default obligation to participate in jury service, and that individuals who refuse to serve on a jury must offer some good reason for their refusal. Of course, there are significant disanalogies between jury service and participation in medical research. However, my key claim is that just as we would not allow people to refuse to serve on a jury without providing us with any good reason for their refusal, so, too, we should not allow people to refuse to participate in research without offering some kind of justification for their actions.

What, though, should we do in the case where someone is unwilling to contribute to medical research in any manner? It seems reasonable to suggest that we ought to censure those who refuse to participate in any research at all. To think that a concern with promoting patients' autonomy – often assumed to be a key value in research ethics – implies that physicians ought not to censure their patients is to confuse respect for autonomy with respect for selfishness. Censure is, of course, an extremely powerful instrument by which we can encourage people to live up to their fairness-based obligations.[19] However, I also suggest that it might be legitimate to go further. If someone consistently refuses to participate in research, then it would not be unreasonable to place limitations on her entitlements to medical care. For example, we might decide that those who consistently refuse to participate in medical research ought not to have access to various kinds of new drugs, or ought to be regarded as less of a priority than those who do participate in research.

One function of these medical care sanctions would be to incentivize participation in research. However, they also serve to express a reasonable attitude towards free-riders: that, where possible, they ought to be made to bear the costs of their selfishness. Furthermore, allowing for such sanctions might prevent one response to the argument that each has a fairness-based obligation to be willing to participate in research, the response that 'I did not ask for these benefits (of a system of medical care and research), so I should not pay for them'. If this is genuinely a principled response to our censure of someone who seems to free-ride on the willingness of others to participate in research, then, I suggest, the medical care sanctions allow for a partial 'opt-out' from the integrated system of research and treatment. If someone really feels that she should not be expected to participate in research, then she is welcome not to do so, as long as she is willing to bear the costs of her actions.[20]

----

[18] Several people, including Charlotte Goodburn, John McMillan, and Onora O'Neill, have suggested this parallel to me in discussion.

[19] I am assuming here, of course, that the physician has made a determined effort to check whether the refusal is pure selfishness. For a useful analysis of the relationship between shame, censure, and breach of imperfect obligation see Sinnott-Armstrong (2005).

[20] Of course, there might be problems with the implementation of this proposal in practice. These problems raise a slightly different issue: should we create complex and costly systems to allow for the selfish to opt out of social services? I am not certain we should, but this is a difficult question.

At this point, it is important to stress the nature of the arguments above. The claim that we ought to remove incentives to free-riding or opportunities to act selfishly is not intended as a response to a perceived problem that 'not enough' people contribute in research.[21] Rather, the claim of this essay is that there is something *morally* problematic with a system for recruiting research volunteers which systematically allows individuals to benefit from the existence of a system of research while consistently refusing to act in accordance with their obligations of fairness, thus creating incentives not to act fairly towards others. It is this 'moral loophole' which, I claim, ought to be closed. My suggestion, then, is not that we ought to institute my proposed alternative scheme because to do so would lead to *more* research being pursued, but that we ought to institute my scheme because this would create a system which better reflects considerations of fairness. Of course, we might decide that if the system is not (in a consequentialist sense) 'broken', then we might reasonably ignore considerations of fairness, perhaps on pragmatic grounds. However, this is a substantive claim about how we ought to balance considerations of fairness and considerations about outcomes in the context of policy-making. Perhaps, then, there might be reasons not to adopt the scheme above, but at the very least, I hope to have clarified what form these responses ought to take.

Having clarified the nature of my arguments, I should also stress that they are limited in scope. I have suggested some sanctions we might impose on those who refuse to participate in research, but these sanctions are far weaker than they might have been. The reasons for this are three-fold. First, a functioning medical system requires contributions other than participation in research, such as financial contributions raised through general taxation, and even those who free-ride on research have usually made this kind of contribution. Therefore, it would be unreasonably harsh to refuse these individuals *any* access to medical resources. It should, however, be stressed that financial contributions should not be thought of as potentially serving to replace contributions as a research subject. Successful research requires both experimentation on subjects and monetary inputs: the one cannot replace the other, and, as such, it is difficult to see how we might calculate 'how much' money is necessary to replace research participation.

Second, refusing some individuals any kind of treatment whatsoever may ultimately generate further social costs for society as a whole. Even though refusing a bird-flu vaccine to someone who has consistently refused to participate in past research might be morally legitimate, it would be likely to have serious costs for other members of society. We might aim to push the costs of the selfish individual's choices on to the individual, but unintentionally push the costs on to innocent others.

Third, and most importantly, it is clear that, important as considerations of fairness are, we often think that even the most indigent ought to enjoy access to health care as a matter of solidarity or of charity. Therefore, even if considerations of fairness actually

---

21 Indeed, it is unclear how we might even decide whether 'enough' people are already agreeing to participate in research given that researchers' choices to pursue various avenues of research are (presumably) partly circumscribed by knowledge of current research ethics protocol.

imply that it might be reasonable to impose very high sanctions on those who refuse to participate in research, I suggest that we may have countervailing reasons to limit the sanctions which we place on those who 'free-ride' on the contributions of others. We might think that it is a mark of a decent society that it allows physicians to act in accordance with the principle of unconditional treatment for those in medical need, according to the 'rescue principle'.[22] However, even if simply denying the selfish *all* access to health care would be contrary to important social values, it does not follow that it would be illegitimate to deny them access to at least some services.[23]

In this section, I have argued for a new account of how we ought to structure medical research and treatment if we think that each has an imperfect fairness-based obligation to participate in (at least some forms of) medical research. As I have shown, there is no easy way in which to argue from the claim that each has a fairness-based obligation to participate in research to the claim that it would be legitimate to enforce participation in research. However, if we think that each does have a fairness-based obligation to participate in medical research, then any refusal to participate in a *particular* piece of research ought to be accompanied by a willingness to participate in some other form of research. Furthermore, it might be legitimate to impose sanctions on individuals who continually refuse to participate in any form of research and cannot offer socially valid reasons for their refusal. These sanctions can range from censure to loss of entitlements to certain kinds of future medical treatments. Underlying these arguments is the thought that if we treat individuals' consent or refusal to participate in research as all that is necessary to make research permissible or impermissible, we risk condoning, or even creating incentives for, acts of selfish free-riding.

7.4 Autonomy and consent

How do these arguments relate to standard justifications for informed consent requirements? To discuss these issues, it is useful to distinguish two broad ways in which we might argue for the necessity of informed consent requirements for ethically permissible research: as reflecting the centrality of 'autonomy' to medical ethics; and as reflecting patients' 'rights' (Beauchamp *et al.* 1986). In this section, I shall focus on the relationship between the arguments above and the 'autonomy' justification for informed consent requirements.

The autonomy justification for informed consent requirements rests on the claim that we ought to promote individuals' 'autonomy', where this is understood in terms of something like our ability to choose to perform actions which are in accordance

---

[22] This tension is not unique to the model I have suggested: see Anderson (1999, 295-6) for discussion of a related problem for 'luck egalitarian' theories of justice.

[23] We might model this tension between demands of fairness and of decency by thinking about National Insurance contributions: we do not think that those who have completely failed to pay any National Insurance contributions ought to bear the costs of their failure completely. Rather, we do provide them with a minimal pension, such that they bear some, but not all, of the costs associated with their decisions.

with our concept of the good life (Faden *et al.* 1986; Beauchamp and Childress, 1994). Proponents of autonomy claim that our ability to make reasoned choices in accordance with our conceptions of the good life is particularly at threat in contexts of medical research and treatment. Mechanisms of informed consent are viewed as tools which respond to this (perceived) problem, by ensuring that we have the full information and the power to make certain sorts of choices, and will not be forced by others to do as they think we ought to do.

The claim that we ought to protect and to promote autonomy can seem self-evident, and it is thus easy to agree with the autonomy justification of strong informed consent requirements on medical research. However, the arguments above suggest that, even if we think consent is important for various reasons, we should be careful of modelling our account of its role in medical research solely on the basis of the claim that autonomy is valuable. In the case of medical research, it might be that policies which we justify in terms of their promotion of the good of autonomy actually serve to create a system where failure to respect our obligations of fairness is 'cost-free'. Normally, we threaten those who would free-ride with various sanctions (we fine the ticketless traveller on the bus). In the case of medical research, we do not. In some ways, then, we create incentives to free-ride: acting fairly has costs – participation in research – which free-riding does not. In effect, we can say that – from an ethical point of view – there is a potential clash between promoting one good (individual autonomy) and promoting a second good (individuals acting in accordance with their obligations of fairness).

When we encounter this clash of values, we can, I think, respond in one of two ways. The first option would be to say that there is no clash, by denying that autonomy (as normally conceived) really is valuable, or by arguing that we do not have an obligation to participate in research (or, perhaps, that this obligation is not relevant to social policy). Alternatively, we might recognize that there is a clash of values, but suggest that this clash can be resolved by constructing a system which balances the good of promoting or preserving autonomy with the good of encouraging people to respect their obligations of fairness.

Evidently, I do not think that we can respond to these problems by denying that individuals have a fairness-based obligation to participate in research, or by saying that this obligation is not a proper concern of social policy. It is, I hope, clear from the arguments above that we do have an obligation to be willing to participate in research. Also, although it is difficult to reflect claims about imperfect obligations in the context of social policy, it is a mistake to think that we can never encourage people to discharge their imperfect obligations. If, for example, we think that charitable giving is an imperfect obligation, it seems reasonable to suggest that those who give money to charity ought to enjoy some 'tax-breaks'. Therefore, I suggest the more reasonable responses to the problem identified above would be either to deny that autonomy (as normally conceived in research ethics) really is valuable or to find some way in which to balance the values of 'autonomy' and 'respect for imperfect obligations'.

Personally, I suspect that many of the kinds of concerns which usually motivate the claim that we ought to respect individuals' autonomy within research ethics – worries, for example, over the conflict between participating in some forms of research and religious observances – might be captured by the kind of scheme outlined above, where we insist that people give some kind of reason for refusal to participate in research. Therefore, I think that we can do without the value of autonomy, at least insofar as its recognition in institutional practices seems to condone selfish behaviour.

However, even if this is too strong a claim, and it seems more plausible to suggest that we ought to balance considerations of 'autonomy' and 'fairness' in the regulation of research, the arguments of this section imply that we should not understand the ethics of medical research solely in terms of the protection and promotion of individual autonomy. Even if we think that 'autonomy' is valuable, such that sometimes it would be wrong simply to impose risks on people without their consent, it seems implausible to claim that there is some free-floating value of autonomy such that we ought *always* to treat individuals' refusal to participate in research as 'final'.[24] Rather, unless we are to conflate respect for autonomy with some more general principle that selfishness is not morally reprehensible, it seems legitimate to claim that consent requirements should be structured in the way outlined above.

7.5 Research, risk, and consent

In this section, I shall clarify the relationship between my arguments and a second way in which we might conceptualize the relationship between research and consent: in terms of individuals' rights. A standard claim in research ethics is that we must seek patients' informed consent to their participation in research because not to do so would constitute a violation of their rights. According to this view, subjects' informed consent to their participation in research is necessary for that research to be ethically permissible because the consent serves to waive one (or various) of their rights. In this section, I shall clarify the relationship between rights, consent, and waiver in the context of medical research, and show how these arguments relate to the conclusions of sections 7.2 and 7.3.

Medical research usually takes place against a backdrop of rights and obligations. We can often best make sense of the claim that we ought to seek subjects' informed consent to their participation in research by reference to features of these general rights and obligations, regardless of questions of autonomy. For example, if research involves cutting someone open with a scalpel, then we might explain the need to gain the subject's consent to her participation in this research by appeal to her more general right to bodily integrity. Further kinds of rights and obligations might also be relevant to understanding the ethical weight we place on consent in research contexts. We often think that physicians have particular, well-defined professional obligations towards their patients, and that, in virtue of this fact, patients have some special claim-right with regard to their physician. If so, then we might understand consent procedures in some contexts in terms of patients waiving their special rights. For example, we might think that physicians have professional obligations to minimize the risks of physical harm that their patients face, and enrolling patients in research

---

[24] For similar worries, see Callahan (1996), Holm (2001), and O'Neill (2001).

trials would involve a breach of these obligations. In these circumstances, then, the patient's consent to enrolment in the research trial can be understood as relieving the physician of her normal professional obligations, and as a waiver of a particular kind of special right patients enjoy *vis-à-vis* their physicians (Manson *et al.* 2007).[25]

These kinds of everyday concerns explain the sense that consent is often necessary for research to be ethically permissible. How, though, do they relate to the conclusions of section 7.3 above? It is clear that there is no necessary conflict between the claim that consent procedures are often necessary to ensure that patients' rights are not violated and the claim that we might legitimately encourage people to participate in research. Again, a comparison with charitable giving is useful here: it would be wrong for a representative of Oxfam to steal your money, but this does not mean that it would be wrong for the state to encourage you to give money to charity.

Of course, there might be a clash between the rights-based account of the role of informed consent requirements in medical research and the conclusions of section 7.3 above, if we could show that the kind of system proposed above would leave people with no real option but to participate in research. If this were the case, then individuals' 'apparent' consent to participation in research would, in Norman Daniels' useful phrase, be quasi-coerced and, thus, not genuine (Daniels 1985). However, although the system suggested in section 7.3 above would make a policy of refusing to participate in research costly, it would seem excessive to say that the proposed system would, in effect, leave individuals with no reasonable choice but to participate in research. Being placed at the bottom of a waiting list for future treatments is a high price to pay. However, I suggest that imposing this cost on those who consistently refuse to participate in research would not be tantamount to *coercing* those individuals to participate in research: it is not as if a reasonable agent might feel she had no reasonable option but to pay this cost. Therefore, I suggest that even if we adopt an account of informed consent which stresses the importance of consent procedures in terms of rights-waivers (rather than merely as expressing some kind of pragmatic requirement), this would not pose problems for the system outlined in section 7.3. There might be good arguments that it would be coercive to threaten individuals with loss of *all* entitlements to medical care if they refuse to participate in research (although even this claim would require defence). However, the recommendations of section 7.3 were far weaker, and, therefore, avoid worries over coercion and rights.

A final point about rights and obligations is also necessary here. Recent work on informed consent, associated with the work of Onora O'Neill, has shifted attention away from understanding consent primarily in terms of subjects' 'autonomy' or 'rights' to a focus on researchers' obligations (O'Neill 2002; Manson and O'neill, 2007). I should stress here that just as my arguments are not, I claim, in tension with the thought that consent procedures are often necessary for purposes of rights-waiver, neither are they incompatible with the thought that consent procedures often

---

[25] note that, following Brownsword (2004) I am assuming here that there is no general 'right not to participate in medical research'. Rather, I assume that different rights will be relevant to understanding the demand for informed consent in different research contexts.

function to ensure that physicians live up to their obligations not to harm or not to deceive others. To say that individuals have an obligation to participate in (at least some forms of) research is clearly not to say that physicians have no obligations towards their patients, or to deny that consent procedures can play an important role in ensuring that physicians fulfil these obligations.

Although my claims are certainly compatible with understandings of consent framed in terms of the obligations of physicians, it is important here to note a topic I have not discussed in this paper: the nature and extent of researchers' obligations of fairness towards patients. In many instances of research, we might feel that researchers are not acting fairly towards research subjects. For example, when researchers are well-remunerated for their work, but research subjects are not we might worry that the researcher is breaching some kind of implicit norm of fairness. Far more generally, and more complex again, we might feel that it is somehow problematic to demand of individuals that they participate in research where choice of research goals or the probable distribution of resultant treatments seems skewed towards certain sectors of the population and, thus, 'unfair'. These topics are complex, however, because there is no reason to suppose that merely because researchers are paid to act as researchers, they must be exploiting (comparatively badly-remunerated) research subjects.

There is, then, a serious danger that we might stress the fairness-based obligations of research subjects while overlooking the fairness-based obligations of researchers or those who fund research. Given the kinds of epistemic and power asymmetries between researchers and subjects which already exist, this may seem particularly problematic. Therefore, it is clear that a fuller account of the role of fairness in research would need to take account not only of research subjects' obligations, but to the obligations of those who fund and pursue research and distribute its benefits. However, this does not blunt the arguments of this paper, but points towards the need for further research which takes seriously the complexity of the obligations which structure the pursuit of research within a system such as the NHS.

7.6 **Conclusion**

The proposal that we might encourage individuals to participate in research and even sanction those who refuse to do so poses a challenge to accounts of consent which would treat research subjects' 'no' as final. However, in most writing on consent, the obligations of patients are absent. As I have just indicated, there may be good reasons for these silences. However, I hope to have shown that current trends in clinical ethics tend systematically to overlook the fact that research subjects are not helpless guinea pigs who must be protected from scientific researchers. Rather, those who are asked to participate in medical research have often benefited – and more importantly, can expect to continue to benefit – from medical research. As such, they have obligations of fairness to contribute to such research. Of course, these obligations are complex, and it would be a serious mistake to think that we can force people to participate in research. However, it would also be a mistake to allow simplistic views of autonomy or rights to create systems which fail to impose any kind of sanction on those who refuse to act fairly towards others. None of this is to deny that gaining individuals' informed consent may be a vital element of research procedures, but it is to suggest that we must be very careful not to overlook the possibility that *encouraging* participation in research may be necessary if we are to create a society where individuals can be said to live up to their moral obligations of fairness.

References

Anderson, E. (1999). What is the point of equality? *Ethics* **109**, no. 2, 287–337.

Beauchamp, T. and Childress, J. (1994). *Principles of Biomedical Ethics* (4th edition). Oxford: Oxford University Press.

Brownsword, R. (2004). The cult of consent: fixation and fallacy. *King's College Law Journal*, **15**, no. 2, 223–53.

Buchanan, D. and Miller, F. (2006). A public health perspective on research ethics. *Journal of Medical Ethics*, **32**, 729–33.

Callahan, D. (1996). Can the moral commons survive autonomy? *Hastings Center Report*, **26**, no. 6, 41–2.

Cullity, G. (1995). Moral free riding. *Philosophy and Public Affairs*, **24**, no. 1, 3–34.

Daniels, N. (1985). *Just Healthcare*. Cambridge: Cambridge University Press.

Evans, H. (2004). Should patients be allowed to veto their participation in clinical research? *Journal of Medical Ethics*, **30**, 198–203.

Faden, R. and Beauchamp, T. (1986). *A History and Theory of Informed Consent*. Oxford: Oxford University Press.

Harris, J. (2005). Scientific research is a moral duty. *Journal of Medical Ethics*, **31**, 242–8.

Hart, H. (1955). Are there any natural rights? *Philosophical Review*, **64**, 175–91.

Holm, S. (2001). Not just autonomy: the principles of American biomedical ethics. In Bioethics, edited by J. Harris. Oxford: Oxford University Press.

Klosko, G. (1987). Presumptive benefit, fairness, and political obligation. *Philosophy and Public Affairs*, **16**, no. 3, 241–59.

Laurie, G. (2002). *Genetic Privacy*. Cambridge: Cambridge University Press.

Macklin, R. (2004). *Double Standards in Medical Research in Developing Countries*. Cambridge: Cambridge University Press.

Manson, N. and O'Neill, O. (2007). *Rethinking Informed Consent*. Cambridge: Cambridge University Press.

Newdick, C. (2005). *Who Should We Treat? Rights, Rationing and Resources in the NHS* (2nd edition). Oxford: Oxford University Press.

O'Neill, O. (1985). Between consenting adults. *Philosophy and Public Affairs*, **14**, no. 3, 252–77.

–ibid.– (1996). *Towards Justice and Virtue*. Cambridge: Cambridge University Press.

–ibid.– (2002). *Autonomy and Trust in Bioethics*. Cambridge: Cambridge University Press.

Pogge, T. (2004). Relational conceptions of justice in Sen, A, Peter, F and Anand, A. Public health ethics and equity, Oxford: Oxford University Press.

Pogge, T. (2006). Human rights and global health: a research program'. In *Global Institutions and Responsibilities*, edited by T. Pogge and C. Barry. London: Blackwell.

Rainbolt, G. (2000). Perfect and imperfect obligations, *Philosophical Studies*, **98**, no. 3, 233–56.

Sinnott-Armstrong, W. (2005). You ought to be ashamed of yourself (when you violate an imperfect moral obligation). *Philosophical Issues*, **15**, no. 1, 193–208.

Weijer, C. (2002). I need a placebo like I need a hole in the head. *Journal of Law, Medicine and Ethics*, **30**, 69–72.

Weijer, C. and Miller, P. (2004). When are research risks reasonable in relation to anticipated benefits? *Nature Medicine*, **10**, 570–3.

Wolff, J. and de Shalit, A. (2007). *Disadvantage*. Oxford: Oxford University Press.

Chapter 8

Consenting older adults: research as a virtuous relationship

Julian C. Hughes, Erica Haimes, Lorraine Summerville, Karen Davies, Joanna Collerton, and Thomas B.L. Kirkwood[1]

8.1 Introduction

In 1785, Immanuel Kant wrote:

> Act in such a way that you treat humanity, whether in your own person or in the person of another, always at the same time as an end and never simply as a means.

> (Kant 1785, 429)

Kant's principle expresses a worthy sentiment and reflects the great emphasis he placed on the autonomy of the will. In turn, this supports the principle in medical ethics of respect for autonomy, which is central to the notion of informed consent. According to Beauchamp and Childress (2001), informed consent represents 'an individual's *autonomous authorization* of a medical intervention or of participation in research' (p. 78).

Research with older people raises particular issues with respect to consent (Barron *et al.* 2004). At the level of theory in medical ethics, the issues emerge because of the increasingly perceived tension between the notions of autonomy and dependency (Agich 2003). At a practical level, the tension is worked out in the context of a relationship: between the researcher and the participant. In this chapter, we shall reflect on the nature of this relationship involving older people. The notion of 'research as relationship', which is immediately sociological, raises a number of

[1] Our reflections stem from our backgrounds in general practice, gerontology, nursing, old age psychiatry, philosophy and sociology but our reflections here are informed by our involvement in specific research projects. The NEWCASTLE 85+ Study (involving K.D., J.C., T.K.), funded by the Dunhill Medical Trust, Unilever, Newcastle Primary Care Trust, and the British Heart Foundation in the pilot phase and the MRC/BBSRC in the main study, seeks to explore the biological, clinical and psychosocial factors associated with healthy ageing. The Genetics of Healthy Ageing study (involving all of the authors) is a pan-European study, funded by the European Union FP6, which aims to determine the genetic factors that contribute to healthy ageing.

clinical and ethical issues, and brings into play a much broader context than the one normally suggested by the basic paradigm, with which our chapter begins. However, the basic paradigm is also challenged by the reality of values diversity. Values are what we prize or regard as important in life. A diversity of values, therefore, will be more problematic when what is valued is highly prized, when it is something we cannot give up. Values-based medicine provides a theory and practical way for values to be negotiated in a careful manner in clinical and research settings.

Whilst our focus is on the notion of research with older people as relationship, this in turn focuses attention, through an appreciation of the textured nature of the sociology of context, on those aspects of practice that ought to help to make research in general more ethical. This comes about when values and the possibility of diverse and conflicting values (which themselves reflect and interact with differences in social status, power, authority, class, resources, knowledge, and the like) are faced square on. What will emerge as ethically crucial will be the idea of the virtues. That is to say, a good relationship must be rooted in a variety of virtues: honesty, compassion, faithfulness, generosity, charity, practical wisdom, and so on. Our discussion will suggest practical implications for research ethics, as well as issues for the underlying moral, philosophical, and sociological theories. Our conclusion is that, beyond valid consent and the legalism of the basic paradigm, consent ought to be regarded as an interactive process of communication grounded in relationship.

8.2 **The basic paradigm of consent**

According to the *Code of Practice* of the Mental Health Act (1983), consent to treatment is defined as:

> … the voluntary and continuing permission of the patient to receive a particular treatment, based on an adequate knowledge of the purpose, nature, likely effects and risks … including the likelihood of its success and any alternatives to it. Permission given under any unfair or undue pressure is not 'consent'.

> (Department of Health and Welsh Office 1999, 67, paragraph 15.13)

In short, the patient must be informed, competent, and non-coerced. Consent must also be continuing. We take this to be the basic paradigm, which reflects the principle of autonomy. However, this legalistic notion of valid consent can be contrasted with the idea that consent involves understanding within the context of a relationship. Crudely, the contrast is between a 'positivistic' notion of consent, where a checklist will do, and the 'social construction' of consent, where consent arises through cultural and social interaction between people.[2] In one sense both stances are true: consent *is* a legal notion, where particular criteria are required, and it also reflects an agreement between people based on interpersonal exchange. But how is it possible for

---

[2] Neither of these phrases (i.e., positivist or social constructionist) is being used in their full sociological sense, but as useful devices through which to draw a practical contrast.

both stances to be true? The answer must be that neither position is quite what it seems at first.

Referring to consent as a positivist or legalistic notion makes it sound as if it is clear-cut. The law specifies clear speed limits for driving. The positivism of scientific statements is similarly clear: the hypothesis that the velocity of sound increases with temperature is susceptible to a scientific test. When we turn to the criteria of the basic paradigm of consent, however, each criterion is corrigible. The extent to which some-one is informed, competent, and non-coerced will always involve judgements that can be both nuanced and (partly for this reason) problematic (Hughes 2000). For instance, the increasing emphasis placed on the need for explicit and specific consent may simply set the standards for consent excessively high (Manson and O'Neill 2007).

Hence, it cannot be said that the criteria for valid consent are clear-cut: albeit they are well established in law, they require judgements in their application and these judgements are essentially evaluative. This does not imply that the law on consent is wholly vague. The law on battery, which underpins the need for consent, is clear enough: to do something to someone's body without his or her consent is an assault. There are also laws to do with negligence that specify that the patient must be informed 'in broad terms', but here the need for evaluative judgements emerges again. So the legalistic, positivistic characterization of consent is misleading inasmuch as it implies that a set of rules can simply be applied, even if consent *is* a matter of law.

Meanwhile, whilst the idea that consent is socially constructed is a useful corrective to the more positivistic notion of consent, social constructionism raises other prob-lems if pushed too far. For instance, the idea that researcher and research participant might co-construct consent has some validity at an heuristic level; and there is no doubt that social exchange is vital to consent. But 'constructed' consent cannot occur in isolation from the normative criteria that constitute it. Social constructionists might argue that the normative criteria are themselves the product of social construc-tion. At some point, however, the grounds for the possibility of social exchange, which must be normative, will need to be adduced. Thornton (2006) has argued, albeit social constructionism has a useful heuristic role, there are doubts that it is coherent to speak of meaning itself being constructed by the social process of discourse. (However, see Velody and Williams (1998) for an elegant exploration of this position.)

Thus, the legalistic notion of consent is subject to evaluative judgements and the social construction of consent in any particular, individual context is bounded by normative criteria. Why, though, is such a seemingly straightforward matter – that of one person consenting to something suggested by another – so complicated? Why is the basic paradigm so prone to complexity? The answers to these questions can be found by an application of the theory of values-based medicine (VBM) to the criteria for valid consent. How to deal with the complexity is then suggested by the principles that inform the practice of VBM.

8.3 Values-based medicine and consent in older people

VBM is the complement to evidence-based medicine (EBM) and it relates to the values that impinge on medical practice in the same ways that EBM is concerned with the pertinent facts. The issue of consent is one in which values readily emerge. Fulford (1989) has shown how the fact-centred 'medical' model has to be transformed into the more balanced, broader view, of the fact + value model. In this section we shall apply the principles that make up the theory of VBM (Fulford 2004) to the criteria for valid consent in the context of research involving older people.

1. *The 'two-feet' principle* simply states that medical practice usually involves both facts and values. Valid consent is also called informed consent. How much information a person requires is a matter of judgement. This will normally involve some sort of weighing up of the person's intellectual and emotional needs, against a background of legal and ethical norms. In the case of research with older people, an immediate issue is that older people are not a homogeneous group. Judgements ought to be made in response to the individual. There will be some older people who might be keen to have a large amount of information because of intellectual curiosity; others may be easily overburdened or simply disinterested. Some older people will feel the pressure of time, others will not; some will be too frail, either mentally or physically, to be bothered with large amounts of information. Some older people will be vulnerable and this vulnerability will extend to the possibility that, whilst the person is happy enough to participate in the research, information could be provided in a way that might be insensitive.

Similarly, a person's capacity can be assessed both sensitively and insensitively. There should be a presumption that the person has capacity. But just as the criteria for consent are value-laden, so too are the criteria for judgements about capacity or competence. In the law governing England and Wales, a person has to be able to understand, retain, and communicate the material information in order to have capacity. In addition, he or she must be able to use or weigh up the information (The Stationery Office 2005). However, the weighing up of the weighing up is clearly a judgement of value, as well as a matter of fact.

It might be thought that at least the last criterion for valid consent, namely that the person's decision should be non-coerced, is one that does not involve values. However, we do allow that people can be *cajoled*: relatives can cajole the person with mild dementia into attendance at the day centre. Might it also be reasonable for a researcher to cajole a slightly reluctant potential participant into a research project? It may indeed be that the person would benefit from the research (perhaps it would lead to closer follow-up, or more socialization), so that a little cajoling or persistence might seem ethically justified. Yet there will be a line beyond which lies coercion. Some factual things can be stated: the person must not be physically forced to participate. But a more mundane situation is that a judgement of value needs to be made concerning when further cajoling might become coercion.

Values diversity is encouraged by the reality of differing attitudes, many of them uncomplimentary, towards older people. This is seen, for instance, in the tendency for older people not to be recruited for certain types of research. Barriers to recruitment encourage the perception, perhaps, that specific treatments are not appropriate to older people (Townsley *et al.* 2005). Researchers might take a paternalistic attitude towards potential participants who are older, whether they be patients or non-patients, which might lead to an over- or under-estimation of the person's ability to handle (or their requirement for) information. They might presume incompetence; or feel they are more or less justified in cajoling the person to participate.

Thus, researchers might put up barriers to older people participating in research; so too can families. This instinct to protect is itself 'paternalistic'. It may mean that the researcher is denied all contact with the potential participant. It is an instinct that reflects deep values of concern; but it inevitably clashes with the values of concern that prompt research.[3]

2. *The 'squeaky wheel' principle* suggests that values become noticed when they are diverse or when they conflict. Take, for example, the possibility of conflicting values between a professor and a more junior researcher. Perhaps the professor is persuaded that scientific knowledge would be importantly advanced by a particular piece of research. This thought may be entirely justifiable. But it could be that the junior researcher sees many of the potential participants as being too old or frail to take part in the project. This may also be true. The junior researcher, therefore, may not be keen to encourage people to participate and might regard fairly modest evidence of cognitive impairment as a sufficient reason to judge that the person lacks the capacity to consent. The end result might then be that recruitment to the study turns out to be sluggish and the research is never properly pursued. Such an outcome, from the moral perspective, may or may not be acceptable.

Things might go in various ways between the junior researcher and the professor. Of course, the roles could easily be reversed. Difference in status is a potent force, as is the need of the junior to pursue research in order to ascend the career ladder. The temptation to cut consent corners may be strong. Agarwal *et al.* (1996) demonstrated that 15 subjects, already enrolled in a drug trial (and, therefore, putatively consented), all failed to meet more rigorous standards of consent. This might have reflected either benign or malign influences. It may be that out in the field things appear differently to how they seem in the research centre. Such differences may or may not reflect different values.

Again, at a more mundane level, the squeaky wheel principle is one that many novice researchers experience. On entering research, particularly from a background of clinical practice, a period of questioning one's purpose and the ethical credibility of a study, which is usually not directed at the good of the individual patient, is not uncommon. These differences in value require explicit recognition through training. For although, like a squeaky wheel, they can be ignored, it is unlikely that they can be ignored indefinitely without either some attention (a drop of oil) or a crisis (the wheel finally jams), which might even show itself in the form of a series of medical scandals to do with consent.

3. *The 'science-driven' principle* recognizes the importance of scientific advance. It is sometimes suggested that such advance, which increases the store of facts, might reduce the need to worry about values. In the case of research with older people there are two points. The first point might be easily allowed: as science drives forward,

---

[3] The need to understand barriers to research, why consent is refused, is discussed further in this volume by Snowdon *et al.* (Chapter Four).

the problems involving values simply multiply. Indeed, ageing research itself raises questions of value. Inasmuch as the aim is to 'square off' the morbidity curve, that is to try to increase the chances that we shall remain fitter for longer and die after only a short illness, there is probably little conflict in terms of values. However, if the aim of ageing research is longevity (without an obvious benefit in terms of decreased morbidity), diverse values readily start to appear (Kirkwood 1999). Similarly, we can now feed people through percutaneous endoscopic gastrostomy (PEG) tubes, but should we? This scientific and technical advance has generated a whole ethics literature of its own (e.g., Gillick 2000). We now have medications that can bring about a modest improvement in the symptoms of dementia, but should they be used (Hughes 2000)? Should stem cells be used to treat Parkinson's disease (Henon 2003)? The number of such questions multiplies as science moves on.

The second point might be regarded as more contentious. Returning to the criteria for valid consent, it might be thought that the process of gaining consent could itself be made more 'scientific'. In particular, it might seem as if the criteria for saying whether or not someone has capacity should be open to operationalized instruments. Increasingly, standard questionnaires are being designed and subjected to scientific tests for their validity and reliability (Fazel 2002). But producing tick-box forms for this or that capacity would seem to downplay the place of values in these judgements. Such forms might allow it to be said, seemingly as a matter of concrete fact, that the person lacks such-and-such a capacity. However, the choice of elements to be tested by the tick boxes itself involves judgements of value; and, in addition, ticking a particular box might also involve a considerable evaluative weighing-up.

To take a specific example, Pucci *et al.* (2001) considered the difficulties of gaining informed consent to pursue research amongst people with Alzheimer's disease and their family caregivers. Both those with Alzheimer's and their family caregivers were assessed for their competency (or capacity) to consent to a clinical drug trial. The researchers found that 70% of the caregivers (who did *not* have dementia) were unable to comprehend basic information about the study. So there is a question about whether carers are able to act as surrogates for patients when it comes to consent. In addition, 70% of the patients with Alzheimer's disease were unable to demonstrate even a minimal understanding of the research procedures. People with a Mini-Mental State Examination (MMSE) score (Folstein *et al.* 1975) of less than 18 were rated as incompetent or marginally incompetent in 95% of cases.

The issues raised by this sort of research are numerous. At one extreme, the issue might be that researchers are simply not well trained enough to gain consent properly. At another extreme, it might be (as the above authors seem to suggest) that the strict application of the criteria for consent in these settings is not feasible, or perhaps not appropriate. In other words, the well-established legal criteria for valid consent are impracticable. Between these two positions, however, values-based practice can gain some purchase. For it may be that the problem is also the solution, namely that evaluative judgements are just an inescapable fact of life when operating in this arena. The solution is to deal with the possibility of diverse and conflicting values in an open way, rather than pretending that the values are not there or can be ignored in favour of a more legalistic, algorithmic process that will (supposedly) deliver valid consent as a fact.

The other point to note in Pucci *et al.* (2001) is the suggestion that the MMSE might in some way be used as a measure of competence or capacity. A score of less than 18 might be regarded as signifying at least a degree of incompetence. This has the air of a scientific statement: tests of competence have been correlated with scores on a well-validated and reliable test of cognitive function. But, rather than eliminating the need for value judgements, it makes them more urgent. As Sabat (2001) has argued, first, failing the MMSE may have nothing to do with the competence that is being judged; secondly, the MMSE mainly tests recall memory and it may be that this is not the most appropriate type of cognitive function to be tested. Thirdly, this seems to suggest that competence (or capacity) is mainly a matter of cognitive function (largely to do with recall), rather than something that can involve an emotional response and a different sort of weighing-up (Charland 1998; Sabat 2005). Finally, the 'scientific' correlation of competence and MMSE ignores the masking effects of group norms: the correlation shows that on average a person scoring below 18 also failed the test of competence, but this does not mean that a particular individual failed. The (in)competence of the individual is covered up by the reliance on a group statistic. This 'scientific' way of establishing competence, therefore, hides and distorts the very values that the law is keen to protect. The law insists on the need to presume capacity, so it would be ironic if in a legal arena a test such as the MMSE were taken to be proof or disproof of competence (Sabat 2005).

So, in a number of ways, scientific advances seem inevitably to raise further examples of diverse and potentially conflicting values; and, in addition, the application of scientific methods to the criteria of consent (and, in particular, capacity) ought not to ignore the inescapable requirement for value judgements to be made.

4. *The 'patient-perspective' principle* implies that the patient should always be heard. When it comes to research, if this principle remains relevant, the potential participants should also have their perspectives recognized. There has been a trend in this direction in recent years. For instance, in England and Wales the Alzheimer's Society – perhaps most notably in the field of research with older people – has a panel of carers and people with dementia who determine which research proposals should be considered for funding. In some places it is increasingly common to have 'user panels' involved in research (Corner 2002). Although the usefulness, the feasibility, and the point of such involvement can be questioned, if we again consider Pucci *et al.* (2001), it is readily apparent that some of our speculations about the significance of the study would be helped if the views of those involved were known. Some years ago, Cotrell and Schulz (1993) made the suggestion that the perspective of people with dementia was not being heard in research. To hear this voice, although perhaps at times difficult, would seem to be a way fully to ensure that the person was used 'as an end and never simply as a means' (Kant 1785, op. cit.).

5. *The 'multi-perspective' principle* continues the theme, but broadens it. The patients' or (in the research setting) the participants' voices must be of central concern. But values diversity means that the possibility of values conflict is real, even though in many regards values will be shared. There may be conflicts between potential participants and research teams in terms of values; or there may be values conflict within teams. Once again, the principles of VBM make it plain that such conflicts

ought to be faced. This principle does not privilege any particular perspective; rather it points towards a process. If there is a conflict, this principle suggests that the right answer will not follow the application of a rule, but will emerge from a process of balanced support for the legitimately held views of others. Hence, most good research will require multi-disciplinary planning. To have the views of lay people or 'users' in some way represented is likely to add to the usefulness of the eventual findings (Haimes and Whong-Barr 2004).

In research with older people, where there is a tendency for a broader range of issues to be pertinent (because there may be physical or mental frailty, social isolation or social pressures, and vulnerability), the broader the base of the research team (and, therefore, the more perspectives represented) the better. This increases the scope for conflicting values, but (providing these are listened to in a supportive and constructive way) is likely to improve methodology and the ethical basis of research. Anecdotal evidence that the multi-disciplinary perspective is useful ought, perhaps, to be supportable by some form of empirical research. But the principle of taking multiple perspectives into account should inform our thoughts about what might or might not constitute a suitable process for gaining consent.

8.3.1 Summary

In this section we have demonstrated how VBM is relevant to valid consent in the context of research with older people. The importance of this goes back to our earlier statement that legal criteria for valid consent require judgements in application and that such judgements are essentially evaluative. That is, consent in practice is a matter of values-based practice; it can never be *just* a matter of fact, even though facts may be crucial. Both the relevant facts *and* values, however, must be understood in the context of relationships, to which we now turn.

8.4 Research as relationship

So the basic paradigm of valid consent is complicated by the ubiquity of values; but the way to handle this is to acknowledge values diversity and the possibility of conflict. The 'multi-perspective' principle suggests the tendency for research to involve teams, partly as a way of dealing with the multifarious values that crop up. Using the language of 'potential participants' helps to emphasize the importance of relationships in connection with research. Not only are there relations between people in the team, but the team (sometimes through a particular researcher) stands in a relationship with the older person participating in the research. In this section we shall consider the notion of research as relationship with respect to work with older people.

The immediate question is whether it actually makes sense to speak of 'research as relationship'. Perhaps the extent to which research is based upon relationship is so small as to be negligible. This raises an important point about different types of research. Some research may involve seemingly little contact between the participant and the researcher. Nevertheless, when we think of consent and the complexity of the consent process, with all of the embedded value judgements that might be required, it becomes reasonable to think of research as relationship, even if the relationship is mediated through a group. In older people, if for instance their social circle is diminished by deaths or their ability to socialize is curtailed by physical infirmity, relationships can become quite significant and are strikingly pertinent to consent. This can be demonstrated by considering an A–G of relationships: Acquaintance, Being with, Contiguity, Dependency, Exchange, Fruitfulness, and Gift.[4]

To gain consent, the researcher and the potential participant must form an *acquaintance*. This requires them to occupy the same space for at least a modicum of time and the very fact of this co-presence establishes the consent process as a social and, therefore, a moral relationship. This acquaintance might be either superficial or genuine. The potential participant might feel the researcher's genuine concern, or might be left with the feeling that he or she was simply being used as a means, with no recognition of his or her individual standing. For older people, this acquaintance might be very significant in the person's life. He or she might be too busy for the research relationship to mean very much. But, equally, it may be that the time spent with the researcher (especially where we are considering long interviews as part of qualitative research) is of considerable importance in terms of decreasing loneliness and vulnerability.

The quality of the relationship will be affected by the extent to which it is a matter of '*being with*' rather than 'doing to'. It is easy for much research to slip into the 'doing to' mode, which causes the Kantian worry that this might amount to using the person as a means and not as an end. Research can be alienating in and of itself (Oliver 1992).

'Being with' requires a greater degree of genuineness. This should mean that the consent process is more meaningful, if the researcher and the potential participant are engaged with one another at a level that is not simply instrumental. For the older person this 'being with' might become an important aspect of his or her life. The relationship, therefore, needs to be carefully considered: how it is established, how it is pursued (which may at times require careful renegotiation), and how it will be ended. For the older person, the ending of the relationship is in danger of being a further loss in a life that has, at least potentially, already witnessed a number of losses. It may be, for this reason, that the follow-up needs to be extended to allow the relationship to be terminated in a gentler way. This is particularly important when the research has involved in-depth interviews over an extended period of time (Mason 1996). Of course, terminating the relationship is not solely a problem in research with older people. The key is to recognize the complexity and the range of the individual's needs.

Contiguity refers to closeness. The research relationship, especially if the research is extended over time, is likely to lead to friendships between the researcher and the participant. From the researcher's perspective, this friendship should be professional,

---

[4] We are grateful to Dr Bernard Jeune who, in reading this paper, suggested that 'confidence' might be another concept relevant to relationships. This suggests the need for experience on the part of the researcher. Our own reflections suggest that the list could be lengthened: for example, Honesty (discussed below), Integrity, Justice, Kindness, Love, etc.

with set boundaries. But it may not appear in this light to the participant who may have revealed intimate details to the researcher. The contiguity may be physical, or it may reflect psychodynamic attractions, for example, between the older (parent or grandparent-like) person and the younger (child or grandchild-like) researcher. Apart from the difficulties of ending such a relationship, consent may, under such circumstances, become more like a favour to the researcher, which would need to be handled with care.

For one thing, there may be a degree of *dependency* in the relationship. This is sometimes the reality for older people and can become increasingly so with frailty. It is the reality that undermines the possibility of the autonomy which, in turn is seen as underpinning the basic paradigm of consent. The older person, being dependent, may feel he or she has to acquiesce to requests from his or her professional caregivers. This may sound like coercion, but it may be that – to some extent – the older person does not mind acquiescing. The extent to which this is true helps to draw the line between coercion and more acceptable cajoling. However, it should be noted that the position of the researcher and the potential participant already sets up a power differential that is potentially coercive.

The older person may be happy to acquiesce because there are benefits to participation, even if these benefits are only marginal. But it may be that both parties in the relationship recognize the mutual *exchange* that is possible, in terms of time and commitment, and closeness. The giving of consent might be regarded as part of this exchange, even in the face of some lack of understanding of the details of the research. But a participant might feel aggrieved if the exchange does not seem to be mutual. In addition, the older person may well be dependent in other ways on his or her family and they may expect something tangible in exchange for their participation at a distance. The suggestion is not that they would necessarily want pecuniary exchange (although this may need to be considered), but it might be that they have played a significant role in encouraging the older person to give consent and they might then feel that they should be kept informed of the results. Or they might feel they have a claim on the researcher's time if there are problems.

This notion of exchange links to the idea that a relationship involves *gift* and this is sometimes used to suggest that people participate in research without any expectation of return; altruistically, in other words. However, the anthropological and sociological research on 'gift exchanges' (Mauss 1925/1997; Titmuss 1970; Tutton 2004) suggests that such exchanges are based on much more complex understandings of the expectations associated with gift-giving, including subtle understandings of reciprocity and solidarity, mediated through key social institutions (such as, given the interests of this chapter, the NHS, universities, and key research funding agencies). And this is as much the case for agreeing to participate in research and to give the gift of one's time, information, energy, and physical samples, as it is the other types of gift exchange (see Tutton 2004) on how this applies to participating in research involving genetic databases). Part of what participants might expect in return is that the relationship should be *fruitful*. They do not want their gift to have been given for no purpose. When they consent, they do so with this expectation (that there will be a useful outcome from the research) in mind. This expectation may be pertinent to the judgement concerning the person's capacity to participate in the research.

There are various ways, then, in which it seems entirely reasonable to talk of research in terms of a relationship. The bonds and shape of this relationship will be fashioned in part by factors that are related to older age: mental and physical frailty, social isolation, decreasing mobility, etc. Moreover, the nature of the relationship will have an effect on the process of gaining consent. This is because, over against the positivistic conceptualization of consent, whether or not one subscribes to the idea of social construction, it is certainly true that consent is gained in a particular context. The context is that of a relationship, which may be more or less strong, but the features of which can be exaggerated in older age.

8.5 **Situated people: from contexts to virtues**

Consent occurs in a context and, to understand what occurs during the consent procedure, the context needs to be understood. This raises practical difficulties, because observation might alter the context. But there are some conceptual points that can be made relevant to older age in particular. A starting point is the recognition that persons are situated embodied agents (Hughes 2001).

Being embodied, for older people, entails the possibility of the sort of frailty, dependency, loneliness, immobility, and vulnerability we have already referred to. This is part of the situated context for many older people and it fashions their abilities and inclinations to consent. Thinking about ageing can also challenge our assumptions about agency. On the one hand, the older person (despite a degree of physical or mental frailty) should be encouraged to exercise this agency. Assessments of capacity, for instance, ought to facilitate the person's ability to make decisions:

> A person is not to be regarded as unable to understand the information relevant to a decision if he is able to understand an explanation of it given to him in a way that is appropriate to his circumstances (using simple language, visual aids or any other means).
>
> The fact that a person is able to retain the information relevant to a decision for a short period only does not prevent him from being regarded as able to make the decision.
>
> (The Stationery Office 2005, 3(2-3))

On the other hand, it may increasingly be that others have to act for the person as she ages. Whilst the family cannot consent for the person, they may be involved in the process, by passing on information, by explanation, by reassurance, and it may be that the consent procedure needs to involve families and main carers more fully.

Older people are situated in a variety of ways. They are situated in their personal histories, which may or may not include physical or mental illness, but they are also situated in a social and cultural context. Consent procedures will take place in these contexts. It may be that consent needs to be gained in the person's own home. Going into the person's domain might shift the power dynamic back in favour of the older person, but is also a potential invasion, which the person may not feel able to resist. Part of the person's situatedness might be precisely the context of dependency.

Should this be the case it might be important for consent to be checked and renegotiated as the person's relationship with the research team progresses.

When VBM turns from theory to practice (Fulford 2004), good communication becomes increasingly important. In a similar way, Moody (1992) called for 'a communicative ethics grounded in practice and lived experience' to replace 'an abstract ethics of rules or principles'. The basic paradigm of consent has to be similarly replaced by an interactive process of communication grounded in relationship. This is the idea of the fiduciary relationship, where consent is based on partnership (Dyer and Bloch 1987). The need for this is more pointedly seen in older people, for whom the issue of dependency and the difficulties associated with autonomous authorization become more apparent. But the change from a basic consent paradigm to the notion of situated, relational consent – where the emphasis is on good-quality communication over time – needs to be generalized to other situations.

Consent has to be negotiated, therefore, between individuals in a particular context. This implies that the researcher needs very specific skills when working with older people. What is required, however, are not simply skills but a set of dispositions to act in certain ways in given contexts. That is, the researcher needs particular virtues to support good practice (May 1994; Hughes and Baldwin 2008). Practical wisdom (*phronesis*), which requires contextualized knowledge and knowing how to negotiate in the space of values shaping the relationship between the researcher and the potential participant are crucial. But there is also a requirement for truthfulness, to self and to others. Consent in research cannot be based on any form of deceit (i.e., the researcher must demonstrate the virtue of honesty).[5] The researcher, especially given the tendency for dependence to emerge in one form or another in later life, must be loyal to the participant. Given how central the idea of relationship is in research with older people, participants, and potential participants deserve kindness and compassion. They in turn may demonstrate generosity of spirit, which ought to be received by the researchers with gratitude. Thus, there is an array of virtues required if consent is to be obtained in a way that does justice to legal requirements and moral considerations.

It is important to notice that, in the classical tradition, virtues are based on training and education. It cannot be assumed that a researcher will possess the necessary dispositions; some form of training in these matters should be possible. Further more the right disposition is everything without attention being paid to practical details. Acting virtuously also requires that people show good governance and keep appropriate records to monitor the process of gaining consent.

---

[5] The virtue of honesty and the avoidance of deceit obviously form the bedrock of the sort of trusting relationship advocated by Miller and Weijer in this volume (see Chapter Two).

8.6 **Conclusion: practical steps beyond the limits of consent**

We have argued in favour of a shift from the basic paradigm of consent to one in which consent is seen as an interactive process of communication grounded in relationship. The constituents of this relationship are potentially broad, for they include not only the research team, but also those other significant people with whom the potential participant interacts. There may then be clashes at the level of values; but it is here that the need for good communication skills emerges, backed up by the exercise of the requisite virtues engendered by experience and training (Widdershoven and Widdershoven-Heerding 2003). With these in place, it should be possible for researchers to negotiate consent even when the criteria for valid consent (according to the basic paradigm) are fuzzy. It may be that some sort of weighing up of values will have to occur before a decision about consent can be reached.

A stronger claim would be that the difficulties surrounding 'valid informed consent' are such that we should drop the whole notion in favour of the new concept of 'negotiated consent'. There are, however, problems with this suggestion. One concerns the need to give content to this concept in such a way as to enable judgements to be made concerning whether or not such consent has been achieved. This takes us back in the direction of legalistic criteria. It seems better, arguably, to acknowledge that whatever criteria are used will lead to practical problems because of the evaluative nature of the concepts under consideration. Hence the need for VBM, with its suggestions about how – in real life – the differences in underlying values must be negotiated through honesty and good communication.

In some cases, valid consent will not be obtainable because the person lacks capacity through very obvious dementia. In which case, researchers would need to consult local guidelines developed over many years (e.g., AGS Ethics Committee 1998; Brodaty *et al.* 1999). In England and Wales, the Mental Capacity Act 2005 now stipulates what must be done under these circumstances (The Stationery Office 2005). In brief, the Act states that actions taken must be in the person's best interests with attention to the possible benefits and harms that might result. We have already seen that this will need to be assessed very broadly because the person is situated in such extensive fields. For instance, we have not touched upon the ethical and spiritual fields that might shape the person's decisions and will be relevant to what might be best. In this regard it is worth recalling Hans Jonas (1989), who is cited by Sachs and Cassel (1990):

> Let us not forget that progress is an optional goal, not an unconditional commitment, and that its tempo in particular, compulsive as it may become, has nothing sacred about it.

When the person with dementia can clearly not consent, it is good practice to seek any possible indication of the person's views. It then becomes necessary to gain assent from a proxy, usually a close family member, as a way of supporting any decisions about what might be best for the person (Ferrucci *et al.* 2004). Proxy assent was initially seen as a way round the problem of not being able to pursue biomedical research in people with dementia because of their inability to give consent (High 1992). The emphasis has shifted in the direction of establishing the quality of proxy consent (Lynöe *et al.* 1998), with increasingly more attention being given to the difficulties and burdens of proxy decision-making (Sugarman *et al.* 2001).

The ethical justification for turning to people who know the person well comes from considering the broad context in which the person is situated, where his or her agentive capabilities are held in place in large measure by others (Aquilina and Hughes 2006). In addition to proxy assent, given the difficulties knowing how much information to impart, it may be that consent could involve explanations beforehand and also some form of post-hoc consent: checking that the person does not object to the research once it is under way.[6]

Our discussions lead to some further practical recommendations. We have already suggested that potential participants (or their main carers) should be part of the process of determining which research should proceed. Given our emphasis on relationships and the need for a virtuous character to perform the research, it is odd that there is no real check on the skills or aptitudes of the main researcher. It may again be that a participants' panel should sit to review research progress and to monitor the work of researchers, bearing in mind that the named principal investigator (perhaps a head of department) is not necessarily the person who will be meeting the potential participants. Such a review need not be too intrusive, but might become a normal part of research governance. In addition, facilitative research mentoring might be set up, with a more senior researcher talking through and demonstrating how to gain consent. It is sometimes, mistakenly, presumed that gaining consent in the research setting is relatively unproblematic. Such instruction would improve skills and increase the practical understanding of where the ethical lines in the sand ought to be drawn. As Kitwood (1995) commented: 'we must attend not only to the content of research, but also to the process'.

For research to be ethical, procedures for gaining valid consent must be in place. There is no way around this, but beyond the limits of consent there is a place for a more careful consideration of the nature of the research relationship. Research with older people emphasizes the importance of such relationships, in which persons are treated as ends in themselves. Hence, attention to the ending of the relationship needs to be built into the research process. Perhaps all research should involve a debriefing session, a contact number (for after the research), and a formal (written) thank you for the person's participation. But these relationships will be nuanced by individual circumstances and textured by context.

Whilst there may be a number of practical implications that stem from a more careful understanding of consent as relationship – e.g., post-hoc consent, participants' panels, facilitative research mentoring with training in consent procedures, feedback, and acknowledgement of the gift given by participation – the notion also implies something about approach and tone. Going beyond the limits of formal (i.e., legal) consent takes us back to Kant. As an end, a situated person must be regarded mutually as a participant in the research. The approach should suggest that

---

[6] The importance of the supportive relationship is also emphasized by Bielby's recommendations for subject counsellors in this volume (see Chapter Nine).

nothing is presumed, that everything is open, that there are no implications in terms of commitment and that there will be no overreaching. The tone should be that of friendship, albeit professional friendship, but friendship none the less, where concern, compassion, honesty, integrity, helpfulness, fidelity, and even love might play a part.

The title of our chapter suggests a *double entendre*. Relationships come in many forms: so too in research. They may be fleeting and are not necessarily diminished by being so. But they may be problematic. They may be casual or even abusive. Or they may be enduring, enriching, and fruitful. Relationships at their best are mutual affairs. Older people naturally bring a whole variety of experiences, attitudes, and values with them into any relationship. Our contention is that the researcher must approach the older person with an openness to the possibilities that might stem from the research relationship. This requires, we have suggested, a range of virtues. According to this view, the researcher must not only be concerned with the knowledge or advantage that will flow from the research, but also with what the experience of the research will do to all involved. The question is not just: What do I gain? It is also: What do we become? Beyond consent, therefore, is the pattern of our lives, shaped by our virtues and values, which impelled us to take consent seriously in the first place.

References

Agarwal, M.R., Ferran, J., Ost, K., and Wilson, K.C.M. (1996). Ethics of 'informed consent' in dementia research – the debate continues. *International Journal of Geriatric Psychiatry*, **11**, 801–6.

Agich, G.J. (2003). *Dependence and Autonomy in Old Age: an Ethical Framework for Long-term Care*. Cambridge: Cambridge University Press.

AGS Ethics Committee (1998). Informed consent for research on human subjects with dementia. *Journal of the American Geriatrics Society*, **46**, 1308–10.

Aquilina, C. and Hughes, J.C. (2006). The return of the living dead: agency lost and found? In *Dementia: Mind, Meaning, and the Person*, edited by J.C. Hughes, S.J. Louw, and S.R. Sabat. Oxford: Oxford University Press.

Barron, J.S., Duffey, P.L., Byrd, L.J., Campbell, R., and Ferrucci, L. (2004). Informed consent for research participation in frail older persons. *Aging Clinical and Experimental Research*, **16**, 79–85.

Beauchamp, T.L. and Childress, J.F. (2001). *Principles of Biomedical Ethics* (5th edition). Oxford: Oxford University Press.

Brodaty, H., Dresser, R., Eisner, M., *et al.* (1999). Consensus statement: Alzheimer's Disease International Working Group for the Harmonization of Dementia Drug Guidelines for research involving human subjects with dementia. *Alzheimer Disease and Associated Disorders*, **13**, 71–9.

Charland, L.C. (1998). Appreciation and emotion: theoretical reflections on the MacArthur Treatment Competence Study. *Kennedy Institute of Ethics Journal*, **8**, 359–76.

Corner, L. (2002). Including people with dementia: advisory networks and user panels. In *The Perspectives of People with Dementia: Research Methods and Motivations*, edited by H. Wilkinson. London: Jessica Kingsley.

Cotrell, V. and Schulz, R. (1993). The perspective of the patient with Alzheimer's disease: a neglected dimension of dementia research. *Gerontologist*, **33**, 205–11.

Department of Health and Welsh Office (1999). *Code of Practice. Mental Health Act*. London: HMSO.

Dyer, A.R. and Bloch, S. (1987). Informed consent and the psychiatric patient. *Journal of Medical Ethics*, **13**, 12–16.

Fazel, S. (2002). Competence. In *Psychiatry in the Elderly*, edited by R. Jacoby and C. Oppenheimer. Oxford: Oxford University Press.

Ferrucci, L., Guralnik, J.M., Studenski, S., Fried, L.P., Cutler, G.B. Jr, and Walston, J.D. (2004). Designing randomized, controlled trials aimed at preventing or delaying functional decline and disability in frail, older persons: a consensus report. *Journal of the American Geriatrics Society*, **52**, 625–34.

Folstein, M.F., Folstein, S.E., and McHugh, P.R. (1975). 'Mini-mental state': a practical method for grading the cognitive state of patients for the clinician. *Journal of Psychiatric Research*, **12**, 189–98.

Fulford, K.W.M. (1989). *Moral Theory and Medical Practice*. Cambridge: Cambridge University Press.

–*ibid.*– (2004). Ten principles of values-based medicine. In *The Philosophy of Psychiatry: a Companion*, edited by J. Radden. Oxford: Oxford University Press.

Gillick, M. (2000). Rethinking the role of tube feeding in patients with advanced dementia. *New England Journal of Medicine*, **342**, 206–10.

Haimes, E. and Whong-Barr, M. (2004). Levels and styles of participation in genetic databases. In *Genetic Databases: Socio-ethical Issues in the Collection and Use of DNA*, edited by R. Tutton and O. Corrigan. London: Routledge.

Henon, P.R. (2003). Human embryonic or adult stem cells: an overview on ethics and perspectives for tissue engineering. *Advances in Experimental Medicine and Biology*, **534**, 27–45.

High, D.M. (1992). Research with Alzheimer's disease subjects: informed consent and proxy decision-making. *Journal of the American Geriatrics Society*, **40**, 950–7.

Hughes, J.C. (2000). Ethics and the anti-dementia drugs. *International Journal of Geriatric Psychiatry*, **15**, 538–43.

–*ibid.*– (2001). Views of the person with dementia. *Journal of Medical Ethics*, **27**, 86–91.

Hughes, J.C. and Baldwin, C. (2008). Ethics and old age psychiatry. In *Oxford Textbook of Old Age Psychiatry*, edited by R. Jacoby, C. Oppenheimer, T. Dening, and A. Thomas. Oxford: Oxford University Press.

Jonas, H. (1989). Philosophical reflections on experimenting with human subjects. In *Contemporary Issues in Bioethics* (3rd editon), edited by T.L. Beauchamp and L.R. Walters, California: Wadsworth, Belmont.

Kant, I. (1785). *Grounding for the Metaphysics of Morals*, (trans. J.W. Ellington). New York: Hackett Publishing Company [3rd edn, 1993].

Kirkwood, T. (1999). *Time of Our Lives: the Science of Human Ageing*. London: Weidenfeld and Nicolson.

Kitwood, T. (1995). Exploring the ethics of dementia research: a response to Berghmans and ter Meulen: a psychosocial perspective. *International Journal of Geriatric Psychiatry*, **10**, 655–7.

Lynöe, N., Sandlund, M., and Jacobsson, L. (1998). When others decide: reasons for allowing patients with Alzheimer's disease to participate in nontherapeutic research. *International Psychogeriatrics*, **10**, 435–6.

Manson, N. and O'Neill, O. (2007). *Rethinking Informed Consent*. Cambridge: Cambridge University Press.

Mason, J. (1996). *Qualitative Researching*. London: Sage.

Mauss, M. (1925/1997). *The gift. The Form and Reason for Exchange in Archaic Societies* (trans. W.D. Halls). London: Routledge.

May, W.F. (1994). The virtues in a professional setting. In *Medicine an Moral Reasoning*, edited by K.W.M. Fulford, G.R. Gillett, and J.M. Soskice. Cambridge: Cambridge University Press.

Moody, H.R. (1992). A critical view of ethical dilemmas in dementia. In *Dementia and Aging: Ethics, Values and Policy Choices*, edited by R.H. Binstock, S.G. Post, and P.J. Whitehouse. Baltimore: The Johns Hopkins University Press.

Oliver, M. (1992). Changing the social relations of research production? *Disability, Handicap and Society*, **7**, 101–14.

Pucci, E., Belardinelli, N., Borsetti, G., Rodriguez, D., and Signorino, M. (2001). Information and competency for consent to pharmacologic clinical trials in Alzheimer disease: an empirical analysis in patients and family caregivers. *Alzheimer Disease and Associated Disorders*, **15**, 146–54.

Sabat, S.R. (2001). *The Experience of Alzheimer's Disease: Life through a Tangled Veil*. Oxford: Blackwell.

–*ibid*.– (2005). Capacity for decision-making in Alzheimer's disease: selfhood, positioning and semiotic persons. *Australian and New Zealand Journal of Psychiatry*, **39**, 1030–5.

Sachs, G.A. and Cassel, C.K. (1990). *Law, Medicine and Health Care*, **18**, 234–43.

Sugarman, J., Cain, C., Wallace, R., and Welsh-Bohmer, K.A. (2001). How proxies make decisions about research for patients with Alzheimer's disease. *Journal of the American Geriatrics Society*, **49**, 1110–19.

The Stationery Office (2005). *Mental Capacity Act 2005*. Norwich: The Stationery Office.

Thornton, T. (2006). The discursive turn, social constructionism, and dementia. In *Dementia: Mind, Meaning, and the Person*, edited by J.C. Hughes, S.J. Louw, and S.R. Sabat. Oxford: Oxford University Press.

Titmuss, R.M. (1970). *The Gift Relationship: from Human Blood to Social Policy*. London: George Allen and Unwin.

Townsley, C.A., Selby, R., and Siu, L.L. (2005). Systematic review of barriers to the recruitment of older patients with cancer onto clinical trials. *Journal of Clinical Oncology*, **23**, 3112–24.

Tutton, R. (2004). Person, property and gift: exploring languages of tissue donation to biomedical research. In *Genetic Databases: Socio-ethical Issues in the Collection and Use of DNA*, edited by R. Tutton and O. Corrigan. London: Routledge.

Velody, I. and Williams, R. (eds) (1998). *The Politics of Constructionism*. London: Sage.

Widdershoven, G.A.M. and Widdershoven-Heerding, I. (2003). Understanding dementia: a hermeneutic perspective. In *Nature and Narrative: an Introduction to the New Philosophy of Psychiatry*, edited by K.W.M. Fulford, K. Morris, J.Z. Sadler, and G. Stanghellini. Oxford: Oxfrod University Press.

Chapter 9

Towards supported decision-making in biomedical research with cognitively vulnerable adults

Philip Bielby

9.1 Introduction

A particular challenge for consent in biomedical research is the participation of adults with mental disorder or intellectual disability to a degree that impinges on but does not necessarily erode decisional competence. This challenge is emphasized by recent developments in neuroscience which have reinvigorated interest in biomedical research with cognitively vulnerable human participants, particularly research into the origins and treatment of mental disorder (see Merkel *et al.* 2007, Part I and Glannon 2007, for discussion). Such individuals may be thought of as 'cognitively vulnerable', as the effects of the condition raise their vulnerability above the baseline existential level shared by all human beings (Kipnis 2004; Karlawish 2007; Bielby 2008). These typify 'borderline' cases of competence, which occupy the 'grey area' between 'obvious' competence and 'obvious' incompetence (Murphy 1979, 174; O'Neill 2002, 42).

This chapter has two connected aims. First, I argue that we can best understand the scope and limits of consent as a 'procedural' principle of empowerment. I ground this argument in a rationalist moral theory of human (or agency) rights devised by Alan Gewirth (1978). Drawing on the recent work of Gewirthian legal theorists Beyleveld and Brownsword (2004 and 2007), I offer a defence of the ethical significance of consent as a procedural human rights value, which does not in itself constitute a substantive human right.

My starting point is to identify two lines of critique consent has received. The first is the risk of over-valuation that occurs when one understands consent as having a value independent of a human rights justificatory framework (Brownsword 2004; Beyleveld and Brownsword 2007). The second is how overly abstracted accounts of consent do not reflect the experience of individuals in everyday research settings (Corrigan 2003). I will show how this rests upon a problematic understanding of the self, which informs such accounts of consent. These critiques epitomize the challenge to which any proponent of consent must respond.

Empirical research suggests that seeking 'first-person' consent to research and treatment with cognitively vulnerable adults is possible (e.g., Wong *et al.* 2000; Dunn *et al.* 2001;

Buckles *et al.* 2003; Lapid *et al.* 2004). Nevertheless, the processes employed in seeking consent require imagination and sensitivity. Using the 'procedural' justification of consent outlined above, my second aim is to propose a theory of supported decision-making in biomedical research that seeks to nurture the abilities of cognitively vulnerable participants to make decisions within the context of a 'helping relationship' (Rogers 1961). This reframes consent as the basis of the empowerment of cognitively vulnerable adults.

In the final section, I assess the legal prospects for supported decision-making, with particular reference to English law. Supported decision-making has already been adopted by certain jurisdictions, notably in Manitoba, Canada (Gordon 2000; Glass 1997).[1] Although no explicit provision for supported decision-making in research currently exists in English law, there appears to be some limited scope for accommodation.

9.2 Two critiques of consent

9.2.1 Over-valuing consent

'Over-valuation' is a threat to the integrity of consent (Brownsword 2004, 224; Beyleveld and Brownsword 2007), a theme which Liddell also explores in her contribution to this volume (see Chapter Five). Brownsword argues that the proper role of consent is a procedural justification to grant or withhold authority for a modification of or interference with the object of the right (Brownsword 2004, 225, 228). Over-valuation occurs where consent ceases to be a value implicated by human rights-based moral theory and takes on an independent justification of its own (Brownsword 2004, 224, 226). This does not diminish the significance of 'under-valuation', of which the history of biomedical research with human beings is replete with examples (e.g., Jonsen 1998, Chapter Five). However, the risk of fixation with consent in societies committed to human rights raises problems of its own (Brownsword 2004, 224).

According to Beyleveld and Brownsword, 'fixation' can take two different forms (2007, 355–7). The first involves claiming that where there is not consent there is a wrong (the fallacy of necessity of consent). Such a claim overlooks the fact that the wrong stems from a violation of a right rather than from a violation of consent, since

---

[1] s.6(1) of Manitoba's Vulnerable Persons Living With a Mental Disability Act 1993 defines supported decision-making as 'the process whereby a vulnerable person is enabled to make and communicate decisions with respect to personal care or his or her property and in which advice, support or assistance is provided to the vulnerable person by members of his or her support network'. s.6(2) goes on to state: 'supported decision-making by a vulnerable person with members of his or her support network should be respected and recognized as an important means of enhancing the self-determination, independence and dignity of a vulnerable person'. Both this definition and claim dovetail with the argument of this chapter. However, as the title of the Act suggests, this provision only covers adults with intellectual disability rather than adults with mental disorder (Gordon 2000, 67–8). Elsewhere in Canada, Prince Edward Island has drawn up the Supported Decision-Making and Adult Guardianship Act 1997 (discussed in Gordon, *ibid.*) but as of February 2008, this has not been proclaimed.

'there is no right to consent as such' (Brownsword 2004, 229). The example of the convicted offender who does not give her consent to the state-imposed sanction she receives (where this sanction is justified on human rights grounds) illustrates this vividly.

The second involves claiming that where the relevant parties have given their consent, there can be no other reason to regulate or prohibit their conduct (the fallacy of sufficiency of consent). Such a claim negates the fact that there may still be a public wrong (similarly justified on Gewirthian human rights grounds) even though no private wrong has been committed. The example of two individuals who consent that one should kill and eat the other (such as in the notorious case of 'consensual cannibalism' in Germany in 2004 (Harding 2004)) provides a clear indication of when the state may have a *prima facie* justification in prohibiting certain conduct that is apparently consensual.

I agree with Beyleveld and Brownsword's taxonomy of misconceptions about consent. However, I would add another fallacy to the taxonomy: the fallacy of validity. This fallacy supposes that the ethical validity of consent by a decisionally competent individual rests simply upon the provision of relevant information and the communication of a voluntary decision. Such an understanding of the conditions for validity may stem from an attempt to distinguish between consent given on one's own behalf at the relevant time ('first person' contemporaneous consent) and that given on one's behalf by a proxy or offered prospectively through an advance directive. But to frame the validity of consent in these terms overlooks the role of supportive interventions by the person seeking consent or by a third party in how the decision-maker engages with the nature of the decision in question.

To deny this as a fallacy would lead us to the view that support and assistance in the decision-making process somehow makes the decision arrived at less the decision-maker's own. At best, this suggests that competent decision-making and support from others are mutually antagonistic, and at worst, implies abandonment to one's autonomy. Support of some kind is necessary if the decision reached is one that is the product of genuine deliberation (Buchanan and Brock 1990; Savulescu 1995; Savulescu and Momeyer 1997; Feenan 1997). The position of participants whose decisional competence is apparent but is fragile or diminishing brings into sharp relief the implications of committing this fallacy. If we take our starting point in human rights thinking, assistance in decision-making serves to galvanize rather than to erode autonomy. Indeed, the relational processes involved reflect the interdependence of most adults in making decisions for whom decisional competence is not an issue (Gordon 2000, 65).

9.2.2 Abstracting the process of consent

Empirical social science studies into patient decision-making in research have called into question the plausibility of overly abstracted accounts of consent. Such accounts tend to marginalize the influence of social relationships of trust and role perception in the process of deciding whether to participate (for a discussion, see Corrigan 2003). This stands at odds with established notions of the biomedical research participant who is autonomous and self-determined (e.g., National Commission for the

Protection of Human Subjects of Biomedical and Behavioral Research 1979; Beauchamp and Childress 2001).

The findings of the US Advisory Committee on Human Radiation Experiments (discussed by Dresser 2001, 56) epitomize this. In follow-up studies, individuals freely admitted to deciding whether or not to participate before they had been provided with relevant information and risks by the researchers involved. One respondent commented that they did not read the consent form fully because they assumed that the benefits and burdens of the research protocol had already been evaluated on their behalf (*ibid.*).

From a UK perspective, Corrigan's empirical study (2003) examined the impact of the social processes involved in several clinical drugs trials. She found that social understandings of the physician–patient relationship, anxieties about treatment, and expectations of care were frequent preoccupations amongst research participants. Corrigan concludes that consent is often 'an important ethical tool' (2003, 788) but proposes that it be freed from its current narrow focus in which inequalities of power and socio-cultural influences are commonly ignored. Addressing the conceptual nature of consent, Corrigan observes:

> the concept of informed consent [is] problematic within its own terms of reference. … ideas of autonomy, freedom and choice belie the extent to which they are both limited and regulated.

> (2003, 789)

We can explain the essence of this critique by tracing it to a tension in the nature of selfhood which underpins the concept of consent. The abstracted, autonomous self, which forms the basis of many influential accounts of consent (e.g., Faden *et al.* 1986) is juxtaposed by the 'situated' self who is constituted by a nexus of roles and relationships, and who forges an identity within a socially rich milieu. Being a patient and being a family member are examples of such roles (Ingelfinger 1972; Lindemann-Nelson and Lindemann-Nelson 1995; Corrigan, *ibid.*). The so-called 'communitarian' critique of liberalism in contemporary political philosophy (see Mulhall and Swift 1997, for a discussion) highlights the shortcomings in the concepts of selfhood inherent in such accounts of informed consent. Of particular relevance here is Michael Sandel's critique of the 'unencumbered self' (1984, 1998).

Sandel takes Rawls' *A Theory of Justice* (1972, rev. ed. 1999) as the epitome of the self in contemporary liberal political thought. He claims that the account of the self articulated by Rawls is artificially separated from its ends and purposes in a way that no real self is. On this account of the self, one can only think of oneself as autonomous and independent provided 'my identity is never tied to the aims and interests I may have at any moment' (1984, 86). By extension, the ends that the person chooses for herself are not capable of becoming part of that person's self-identity (1984, 86, *passim*; 1998, 15–24; Mulhall and Swift 1996, 51). Several feminist commentators (e.g., Gilligan 1982; Benhabib 1992; Noddings 2003) develop the essence of Sandel's critique by emphasizing the impersonal moral reasoning found in such understandings of the self. This reasoning tends to valorize a 'masculinist' self-concept, which marginalizes the influence that situation, empathy, and context have on moral choice and personal identity.

The central problem with an understanding of the self defined along these lines is that it defines the nature of the self prior to what the self is actually like or what it is good for it to be like. Grounding informed consent on such a concept of the self risks both ignoring the particularities of human experience and the challenges that seeking consent faces at a practical level. Research participation by cognitively vulnerable individuals may increase our scepticism towards a notion of the self characterized by its independence or self-determining character, as it confronts us with a vivid example of its antithesis – selves which are especially dependent upon others for their support.

Viewed together, these two critiques raise a powerful objection to predicating consent as a free-standing value on a model of the self which is defined independently from its relational context. We should also not overlook the fact that these are problems which extend beyond seeking consent with cognitively vulnerable populations to the process of seeking informed consent with 'healthy' populations. This reminds us that it is not only in borderline cases that consent is problematic (O'Neill 2002, 42).

9.3 **Cognitive vulnerability**

It is quite plain that all human beings share a similar level of baseline vulnerability – that vulnerability which is bound up with the threat to our continuing existence. Cognitive vulnerability, however, is best understood as a form of *heightened* vulnerability (Bielby 2005a, 235–6). Heightened vulnerabilities may not be exclusively cognitive, they may also be circumstantial (Berg *et al.* 2001, 266), and these two types of vulnerability may overlap. It is helpful to first identify in which sense an individual primarily experiences heightened vulnerability, particularly so we can identify the locus of vulnerability in cognitively vulnerable research participants.

Individuals experiencing mental disorder and adults with intellectual disabilities are primarily cognitively vulnerable, albeit to different degrees, and in different ways. This is due to incompleteness, imbalances, or immaturities of their ratiocination and affective responses that limit or undermine decisional and task competences. They may also be circumstantially vulnerable insofar as their lived experiences, such as within a psychiatric hospital, generate power relationships within the institution responsible for their care (e.g., Goffman 1961; Moreno 1998).

For individuals with mental disorder and intellectual disbalities who reside in the community, their lack of educational opportunities and/or employment along with an absence of a social network may predispose them to poverty, ill health, and social exclusion. This coalescence of cognitive and circumstantial vulnerabilities exacerbates the overall degree of heightened vulnerability they experience. I refer to individuals experiencing mental disorder and intellectual disabilities as being primarily cognitively vulnerable because the principal source of their vulnerability arises from impairment to ratiocination and affect. Indeed, in many cases, their circumstantial vulnerability would not exist were it not for the antecedent cognitive vulnerability.

An ascription of cognitive vulnerability may connote permanence in an individual's mental state, but need not do so. It is sufficient to recognize that she either currently is or has been previously affected by a condition that could lead to cognitive vulnerability. Also, cognitive vulnerability is not merely an abstract concept. Rather, it is a lived experience that can be described and explained in terms of the normative criteria that supply the basis of psychiatric diagnosis (see Sadler 2005) or alternatively according to 'narrative' approaches that proceed from the viewpoint of the person experiencing the condition (Harré 1998, 141–3). It is, of course, possible that circumstantial vulnerabilities could exacerbate or even create cognitive vulnerabilities, to an extent where the line between circumstantial and cognitive vulnerabilities blurs. Consider, for instance, the case of a terrorist suspect subject to indefinite detention who experiences clinical depression as a result. Even here, though, the distinction between cognitive and circumstantial vulnerability does not dissipate entirely as it is still possible to identify the origin of the vulnerability in question.

9.4 **Cognitive vulnerability, consent, and research**

Empirical studies of seeking consent with cognitively vulnerable adults amplify the critiques of consent identified earlier. Eckstein (2003) identifies several obstacles in the context of research on the elderly, which explain why vulnerability may undermine the likelihood of obtaining informed consent. These are willingness to defer to authority; dependence on others (which could lead to the use of coercive practices); and a concept of themselves which departs from how someone different or younger (such as the researcher) may view themselves (*ibid.*, 107). It is conceivable that these obstacles could arise in relation to research participants who do not experience a form of heightened vulnerability. However, participants whose vulnerabilities arise primarily because of cognitive factors incur a greater risk that such vulnerabilities will erode decisional competence.

As Berghmans *et al.* (2004) acknowledge, the significance of mental capacity becomes more evident when considering vulnerable groups (*ibid.*, 251). A survey of the existing literature relating to the consent of cognitively vulnerable individuals in biomedical research, however, reveals a difference of opinion. Elliott (1997), for instance, argues that severely depressed persons are unlikely to retain any decisional competence to give consent on their own behalf. Alternatively, Appelbaum *et al.* (1999) suggest that, whilst the experience of depression has repercussions for decisional competence, it does not displace it altogether.

Elsewhere, studies indicate that particular efforts to improve understanding of research procedures may be successful. These apply both in relation to cognitively vulnerable individuals and in relation to healthy volunteers. Flory and Emanuel (2004) surveyed a selection of research projects conducted between 1966 and 1994, which compared enrolment through a standard informed consent process and enrolment using efforts to improve patient understanding. These included multimedia, enhanced consent forms, counselling, and 'neutral educators' across a range of participant populations, including people with mental disorders and psychiatric patients. Of the various efforts undertaken, the authors found that time spent talking on a one-to-one basis (whether through neutral educators or from a member of the research team) was proven to be the most effective way of raising potential participants' understanding about the nature of the research. They concluded that:

> direct human contact tends to be more successful in improving understanding ... [this] has more potential for active engagement and responsiveness to the individual needs of the research participant.

> (*ibid.*, 1599)

In a separate study, Carpenter *et al.* (2000) assessed the decisional competence of 30 research participants with schizophrenia and 24 healthy comparison participants to consent to clinical research. The authors compared the cognition of the participants with schizophrenia against those of the healthy volunteers, and measured the decisional competence of all using Appelbaum and Grisso's *MacArthur Competence Assessment Tool for Clinical Research* (Appelbaum and Grisso, 2001). The authors concluded that the participants with schizophrenia did demonstrate significantly poorer performance in respect of decisional capacities relevant to consent to research. However, this did not reflect a persistent inability to understand the information relevant to a research study:

> When offered additional opportunities to learn the necessary data, most subjects with scores below an *a priori* cut-off were able to bring their scores into the range of a comparison group of people without schizophrenia. This suggests that people with severe forms of schizophrenia may be able to give informed consent for research, although a single-session brief presentation of research procedures may not be sufficient. Rather, an informed consent process that engages potential subjects over time and is sensitive to the negative impact of cognitive impairment may be essential for adequate informed consent.

> (*ibid.*, 536)

These two studies suggest possible directions to make the process of seeking consent more responsive to the needs of cognitively vulnerable individuals. In doing so, they echo Roth *et al.*'s (1982) forewarning against the belief that mentally disordered persons and psychiatric patients as a group are necessarily disadvantaged in making competent health care decisions. However, this still leaves two open questions. The first concerns why it is ethically significant that seeking first-person consent may be possible in such situations and why it should be preserved. The second is how to improve the process of seeking consent in a way which is sensitive to cognitive vulnerability.

9.5 **The ethical value of consent in biomedical research**

If we are to avoid the pitfalls of over-valuing and under-valuing consent in research, we need to ensure that we do not frame its ethical significance arbitrarily. An appreciation of the scope and limits of consent first requires that we can provide a robust philosophical justification for its existence. Alan Gewirth's theory of agency rights (which incorporates human rights) provides a particularly powerful account. Gewirth painstakingly argues that all agents have a moral right claim to the generic features of action – freedom and wellbeing – simply by virtue of being agents (1978, 65, 110–19).

He calls this the Principle of Generic Consistency (hereafter PGC) (Gewirth 1978). The theory of rights derived from the argument establishes both positive and negative rights to the objects of one's freedom and wellbeing consistent with a similar right for all other agents (Gewirth 1978, 67, 137, 217–30). In practical terms, the effect of Gewirth's theory is to reconcile liberal–egalitarian thought with communitarian considerations (Gewirth 1996). Beyleveld (1991) has defended Gewirth's argument in considerable detail from an exhaustive range of criticisms, to which I refer the interested reader. Here, my intention is to offer a justification of consent from a Gewirthian standpoint and to show how such justification leads to a more responsive and nuanced approach.

Consent serves a twofold function under the PGC. First, it protects the individual from an unwilled interference in her life, unless there is an overriding human rights-based justification for this interference (such as in cases of indefinite psychiatric hospitalization for psychopathic murderers). Second, the right of choice that consent offers gives expression to human dignity (Beyleveld and Brownsword 2001, 242). This is because being a dignity-holder is derivative from being an agent (Gewirth 1998, 208), which supposes a capacity to pursue freely chosen purposes (Gewirth 1978, 31–42). As Brownsword acknowledges (2004, 229), consent is not itself a human right but instead 'parasitic upon' a morally prior framework of rights and duties. The role of consent is as a procedural justification to grant or withhold authority for interference with the object of the right (e.g., not to have one's bodily or psychological integrity interfered with) where no over-riding human rights-based justification is engaged (Brownsword 2004, 225, 228; Beyleveld and Brownsword 2007, 335–6). Consent is, therefore, a process that legitimizes the waiver of the benefits of the rights at stake on the sufficient and necessary condition that (a) the individual concerned can understand the full implications of waiver and (b) this does not jeopardize the rights of other agents.

To be compliant with the PGC, consent is invoked at the level of defining biomedical research with human participants and informs its ethical character. This separates biomedical research from a notion of physical or psychological violation in the name of medical progress (Bielby 2005a, 222). It is similar to how consent forms part of the definition of sexual intercourse (without which the definition of the act would become that of another, namely rape). Unlike sexual intercourse, however, the scope of consent is not limited to the person who is to participate (i.e., 'first-person' consent) but extends to proxy consent if the individual concerned is decisionally incompetent. The same ethos underpins consent provisions in the earliest codes of research ethics of the post-Second World War period, such as the Nuremberg Code and the World Medical Association Declaration of Helsinki. However, it would appear that to take this approach risks a return to the source of the original problem – founding consent on a notion of the self, which is unrealistically abstracted. If this is so, then the PGC can do nothing more than offer another ethical justification of informed consent upon this same premise.

I believe that the PGC does much better than this. The generation of a positive rights claim from the substance of the argument means that consent – as a procedural justification behind the modification or waiver of a substantive right – places a duty of assistance on the part of others to help the person understand the implications of waiving the benefit of that right. This is a corollary of the positive-rights claim to the object of the right itself. It follows from the PGC-protected right to have knowledge of circumstances relevant to the particular context of action (Gewirth 1978, 250–2, 258, 260). To deny this amounts to a breach of the ethical duty that follows from the positive dimension to the right. This duty of assistance requires responsiveness to the needs of the agent in question if we are to make a sincere effort to assist her to understand, even if it transpires that she apparently cannot understand, due to decisional incompetence. Common forms of assistance include education and information provision that is appropriate to the developmental stage that the person has reached. This makes the processes leading up to offering or withholding consent sensitive to the psychological needs and dispositions that accompany the experience of cognitive vulnerability in particular and of existential vulnerability in general.

The consequences of this for consent in biomedical research are wide-ranging. It follows that there is an ethical duty incumbent upon anyone undertaking research and those responsible for its oversight to be mindful of the cognitive and/or circumstantial vulnerabilities of the individuals approached to participate. The ethos, therefore, shifts from obtaining consent to empowering the potential participant to decide (see Feenan 1997 for a discussion of empowerment in relation to assessment of competence to consent to treatment). On a practical level, this involves putting in place mechanisms to assist actively the potential participant's understanding and appreciation of the research process. As a minimum, this includes explanation of its objectives, the nature, and consequences of participation and the rationale upon which she is being approached to have her consent sought in the first place. There should also be scope to identify a person or persons with whom the potential participant would wish to make the decision if she was not prepared to reach a decision alone (such as a family member or a physician, assuming she has the decisional competence to do this).

This has two consequences. First, the Gewirthian approach to consent moves the bioethical debate away from unhelpfully bifurcated thinking about autonomy and paternalism. Instead, it recognizes that individuals should receive assistance in making decisions for themselves and that this is not something that is likely to happen without active interpersonal support. Such interventions are best articulated as duties, which attach to particular roles (e.g., physician, researcher, or counsellor), although we can also imagine them arising in everyday contexts that do not involve the seeking of consent, such as where a person reads out the bus timetable to a partially sighted person in order to help her plan her journey. These represent interventions that seek to promote the autonomy interests of the individual concerned, and elicit her decisional independence, motivated by a sincere concern for her dignity and capability as an agent. They are entirely consistent with an individual subsequently expressing a wish that she would like someone else to help her make the decision or even to make it on her behalf – this, after all, is just another example of a freely made decision.

Second, where an individual has a questionable ability to make decisions about participation, this warrants further and more specialized assistance, ideally from someone who does not have a direct interest in the research project going ahead. The case of individuals with cognitive vulnerability epitomizes the importance of appropriate assistance. The provision of simplified consent forms, greater explanation of research procedures, or provision of information in alternative formats is, by itself, unlikely to offer an improved decision-making situation relevant to their needs (see, for example, Stiles *et al.* 2001).

If we accept the importance that the PGC attaches to the justification of consent and the way in which it should be sought, then we have a reason for preserving the decisional competence of potential research participants as far as possible (an idea endorsed in Recommendation No. R (99) 4 1999 of the Council of Europe concerning the legal protection of incapable adults). There may be fewer negative consequences following from a 'false-positive' judgement of competence to consent, as in any event the potential participant would not simply be 'left alone' to decide for herself but supported in making a decision. Indeed, erring on the side of competence preservation may be preferable (Breden and Vollmann 2004, 279). The more that we treat competence as a dynamic (developable) rather than a fixed (given) quality of an agent (where the evidence suggests that the competence can develop with appropriate support), the more scrupulous a competence assessment must be and the more ethical is our resulting judgement of competence or incompetence. This is because a rigorous assessment process will yield more evidence on which to base a judgement of competence or incompetence, reducing the margin of error and the potential for social bias. In the following sections, I return to the principal focus of the chapter, and examine first the theoretical and second the legal prospects for supported decision-making when seeking informed consent to research with cognitively vulnerable adults.

9.6 **Towards a theory of supported decision-making**

Supported decision-making dovetails with a growing view on capacity assessment which emphasizes that what is important is not how capacity is assessed but how capacity can be developed through 'interaction and dialogue.' (Benaroyo and Widdershoven 2004, 298). Given the range of possibilities this opens, it is helpful first if we identify what supported decision-making is not. Supported decision-making does not correspond to the more widely known phenomenon of 'genetic counselling' (Clarke 1994), which also frequently has a bearing on the conduct of research but less on the consent-seeking process. It is also different from the notion of a 'consent auditor', appointed in the US to provide oversight of the consent process under the provisions of the Common Rule (Berg *et al.* 2001, 266). The language of audit fails to capture the caring and supportive aspects of supported decision-making, and instead concentrates on assuring that researchers adhere to certain protocols in seeking consent rather than enhancing the experience of seeking consent. Supported decision-making is also different from conventional understandings of patient or research participant advocacy, which typically involve patient representative groups campaigning on policy issues related to research priorities at the macro-level (Dresser 2001; Morreim 2004). To subsume supported decision-making within these advocacy initiatives would not give it a sufficiently clear identity, given the multitude of activities which advocacy connotes (Morreim, *ibid.*).

The form of supported decision-making I propose has parallels with the 'neutral educator' mentioned above in the empirical study by Flory and Emanuel. I define it as where an individual, suitably trained, and with sufficient knowledge of contemporary biomedical research practices, facilitates impartial information presentation and discussion in a way that takes the greatest possible account of the potential participant's cognitive abilities, affective state, level of comprehension, values, and personality traits. The effect of this is to tailor the decision-making process to her needs, making it participant-centred.

The work of humanist psychologist Carl Rogers (1961) offers a compelling theoretical basis for the practice of supported decision-making. Rogers defined a 'helping relationship' as 'one in which one of the participants intend that there should come about, in one or both parties, more appreciation of, more expression of, more functional use of the latent inner resources of the individual' (*ibid.*, 40). Rogers' account of a helping relationship resonates with the idea of facilitating the autonomy interests of the potential participant without abandoning her to the decision-making process. As Glass observes:

> [a] model for competence that provides assistance to individuals to exercise their intellectual capacities recognizes that noninterference with liberty and autonomy does not necessitate neglect.

> (1997, 30)

When used to inform the practice of supported decision-making, the idea of the helping relationship could take place on an individual or on a group basis depending upon the nature of the research project, the confidentiality issues involved, and the willingness of the potential participant to have her decision-making supported in this way.

The commitment to help the potential participant furthers the notion of 'relational equality' in research, a principle which aims to reduce power imbalances between the researcher and the potential participant (Bielby 2005a, 224–6). To this end, the dialogue would be accessible and pitched at an appropriate level, with the emphasis on shaping the discussion to minimize the effects that the mental disorder or intellectual disability has on the decisional competence of the individual concerned. Whilst not all forms of relational inequality can be reduced through supported decision-making, nonetheless, there remains a greater chance that the potential participant is likely to be empowered through this experience.

Specifically, the person(s) responsible for supported decision-making would:

(a) be present throughout the whole of the decision-making process or as much of it as the potential participant wished;

(b) help explain difficult ideas and concepts to the potential participant;

(c) reassure the potential participant and listen to her concerns;

(d) respect the confidence of the potential participant and only bring information she divulges to the attention of the researcher or the participant's physician if this were essential to advancing the potential participant's level of understanding and awareness, or if there was a legal duty to do so;

(e) inform the potential participant that if she did not want to make the decision herself, it would be possible for her to share the decision-making process with a willing companion, or possibly even delegate the decision about participation to that person entirely, subject to any legal constraints about proxy decision-making that may apply in that jurisdiction;

(f) establish whether the potential participant wishes to be aware or unaware about information gathered about her on completion of the research (a matter already accommodated by Article 27 of the Additional Protocol to the Convention on Human Rights and Biomedicine, concerning Biomedical Research (Council of Europe 2005a) and discussed in paragraphs 57 and 131 of its Explanatory Report (Council of Europe 2005b)); and

(g) in light of (d), maintain an appropriate record of the discussion (e.g., written notes or audio recording) which could be kept in the potential participant's medical notes.

The schema proposed is different from a model of 'informing decision-making' insofar as the ethos shifts from obtaining consent to empowering the potential participant to decide (see Feenan 1997 and McMillan and Gillett 2002, 225 for a discussion). In a model of 'informing decision-making', (a), (g), and certainly (c) would receive less emphasis or be overlooked altogether in favour of (b) and (d). A model of informing decision-making is perhaps better thought of as an *instance* of obtaining consent, whereas the schema presented above represents a *process* of facilitating consent. This serves to make the information on which one makes the decision more accessible, and with it, reduces the stress placed upon individuals whose circumstances may already cause them a great deal of anxiety (McMillan and Gillett, *ibid.*, 227, discuss this in relation to treatment). A model of informing decision-making would not be as well equipped to emphasize these supportive aspects and would be more likely to invite critiques of consent of the second kind discussed above.

Some researchers have offered recommendations that are more specific. In a study pertaining to a research programme to investigate HIV transmission in Haiti, Fitzgerald *et al.* (2002) found participants' understanding to have increased substantially because of having spent three sessions with a counsellor. The authors recommend specifically that inclusion of a counsellor may raise potential participants' understanding of the consent process and reduce feelings of intimidation and undue influence (2002, 1302).

Supporting decision-making through counselling may seem an attractive idea. However, the provision of counsellors in the research setting gives rise to two practical problems. The first relates to supply and funding, which in the UK at least would have to be provided by the voluntary sector, by the NHS, or by private practices. The source and extent of funding would have a bearing on the national availability and distribution of counsellors, and their ability to be present at the right times in biomedical research projects. Were counsellors to come from the voluntary sector, such as patient support groups, there is a greater risk of an unequal distribution. To attach them to the NHS or to teaching hospital trusts could be economically unfeasible in light of existing budgetary constraints. To have them sourced from private counselling practice may exceed current levels of expertise. If pharmaceutical firms responsible for large-scale biomedical research projects, including clinical drug trials, employed research participant counsellors, this could create conflicts of interests between counsellors and research sponsors, leading to possible bias towards corporate interests at the expense of professional integrity.

A more general reservation concerning the involvement of counsellors is that they would add another layer of bureaucracy to the research process. There is a risk that any increase in the probity of medical research with adults with mental disorder and intellectual disabilities would undermine its efficiency to a degree that may deter the sponsors of small-scale research projects from proposing new studies. Moreover, in the clinical setting, some psychiatrists and clinical researchers experienced in counselling and psychotherapy may see research participant counsellors as an unwarranted encroachment on their field of expertise. This is suggestive of a broader concern about a particular profession monopolizing the techniques of supported decision-making (see also Feenan 1997, 230). These present considerable impediments to the realization of such counselling on a political-administrative level.

Of course, attempts at supporting decision-making cannot elicit decisional competence which an individual has no capability to develop. After an assessment of decisional competence, it may well be that there are those who are uncontroversially incompetent and would require either appropriate decision-making to be made on their behalf by a proxy or possibly being left out of the pool of potential participants altogether. Other potential participants with mental disorder may fail to understand the role of supported decision-making and impute delusional motives to the individuals involved (especially in cases of psychosis and paranoid schizophrenia). Cases such as these present realistic although not insurmountable challenges to the idea of supported decision-making. If there were doubts as to the decisional competence of a potential participant, it would be possible to integrate an understanding of the role of the supported decision-making into the competence assessment process as a preliminary stage, or first assess how well the potential participant responds to supported decision-making before assessing decisional competence to consent to research. The extension of supported decision-making techniques to advise individuals with fluctuating or deteriorating capacity on the consequences of research participation during a time where decisional competence is present (Stroup and Appelbaum 2003) suggests a further possibility along these lines.

9.7 Legal accommodation of supported decision-making

A principal advantage of supported decision-making is that it maximizes the extent to which cognitively vulnerable individuals both possess and exercise legal capacity, as opposed to having legal capacity exercised through a surrogate decision-maker (see Bielby 2005b, 359–61, for a discussion of types of legal capacity). In the final section of the chapter, I will consider the ways in which the current statutory legal framework in England and Wales could accommodate supported decision-making.

The Mental Capacity Act 2005 (hereafter MCA 2005) and its accompanying Code of Practice provide a statutory framework for regulating research that does not involve clinical trials (ss. 30–34). The Medicines for Human Use (Clinical Trials)

Regulations 2004 (hereafter 'the Clinical Trial Regulations') regulates clinical trials (ss. 28–31 and Schedule 1). There is no general exclusion of tissue-based research in either the MCA 2005 or the Clinical Trial Regulations; however, the Human Tissue Act 2004 more comprehensively regulates the removal, storage, and use of human tissue samples.

Schedule 1 Parts 1–5 of the Clinical Trial Regulations outline legal protections for adults, incapacitated adults, and children involved in clinical trials. However, there is no guidance on what approach should be taken if the potential participant's decisional competence to consent is questionable. The Human Tissue Act 2004 makes provisions relating to 'appropriate consent' for the removal and storage of tissue from children and adults (ss. 2 and 3 respectively), although nowhere in this Act is there reference to steps that must be followed to preserve or enhance decisional competence.

The MCA 2005, alternatively, provides in s. 1(2) a clear presumption in favour of the existence of decisional competence (referred to in the Act as 'capacity'). There is a requirement in s. 1(3) of the MCA 2005 that an individual should not be treated as incapable of making a decision 'unless all practicable steps to enable him to do so have been taken without success'. No case law has yet considered the question of what constitutes 'practicable steps', due to the Act only recently having fully come into force. The MCA 2005 Code of Practice, alternatively, suggests establishing the ways in which the individual is already familiar with communication, using a qualified interpreter, employing 'mechanical devices' (such as a voice synthesizer), engaging in non-verbal communication or offering speech or language therapy as examples of assistance in relation to maximizing capacity (Department of Constitutional Affairs (2007), para. 3.11 and para. 2.7). The core objectives of supported decision-making could fall within a broad interpretation of any of these examples of assistance. However, the MCA 2005 does not allow an individual to delegate in law the ability to make health care decisions (including research) to another individual whilst the individual still retains decisional competence (although this is possible in relation to property and affairs). This militates against the possibility of (e) in the schema for supported decision-making presented above.

By way of comparison, s. 1(6) of the equivalent Scottish provision, the Adults with Incapacity (Scotland) Act 2000, stipulates that:

> a person shall not fall within this definition [the definition of incapability of engaging in the decision-making process] by reason only of a lack or deficiency in a faculty of communication if that lack or deficiency can be made good by human or mechanical aid (whether of an interpretative nature or otherwise).

Although s. 1(6) does not suggest that the Scottish legislation is premised necessarily on a concept of supported decision-making, the wording of this section strongly indicates that supportive interventions are of utmost importance when a determination of mental capacity is at stake. Indeed, the emphasis upon remedying shortcomings of communication by an unspecified range of interpretative devices would seem to catalyse such supportive interventions. If a permissive interpretation of the duties upon health care professionals is adopted in relation to the MCA 2005 – and the Scottish legislation may prove a persuasive referent for the English courts – then there is greater potential for a legal accommodation of supported decision-making in English law.

It is important to emphasize that the MCA 2005 could not accommodate supported decision-making by way of the role of the Independent Mental Capacity Advocate (IMCA, set out in ss. 35–41 of the MCA 2005). The function of the IMCA is qualitatively different in two respects from the concept of supported decision-making. First, the IMCA pertains only to individuals who have already been found to be incompetent to make decisions of that particular type. It does not encompass individuals with questionable capacity who may still be able to make decisions of that type. The use of IMCAs is restricted to scenarios where the person for whom the intervention is designed to benefit does not have a Lasting Power of Attorney or a Deputy appointed. Unlike the supported decision-making approach, then, the IMCA becomes operative only where an individual already has been found to lack decisional competence and where no other authorized surrogate exists.

Second, the role of the IMCA is limited to certain specified scenarios: provision of serious treatment by an NHS body and provision of accommodation by an NHS body or by a local authority (MCA 2005, ss. 37–39). This adds weight to the terminological preference for 'supported decision-making' rather than 'advocacy', which has a distinct legal meaning as a result of the implementation of the MCA 2005. The former thus more easily extends to encompass the idea of provision of information and advice to an adult who is still competent, in spite of experiencing a mental disorder or intellectual disability. In the *Consultation on the Independent Mental Capacity Advocate Service* (UK Department of Health 2005), the Government signalled their willingness to consider expanding the service to include individuals who are not suffering from mental incapacity for the purposes of the Act and intimated that the service could expand to include research (*ibid.*, 38). However, the significant costs associated with expanding this service and the lack of enthusiasm for it in the consultation means that this was not carried forward in the Department of Health's 2006 response to the consultation or in The Mental Capacity Act 2005 (Independent Mental Capacity Advocates) (Expansion of Role) Regulations 2006. It is also worth noting that research does not fall within the remit of independent mental health advocates recently created by s. 30 of the Mental Health Act 2007 (but not yet in force at the time of writing).

9.8 **Conclusion**

There is a disjuncture between how the principle of consent is framed as an abstract concept and the practical experience of seeking consent. We have seen how overly abstracted understandings of informed consent are premised upon a problematic account of a disinterested self and risk marginalizing the nature of vulnerability, the need for potential participants to be supported in their decision-making and the consequent challenges this poses for the practice of consent. In light of this, consent has perhaps suffered less at the hand of its critics than from the limitations imposed on it by its own exponents.

I have argued, following Gewirth, Beyleveld, and Brownsword, that the proper place of consent is as an important procedural safeguard of rights to bodily and psychological integrity. Nevertheless, we should not exaggerate the significance of consent as though it were a substantive right itself. Difficulties arise when capacities for autonomous decision-making are assumed which marginalize or exclude the role of practices which assist in autonomous decision-making. Cases where the participants themselves experience cognitive vulnerability that could undermine decisional competence epitomize these difficulties.

To this end, supported decision-making as proposed in this chapter offers a promising strategy to nurture cognitively vulnerable participants' abilities to make decisions. This would take place within a helping relationship that is non-hierarchical and supportive. It moves the debate away from the traditional dichotomy between autonomy and paternalism to refocus attention on the idea that in order to make an autonomous decision – or to decide to delegate such decisions to anyone else for that matter – the decision-maker first needs to receive support to be able to do so. This idea is particularly important where the presence or absence of decisional competence is open to doubt. In this situation, judgements of decisional incompetence would only apply to those individuals who are clearly not amenable to having their decision-making abilities supported, or once reasonable attempts at supported decision-making have failed.

I do not suppose that supported decision-making offers a panacea. Additional arguments are required to apply these recommendations to informed consent for types of research that give rise to novel ethical implications, such as genetic testing (Boylan 2002), biobanking (Corrigan and Tutton 2004), genetic pedigree research (Parker 2002), or brain research (Glannon 2007). To this end, there is also a need for extensive empirical research on the issue of supported decision-making to ascertain how best the idea would operate in practice. Furthermore, any subsequent, explicit acceptance of supported decision-making in English law would require concerted attention both within and beyond the legislative chamber or courtroom. As Gordon rightly remarks:

> [s]upported decision-making is more than a formal legal status granted by a court; it is a process that occurs over time and that will invariably require more than a short-term commitment to address a particular and temporary need.

(2000, 73)

Even with much work still to do, we have nonetheless gone some way to recast consent as a value and practice that is sensitive to the experience of cognitively vulnerable participants. We have good reason to reflect on this as a means to make progress in biomedical research ethics with consent rather than as a way to move beyond it altogether.

Acknowledgements

My particular thanks go to Kathleen Liddell and Tony Ward for their invaluable comments on earlier drafts of this chapter. The conference participants in Hinxton in July 2005 discussed a first draft of the chapter and made numerous suggestions, which were most helpful. In addition, I am grateful to Don Carrick for his diligent research assistance and to Susan Bielby for having introduced me to the work of Carl Rogers.

References

Adults with Incapacity (Scotland) Act (2000) (2000 asp 4). Available at: http://www.opsi.gov.uk/legislation/scotland/acts2000/asp_20000004_en.pdf [accessed 28/02/08].

Appelbaum, P.S. and Grisso, T. (2001). *The MacArthur Competency Assessment Tool for Clinical Research*. Sarasota: Professional Resource Press.

Appelbaum, P.S., Grisso, T., Frank, E., O'Donnell, S., and Kupfer, D. J. (1999). Competence of depressed patients for consent to research. *The American Journal of Psychiatry*, **156**, no. 9, 1380–4.

Beauchamp, T. and Childress, J.F. (2001). *Principles of Biomedical Ethics* (5th edition). New York: Oxford University Press.

Benaroyo, L. and Widdershoven, G. (2004). Competence in mental health care: a hermeneutic perspective. *Health Care Analysis*, **12**, no. 4, 295–306.

Benhabib, S. (1992). *Situating the Self: Gender, Community and Postmodernism in Contemporary Ethics*. London: Polity Press.

Berg, J.W., Appelbaum, P.S., Lidz, C.W., and Parker, L.S. (2001). *Informed Consent: Legal Theory and Clinical Practice*. New York: Oxford University Press.

Berghmans, R., Dickenson, D., and Ter Meulen, R. (2004). Mental capacity: in search of alternative perspectives. *Health Care Analysis*, **12**, no. 4, 251–63.

Beyleveld, D. (1991). *The Dialectical Necessity of Morality: An Analysis and Defense of Alan Gewirth's Argument to the Principle of Generic Consistency*. Chicago: The University of Chicago Press.

Beyleveld, D. and Brownsword, R. (2001). *Human Dignity in Bioethics and Biolaw*. Oxford: Oxford University Press.

–ibid.– (2007). *Consent In The Law*. Oxford: Hart Publishing.

Bielby, P. (2005a). Equality and vulnerability in biomedical research on human subjects. *Imprints: Egalitarian Theory and Practice*, **8**, no. 3, 219–48.

–ibid.– (2005b). The conflation of competence and capacity in English medical law: a philosophical critique. *Medicine, Health Care and Philosophy*, **8**, no. 3, 357–69.

–ibid.– (2008). *Competence and Vulnerability in Biomedical Research*. Dordrecht: Springer.

Boylan, M. (2002). Genetic testing. *Cambridge Quarterly of Healthcare Ethics*, **11**, 246–56.

Breden,T.M. and Vollmann, J. (2004). The cognitive based approach of capacity assessment in psychiatry: a philosophical critique of the MacCAT-T. *Health Care Analysis*, **12**, no. 4, 273–83.

Brownsword, R. (2004). The cult of consent: fixation and fallacy. *Kings College Law Journal*, **15**, 223–51.

Buchanan, A E. and Brock D.W. (1990). *Deciding for Others: The Ethics of Surrogate Decision-making*. New York: Cambridge University Press.

Buckles, V. D., Powlishta, K.K., Palmer, J.L., *et al.* (2003). Understanding of informed consent by demented individuals. *Neurology*, **61**, 1662–6.

Carpenter, W..T, Gold, J.M., Lahti, A.C., *et al.* (2000). Decisional capacity for informed consent in schizophrenia research. *Archives of General Psychiatry*, **57**, no. 6, 533–8.

Clarke, A. (1994). Introduction. In *Genetic Counselling*, edited by A. Clarke. London: Routledge.

Corrigan, O. (2003). Empty ethics: the problem with informed consent. *Sociology of Health and Illness*, **25**, no. 3, 768–92.

Tutton, R. and Corrigan, O. (2004). *Genetic Databases: Socio-Ethical Issues in the Collection and Use of DNA*. London: Routledge.

Council of Europe (2005a). *Additional Protocol to the Convention on Human Rights and Biomedicine concerning Biomedical Research,* Treaty Series No. 19, Strasbourg: Council of Europe. In *Texts of the Council of Europe on Bioethical Matters: Volume 1,* edited by Directorate General I – Legal Affairs Bioethics Department. Strasbourg: Council of Europe. Available at: http://www.coe.int/t/e/legal_affairs/legal_co-operation/bioethics/texts_and_documents/INF_2005_2e%20vol%20I%20textes%20CoE%20bioethique.pdf [accessed 28/02/08].

–ibid.– (2005b). *Explanatory Report to the Additional Protocol to the Convention on Human Rights and Biomedicine concerning Biomedical Research*. Strasbourg: Council of Europe. Available at: http://conventions.coe.int/Treaty/EN/Reports/Html/195.htm [accessed 28/02/08].

Department of Constitutional Affairs. (2007). *Mental Capacity Act 2005 Code of Practice*. London: TSO. Available at: http://www.justice.gov.uk/docs/mca-cp.pdf [accessed 28/02/08].

Dresser, R. (2001). *When Science Offers Salvation: Patient Advocacy and Research Ethics*. New York: Oxford University Press.

Dunn, L.B., Lindamer, L.A., Palmer, B.W., Schneiderman, L.J., and Jeste, D.V. (2001). Enhancing comprehension of consent for research in older patients with psychosis: a randomized study of a novel educational strategy. *American Journal of Psychiatry*, **158**, 1911–13.

Eckstein, S. (2003). Research involving vulnerable participants: some ethical issues. In *Manual for Research Ethics Committees,* edited by S. Eckstein. Cambridge: Cambridge University Press.

Elliott, C. (1997). Caring about risks: are severely depressed patients competent to consent to research? *Archives of General Psychiatry*, **54**, 113–16.

Faden, R.R., Beauchamp, T.L., and King, N.M.P. (1986). *A History and Theory of Informed Consent*. New York: Oxford University Press.

Feenan, D. (1997). Capable people: empowering the patient in the assessment of capacity. *Health Care Analysis*, **5**, no. 3, 227–36.

Fitzgerald, D.W., Marotte, C., Verdier, R.I., Johnson Jr, W.D., and Paper, J.W. (2002). Comprehension during informed consent in a less developed country. *Lancet,* **360**, 1301–2.

Flory, J. and Emanuel, E. (2004). Interventions to improve research participants' understanding in informed consent for research: a systematic review. *Journal of the American Medical Association*, **292**, no. 13, 1593–601.

Gewirth, A. (1978). *Reason and Morality*. Chicago: The University of Chicago Press.

–ibid.– (1996). *The Community of Rights*. Chicago: The University of Chicago Press.

–ibid.– (1998). *Self-Fulfilment*. Princeton, NJ: Princeton University Press.

Gilligan, C. (1982). *In a Different Voice: Psychological Theory and Women's Development*. Cambridge, MA: Harvard University Press.

Glannon, W. (2007). *Bioethics and the Brain*. New York: Oxford University Press.

Glass, K.C. (1997). Refining definitions and devising instruments: two decades of assessing mental competence. *International Journal of Law and Psychiatry*, **20**, no. 1, 5–33.

Goffman, E. (1961). *Asylums: Essays on the Social Situation of Mental Patients and Other Inmates*. Harmondsworth: Penguin.

Gordon, R.M. (2000). The emergence of assisted (supported) decision-making in the Canadian law of adult guardianship and substitute decision-making. *International Journal of Law and Psychiatry*, **23**, no. 1, 61–77.

Harding, L. (2004). Cannibal who fried victim in garlic is cleared of murder. *The Guardian*, 31/01/04. Available at: http://www.guardian.co.uk/print/0,3858,4848810–103681,00.html [accessed 28/02/08].

Harré, R. (1998). *The Singular Self: An Introduction to the Psychology of Personhood*. London: Sage.

House of Lords and House of Commons Joint Committee on the Draft Mental Incapacity Bill (2003). *Draft Mental Incapacity Bill, Volume I - Report Together with Formal Minutes*. London: TSO. Available at: http://www.publications.parliament.uk/pa/jt200203/jtselect/jtdmi/189/189.pdf [accessed 28/02/08].

Human Tissue Act (2004 (c. 30). London: TSO. Available at: http://www.opsi.gov.uk/acts/acts2004/pdf/ukpga_20040030_en.pdf [accessed 28/02/08].

Ingelfinger, F.J. (1972). Informed (but uneducated) consent. *New England Journal of Medicine*, **288**, 465–6.

Jonsen, A.R. (1998). *The Birth of Bioethics*. New York: Oxford University Press.

Karlawish, J. (2007). Research on cognitively impaired adults. In *The Oxford Handbook of Bioethics*, edited by B. Steinbock. Oxford: Oxford University Press.

Kipnis, K. (2004). Vulnerability in research subjects: an analytical approach. In *The Variables of Moral Capacity*, edited by D.C. Thomasma and D.N. Weisstub. Dordrecht: Kluwer Academic Publishers.

Lapid, M.I., Rummans, T.A., Pankratz, V.S., and Appelbaum, P.S. (2004). Decisional capacity of depressed elderly to consent to electroconvulsive therapy. *Journal of Geriatric Psychiatry and Neurology*, **17**, no. 1, 42–6.

Lindemann-Nelson, H. and Lindemann-Nelson, J. (1995). *The Patient in the Family*. New York: Routledge.

McMillan, J. and Gillett, G. (2002). Consent as empowerment: the roles of postmodern and narrative ethics. In *Health Care Ethics and Human Values*, edited by K.W.M. Fulford, D.L. Dickenson and T.H. Murray. Oxford: Blackwell.

Mental Capacity Act 2005 (c. 9). London: TSO. Available at: http://www.legislation.gov.uk/acts/acts2005/pdf/ukpga_20050009_en.pdf [accessed 28/02/08].

Mental Health Act 2007 (c. 12). London: TSO. Available at: http://www.opsi.gov.uk/acts/acts2007/pdf/ukpga_20070012_en.pdf [accessed 28/02/08].

Merkel, R., Boer G., Fegert, J., et al. (2007). *Intervening in the Brain: Changing Psyche and Society*. Berlin: Springer.

Moreno, J. (1998). Convenient and captive populations. In *Beyond Consent: Seeking Justice in Research*, edited by J.P. Kahn, A.C. Mastroianni, and J. Sugarman. New York: Oxford University Press.

Morreim, E.H. (2004). By any other name: the many iterations of 'patient advocate' in clinical research. *IRB: Ethics and Human Research*, **26**, no. 6, 1–8.

Mulhall, S. and Swift, A. (1996). *Liberals and Communitarians* (2nd edition). Oxford: Blackwell.

Murphy, J.G. (1979). Incompetence and paternalism. In *Retribution, Justice and Therapy: Essays in the Philosophy of Law*, edited by J.G. Murphy. Dordrecht: D. Reidel Publishing.

National Commission for the Protection of Human Subjects of Biomedical and Behavioral Research (1979). *The Belmont Report: Ethical Principles and Guidelines for the Protection of Human Subjects of Biomedical and Behavioral Research*. Washington, DC: US Government Printing Office. Available at: http://www.hhs.gov/ohrp/humansubjects/guidance/belmont.htm [accessed 28/02/08].

Noddings, N. (2003). *Caring: a Feminine Approach to Ethics and Moral Education* (2nd edition). Berkeley: University of California Press.

O'Neill, O. (2002). *Autonomy and Trust in Bioethics*. Cambridge: Cambridge University Press.

Parker, L.S. (2002). Ethical issues in bipolar disorders pedigree research: privacy concerns, informed consent, and grounds for waiver. *Bipolar Disorders*, **4**, 1–16.

Rawls, J. (1972, rev. ed. 1999). *A Theory of Justice*. Oxford: Oxford University Press.

Rogers, C.R. (1961). *On Becoming A Person*. London: Constable.

Roth, L.H., Lidz, C.W., Meisel, A., *et al.* (1982). Competency to decide about treatment or research: an overview of some empirical data. *International Journal of Law and Psychiatry*, **5**, 29–50.

Sadler, J.Z. (2005). *Values and Psychiatric Diagnosis*. Oxford: Oxford University Press.

Sandel, M.J. (1984). The procedural republic and the unencumbered self. *Political Theory*, **12**, no. 1, 81–96.

–ibid.– (1998). *Liberalism and the Limits of Justice* (2nd edition). Cambridge: Cambridge University Press.

Savulescu, J. (1995). Rational non-interventional paternalism: why doctors ought to make judgments of what is best for their patients. *Journal of Medical Ethics*, **21**, no. 6, 327–31.

Savulescu, J. and Momeyer, R.W. (1997). Should informed consent be based on rational beliefs? *Journal of Medical Ethics*, **23**, no. 5, 282–8.

Stiles, P.G., Poythress, N.G., Hall, A., Falkenbach, D., and Williams, R. (2001). Improving understanding of research consent disclosures among persons with mental illness. *Psychiatric Services*, **52**, no. 6, 780–5.

Stroup, S. and Appelbaum, P. (2003). The subject advocate: protecting the interests of participants with fluctuating decision-making capacity. *IRB: Ethics and Human Research*, **25**, no. 3, 9–11.

The Medicines for Human Use (Clinical Trials) Regulations (2004). SI 2004/1031, London: TSO. Available at: http://www.opsi.gov.uk/si/si2004/20041031.htm [accessed 28/02/08].

The Mental Capacity Act 2005 (Independent Mental Capacity Advocates) (Expansion of Role) Regulations 2006. SI (2006/2883. London: TSO. Available at: http://www.opsi.gov.uk/SI/si2006/uksi_20062883_en.pdf [accessed 28/02/08].

The Vulnerable Persons Living With a Mental Disability Act (1993 (Man.), S.M. (1993 (c. 29). Available at: http://web2.gov.mb.ca/laws/statutes/ccsm/v090e.php [accessed 28/02/08].

UK Department of Health (2005). *Consultation on the Independent Mental Capacity Advocacy Service*. London: Department of Health. Available at: http://www.dh.gov.uk/prod_consum_dh/idcplg?IdcService=GET_FILEanddID=22394 andRendition=Web [accessed 28/02/08].

–ibid.– (2006). *Consultation on the Independent Mental Capacity Advocate (IMCA) Service (2005: Summary of Responses*. London: Department of Health. Available at: http://www.dh.gov.uk/prod_consum_dh/groups/dh_digitalassets/@dh/@en/documents/digitalasset/dh_4133915.pdf [accessed 28/02/08].

Wong, J.G., Clare, I.C.H., Holland, A.J., Watson, P.C., and Gunn, M.J. (2000). The capacity of people with a 'mental disability' to make a health care decision. *Psychological Medicine*, **30**, 295–306.

Chapter 10

Is consent sufficient?
A case study of qualitative research with men with intellectual disabilities

Margaret Ponder, Helen Statham,
Nina Hallowell, and Martin Richards

10.1 Introduction

The triumph of autonomy in western bioethics (Callahan 1994) is illustrated by the prominence given to informed consent in the deliberations of research ethics committees (RECs), institutional review boards (IRBs) and other ethical oversight bodies (e.g., Ethics and Governance Council of UK Biobank). Indeed, one could be forgiven for thinking that obtaining research participants' consent is all that is required to make research ethical in some cases.

The salience of informed consent within research ethics has grown in recent years (Corrigan 2003; Faden and Beauchamp 1986). From the Nuremberg Trials (Nuremberg Code 1949) through to the Belmont Committee's deliberations (The National Commission for the Protection of Human Subjects of Biomedical and Behavioral Research 1979), there has been a recognition that research participants' autonomy can be protected through the mechanism of informed consent. Consent is necessary to ensure research participation is voluntary (Nuremberg Code 1949) but while voluntariness is an important aspect of consent, it is not sufficient to protect autonomy. Arguably, autonomy can only be safeguarded if consent is informed, that is, if research participants understand that to which they are consenting. Guaranteeing that research participants understand the procedures involved in research and the risks they entail is difficult and raises a number of practical issues for researchers. RECs and IRBs commonly require that potential participants should receive information about: the research aims, what the research participation entails, the risks and benefits to self and others, the right to withdraw, the right to compensation, and the right to standard care following withdrawal, *etc.* Thus, ensuring that consent is informed involves not only giving research participants a great deal of complex information about the research and their role within it, but also ensuring that they understand it. Any failures in research participants' understanding of any aspect of the research – the risks, benefits, processes, or goals (e.g., Appelbaum *et al.* 1982) raises questions about the validity of their consent (Corrigan 2003).

In this chapter, we describe a research project involving persons with intellectual disabilities that we recently completed. The project raised a number of ethical issues for us, but the most vexing were to do with consent. In what follows, we will address the question of whether having an individual's consent is sufficient justification for including them in research.

The research in question examined some of the consequences for families of being part of a molecular genetics research study which set out to find the genetic cause for a condition – moderate to severe intellectual disability (ID) – which had affected some male family members (Ponder *et al.* 2008). While the cause for the ID was unknown, the pattern of its occurrence in male family members over generations strongly suggested an X-linked genetic condition.[1] However, genetic testing had failed to reveal any diagnosis; so, genetic researchers had assembled a group of these families and set out to try to identify gene mutations that might cause the condition (Raymond 2006). That research study was called the Genetics of Learning Disability or GOLD study (http://goldstudy.cimr.cam.ac.uk/). This type of research ('gene hunting') has revealed the genetic basis of a large number of Mendelian genetic diseases over the last 20 years (e.g., Huntington's disease, inherited forms of breast and ovarian cancer – BRCA 1 and 2).

As social scientists, we were interested in the ways in which family members experienced their involvement in such genetic research and what it might mean for them if gene mutations were found, or indeed, not found.

Finding the genetic cause of a disorder is important for understanding the basic biology of the disorder, but it also has other implications. In X-linked conditions, women who are found to be carriers of the gene mutation can have affected sons. Thus, when a gene mutation is found, one of the consequences is that it will give some family members the opportunity to make reproductive decisions based on genetic tests. Prenatal genetic diagnosis can be used to identify affected fetuses and women can choose to terminate the pregnancy. In the future it is possible that pre implantation genetic diagnosis[2] may be used as an alternative to avoid births of affected boys. Family members were often aware of these possibilities when they joined the GOLD study.

Our original research plan was to interview family members, in particular, sisters (who might be healthy carriers of the gene mutation) and the mothers and fathers

---

[1] An X-linked condition is one that is generally passed from mother to son. Males have one X and one Y chromosome while women have two X chromosomes. Thus men inherit their X chromosome from their mother. If a woman has a mutation in one of the genes in her X chromosomes, on average she will pass it to 50% of her children. As women have two X chromosomes, inheriting one with a gene mutation will not normally cause disease, as the normal gene on the other X chromosome will usually override the effect. However, in some X-linked conditions, the female carriers may have mild symptoms. A female with a disease-causing gene mutation on her X chromosome is known as a carrier.

[2] Pre implantation genetic diagnosis involves a woman having IVF to produce a number of embryos. These embryos are then tested at a very early stage so that only those found to be free of the genetic fault are implanted into the woman.

of affected boys and men, but not the affected men themselves. We had considered including these men, but decided that, given the severity of the disorder for most of them, they would be unlikely to be able to tell us very much about their experiences of participation in the GOLD study or what successful gene hunting might mean for them or their relatives. We knew that the participation of the affected men in the GOLD study by providing blood samples for DNA analysis was essential to that study, but we felt it would be better not to include them in our interview-based research. However, when we applied for a research grant, a referee of the research proposal argued strongly for interviewing the affected men and commented that it would be discriminatory to exclude them. The funders suggested that we should follow this advice so we did.

It is perhaps relevant to say here that we are not part of a specialist ID research group. Rather our expertise lies in undertaking research with families about sensitive issues in their family life and especially with those who carry serious genetic disorders (e.g., inherited breast cancer, Huntington's disease, cystic fibrosis, etc.). We were particularly interested in the GOLD study because it allowed us the possibility of a prospective study of the experience of gene hunting, which had never been done before. Social scientists, like ethicists, often seem to follow events rather than watch them unfold. But here was an opportunity to talk to family members before the gene hunting produced any results. We were also very aware that of the many genetic disorders that had been studied (by geneticists or social scientists), relatively little attention had been paid to ID. However, the intellectual disability was not the focus of this aspect of our research.

10.2 **Background**

Our research set out to investigate the impact and experience of participation in a molecular genetic study, specifically looking at the experiences of research participation from the initial point of consent through to the end of the project 3–5 years later. We wanted to explore (a) family members' motives for participation, (b) their understanding of the consent process, (c) their knowledge, expectations, and understanding of the research aims and objectives of the GOLD study, (d) experiences of the feedback of genetic research results, (e) impact on family members of receiving, or not receiving, a molecular genetic diagnosis as a result of the research, (f) their perceptions of the disorder and the communication of information within the families, and (g) these families' views about genetic research more generally. We chose to study participants in this particular molecular genetic study because it offered us the possibility of engaging family members in a study before and after they might receive a genetic diagnosis of the condition running in their family.

10.3 **The GOLD study**

The aim of the GOLD study was to find genetic mutations that are associated with ID. All participant families had two or more male relatives with moderate or severe ID. All had been investigated for known genetic causes of ID and none had been found. All the families based in the British Isles[3] were known to clinical genetics services. They had initially been approached to take part in the GOLD study by a local clinical geneticist. After consent or proxy consent (in the case of the more severely disabled and those who were children) had been given, blood samples for the genetic analysis were taken from family members including affected males, their mothers, and selected unaffected people. Ninety families who had taken part in the GOLD study were approached to take part in our interview study.

As we have discussed already, we had not originally planned to interview any men with ID as we had felt that most would be too disabled to participate actively. A reviewer of the grant application (and our funders) felt that we should attempt to include them, arguing that 'by excluding them we might reinforce existing stereotypes' and that 'including them may be a positive experience for the men/boys that might offer new insights whilst allowing them to feel included and respected'. It is our experiences of attempting to do this that we describe here.

10.4 Planning and developing the interviews

The two research interviewers (H.S. and M.P.) have significant experience in interviewing individuals and families about genetics, ill health, disability, and reproductive choice. We had personal and prior professional experience of people with ID, but had not previously interviewed people with ID as part of a research project. In order to develop an appropriate research approach, we read widely, talked to and met people working in the field, including people with ID who were active advocates of inclusion. We then approached the Fragile X Society (a UK charity that supports, and works with and on behalf of, families affected by Fragile X[4]) and developed a pilot study with a small number of families who had used DNA testing to confirm a diagnosis of Fragile X. We told the Society that we had been encouraged to include people with ID in our research and while they continued to support our research plans they voiced some concerns about the usefulness of such an endeavour. The pilot study was approved by the Cambridge Psychological Research Ethics Committee and the main study was approved by the London Multi Centre Research Ethics Committee.

10.5 Pilot phase

A number of families were approached by the Fragile X Society and asked if they would be willing to take part in an interview study which aimed to explore their

---

[3] The GOLD study included families from several countries across the world but only those from the UK or Ireland were included in our study because of the complications and costs of including those from other countries.

[4] Fragile X Syndrome is the most common cause of inherited ID. It is caused by an abnormality of the X chromosome and may result in a wide range of difficulties with learning, as well as social, language, attentional, emotional, and behavioural problems. It accounts for about 3% of all ID in males. Some female carriers are affected, but usually more mildly than males.

Box 10.1 Extract of information sheet to be read to person with Fragile X

Why do they want to talk to us?
Because they want to find out what people like you and families like ours understand about how you are and about what sort of things we need.

What will they ask about?
They will ask about school, what you like doing, about yourself, and about things that you feel are important in your life.
They will ask about how you feel about having a learning difficulty.

Why are they talking to us?
They want to know what is important for you and your family/all of us [Mum, Dad, brothers, and sisters]. It will show them more about how doctors and nurses should talk to us and how families like ours can best be helped.

experiences of receiving a diagnosis through a genetic test. Those agreeing sent back a consent form with contact details. We explained our research further on the telephone when we were arranging interviews and introduced the idea that we would like to talk to some affected men if possible. If the family thought their son/brother might be willing to participate, we sent them a simplified version of the information sheet that was designed to be read to the person with ID by their carer along with a consent form that could be signed by the person themselves or their proxy.[5] The information sheet explained who the researchers were, what participants would have to do, that tape recordings would be used, that participants could have someone with them in the interview and that they did not have to take part if they did not want to. (See Box 10.1 for an extract of the information sheet to be read to the person with Fragile X.) It also contained sections emphasizing confidentiality and the freedom to withdraw from the research at any time.

We interviewed 27 people from 11 families. This included five men/boys who had moderated to severe ID as a result of Fragile X (ages ranged from teens to 50+) and

---

[5] At the time of these interviews, it was held that a person who lacked capacity to consent could be involved in research if the research was consistent with their best interests. To help ascertain this, it was usual to ask a family member or carer for proxy consent, although strictly speaking this was not itself valid consent. The Mental Capacity Act 2005 came into force in 2007. Since then, there is no longer a requirement to show that a research intervention is in the best interests of the incapacitated person, but the research must involve a benefit to the individual proportionate to the risks, or if it offers no benefit, it should not involve anything more than a negligible risk and should not be unduly invasive or restrictive. A carer or nominated consultee must be consulted, and if they believe the individual would be likely to decline to participate in the research (or wish to withdraw from it), the research cannot proceed.

four women who were mildly affected gene carriers. The four mildly affected women were able to use the standard information sheet and consent form and were treated exactly as those without ID: none of these interviews will be discussed here.

10.5.1 Consent from men/boys with Fragile X

Five of the 11 families had given assent for their sons/brothers to be approached. Those with ID were then approached to give their consent. In one case, the man did not want to participate on the day and that interview was not attempted. In a second case, although the man had already signed his own consent form, he indicated on the day that he did not want to talk to us. The researcher told the carer not to persist but the carer was very keen that the interview should take place because s/he felt it would be a useful experience for the young man in circumstances that s/he considered to be unthreatening. After much discussion, the interview took place. The man was given the tape recorder to control and most of the interview was about football and TV programmes, although some attempt to cover the planned interview topics was made once it was clear he was happy to talk. In one interview, in which two brothers were seen together, there was no hesitation and the researcher felt that consent had been freely given. Another interview took place in a residential home after agreement to ask the affected man had been obtained from several family members and the staff at the care home. The man had signed a form prior to the interview, was waiting for the interviewer to arrive, seemed to understand, and was clearly willing to talk. While talking to the interviewer, he appeared increasingly anxious but declined offers to stop and the interviewer felt it might undermine him if she ended the conversation prematurely. However, very few interview topics were covered. At the end of the interview, it became apparent that he had soiled himself. Although this confirmed to the interviewer that he had been made very uncomfortable, later telephone calls to the care staff on two occasions to check this indicated that in their opinion he had not been upset by the experience in any way. In the final family, the young man was interviewed in the presence of his parent/carer who helped him to answer questions and although he appeared happy, he had very little to say. The parent/carer in this case had been happy for the young man to participate, but had voiced doubts as to how useful we would find it.

These examples suggest that families/carers might have inadvertently cajoled individuals to take part. In the case where the carer insisted on the interview going ahead, clearly there was 'pressure' but the man being interviewed appeared happy once it had started. Maybe this interview should not have been undertaken? However, to refuse to continue would have undermined the authority of the carer who knew the man well. Where the parent/carer was present and participating the young man had little to say and it was hard to judge whether or not he was participating freely. The researcher's concern about the man in the residential home was dismissed by the care staff. However, the researcher still has grave misgivings about that interview and while the discomfort may not have been lasting, it was clear that it had happened.

10.6 The style and content of interviews

The men we spoke to understood that they had agreed to chat with someone; however, we do not believe that they understood what they were going to be asked to talk about even though we had tried to make sure that they had been fully informed (see Box 10.1). We adapted the interview we had conducted with non-disabled family members both in terms of content and style, using a very gentle and non-confrontational style. In all cases, extra time was taken at the beginning and throughout, to make sure participants were comfortable. We were interested in people's experiences of having an intellectual disability and of getting a diagnosis through a genetic test. We were assured by all the families that the people we were interviewing knew about their diagnosis of learning problems. We approached the topic by first trying to ascertain as spontaneously as possible individuals' awareness and understanding of their disability. We approached the topic by asking them to talk about their everyday lives and to compare themselves with family members or friends. We also asked about college, school, work, and about family likenesses (colour of eyes, hair, etc.). In one interview, we talked about drawings that the young men had done. However, responses were mostly very short and unrelated to our research questions. Trying to explore their experiences of getting a diagnosis or opinions about genetic testing was not possible and it was clear from these interviews that we would be unable to answer our research questions about receiving a genetic diagnosis with people as impaired as these people were.

10.7 The main study

10.7.1 Severity of ID in the GOLD study families

Of the 90 UK families from the GOLD study that we approached, 120 members of 37 extended families took part in our study. Within these families there were only 28 men with ID aged 16 years or over. Fifteen of these men lived independently, six with minimal help (i.e., help managing their money and with major decisions), and nine with considerable support from others (these men needed help with many every-day tasks). The other 13 were severely affected and needed full-time care: most of these were unable to communicate verbally.

As a result of our experiences in the pilot phase we decided that we should only include less disabled men who could answer some of the same questions as their non-disabled relatives. We expected to simplify the interview schedule, but we did not have the time or resources to modify the methods, for example, arranging to meet with the men on a number of occasions prior to the interview (Ward *et al.* 2002). This reduced the number of possible participants with ID to 15.

In all the families, non-disabled people had been interviewed before we approached those with ID. As with the pilot study, we relied on non-disabled family members to facilitate access to their disabled relatives. The information sheet for those with ID was similar to that used in the pilot study. It emphasized: the voluntary nature of the research, the freedom to withdraw at any time, and the use of tape recording and also included some specific information relating to the GOLD study (see Box 10.2 for an extract of the information sheet).

Our interviews with the non-disabled people included: an introductory discussion about their experiences of having a relative with ID, memories of being recruited to the GOLD study, the consent procedure, knowledge of the research project, understanding of genetics, and opinions about the use of genetic technology

---

Box 10.2 Extract of information sheet for all participants in the main study

Why have I been approached?

You are being asked to take part in the study because you have a relative who has a learning disability and some members of your family are taking part in a genetics research study, the GOLD study.

What is the purpose of this new study?

The study will look at:

◆ family life where a boy has a learning disability;

◆ what it is like to become part of a genetics research study; and

◆ what may change for families when the results of the genetic research are known.

This study will help us to find out what is important for families – parents, the boys/men with learning disabilities, and their brothers and sisters. It will show us more about how doctors and scientists should explain their research and what support families like yours might want.

(Ponder *et al.* 2008). For the men with ID, we hoped to cover the same ground but modified the introductory discussion to ask about their experiences of growing up and living with ID.

10.8 Interviews with men who had intellectual disability

Following interviews with non-disabled family members, we identified an initial nine men/boys with ID who we thought would be able to participate. Their relatives indicated that they thought their son/brother would be able, and might like, to take part in our study. However, two of them were absent when we expected to meet them, which we understood to be an indication that they did not want to participate. We, therefore, obtained consent from, and interviewed, seven men with ID. All appeared able to read our information sheet and all gave consent themselves. Two were very mildly affected (A and B) and required very little help and support from their families. The other five (C, D, E, F, G) were slightly more disabled. Although some of these men lived away from home they needed help with organizing their lives and managing money and had limited social interactions other than with their family and with people with similar disabilities. One of the mildly affected men was interviewed with his non-disabled partner and one of the more disabled was interviewed with his wife who also had moderate ID. Ages ranged between 18 and 60, three were married, two lived with their parents, and two lived on their own (one has since returned to his parents).

The interviews with A and B followed the same pattern as the interviews with their non-disabled relatives. They were less expansive than most of the other interviewees in our study, but we were able to cover all the topics on our interview schedule.

Both had relatives with more severe ID and had they not been part of a family identified as having inherited ID they might not have been given this label.

In the other five interviews with the men who were less able, we frequently departed from our interview schedule in an effort to make the interviewee feel more comfortable. Thus, we often retreated from our main research questions and allowed them to talk about issues that they found more interesting, such as their experiences of childhood, jobs, friendships, and their lives more generally. These five interviewees acknowledged that they had some form of learning disability although they used different terms to describe this such as 'a bit slow' (C), 'this slow learning' (D), and 'backwards' (E).

In all the interviews, we asked about their memories of consenting to, and taking part in, the GOLD study and giving a blood sample. These men had clear memories of giving a blood sample but, like their non-disabled relatives, had poor recall of the consent procedures (Ponder *et al.* 2008). However, all could remember that the focus of the research was about their learning disability and obtaining a diagnosis. Like many of their non-disabled relatives they said that they had taken part because they were pleased to help. However, as with some of their non-disabled relatives (Ponder *et al.* 2008), it was difficult to know whether or not they felt they had been cajoled or pressurized into participating in GOLD, or indeed, our research, in any way.

Trying to find out whether they understood the aims of the GOLD project, or what they expected would happen, was much more difficult, and was more likely to cause embarrassment as they were unsure of their answers. We responded to non-verbal indications of embarrassment (e.g., long pauses, coughs, sighs, and laughs) by altering our questions:

I: Did you have to sign anything?

E: [very high tone, quite laughingly] No, no.

I: And have they told you anything about …?

E: [very high tone, quite laughingly] No, no. I'm in the dark. I do these things like.

I: Have you given blood lots of times before?

E: I'm a blood donor.

A conversation followed about blood donation. The answers the men gave were often very short; there were many awkward pauses which conventional transcription techniques cannot adequately represent. Moreover, there was evidence that our study questions failed to engage this group of men.

I: Do you know what they will do when they find the results, if they get a result?

E: They'll probably let Dad know and Dad'll let me know.

I: … learning disabilities can happen in more than one person in a family? Do you know how it works at all?

G: Haven't got the foggiest.

I: Would you like to know at all?

G: Not really ha ha …

Except for the interviews with the two mildly affected men, we felt those with men with ID were unsatisfactory on two counts. First, although we struggled to make sure the men did not feel disadvantaged or embarrassed because they could not answer some of our questions, we felt that the interviews had not been a positive experience for them. The men's attitude to being interviewed was very passive, suggesting that participation in our study was not experienced as rewarding. However, it must be noted that in contrast to the pilot study, there was no evidence that the men found the interview disturbing, although some were clearly embarrassed at being unable to answer our questions at times. Second, the data we collected in these interviews failed to answer the study questions; it provided no new information or insights into this group of participants' experiences of the GOLD study. Thus, while there was no evidence that participation in our interview study had explicitly harmed these men, their participation did not further the study's aims and objectives either.

10.9 Discussion

Because of the reactions of this group to being interviewed we decided not to approach the families of the remaining six men with ID who we had originally felt we would like to include. This decision was informed by our experience as interviewers who have tackled subjects that are often sensitive, complex, and occasionally difficult. Although we had not interviewed people with ID as part of a research study before, we both had experience of communicating with and being with people who have ID in other capacities and, thus, recognized that those who had taken part in our study had found the interviews challenging at times.

We have reflected on the question as to whether or not we should have gone ahead and included the men with ID in this study. We had taken care to make their inclusion as pleasant as possible, and we believed that we had acted responsibly and ethically when recruiting them, for we had: discussed our wish to interview the disabled men with their carers, provided tailored information which 'appeared to be understood' by the men with ID, at least in part, and we had asked for and gained their consent. But despite all this, when reflecting upon our experiences we still have doubts about the extent to which their consent was valid or meaningful. While we were sure, in the case of the main study, that all the men with ID had participated voluntarily, it was not really clear to us that they had really understood what they had volunteered to do and, thus, that their consent was informed.

Our initial approach to carers, who were all close family members, was in line with the guidelines that will soon be in place to accompany the Mental Capacity Act 2005 in England and Wales. The Act sets out clear rules for involving adults who lack capacity in research. There is separate legislation for Scotland (Scottish Executive 2001), but both pieces of legislation provide similar provisions for research participation (see Box 10.3).

The provisions of the MCA governing research cover a variety of different types of clinical and social research, including research like the interview study which is the focus of this paper. As the Act has only recently come into force, guidelines concerning who should be involved in the decision to recruit someone who lacks capacity

---

Box 10.3 Information from the Mental Capacity Act 2005 for England and Wales: summary of conditions concerning research participation

- Research involving, or in relation to, a person lacking capacity may be lawfully carried out if an 'appropriate body' (normally a research ethics committee) agrees that the research relates to the person's condition and cannot be done as effectively using people who have mental capacity. The research must produce a benefit to the person that outweighs any risk or burden. Alternatively, if it is to derive new scientific knowledge, it must pose negligible risk to the person and be carried out with minimal intrusion or interference with their rights.

- Carers or nominated third parties must be consulted and agree that the person would want to join an approved research project. If the person shows any signs of resistance or indicates in any way that he or she does not wish to take part, the person must be withdrawn from the project immediately.

---

were in preparation during our study. It is proposed that nominated consultees, who ideally would be relatives or close friends, should be consulted about whether or not someone lacking capacity should be a research participant. Where family members may be unable, or unavailable, to support the person who lacks capacity, this role is to be undertaken by members of specially established independent panels of consultees.

The MCA covers all of those who lack capacity, the majority of whom are persons who through illness, age-related degenerative processes, or injuries have lost their capacity, usually in later life. In such cases, family and friends who are consenting on their behalf will often have a good idea about what the person would have chosen when they had capacity and been able to decide for themselves. The men with ID that we interviewed in our study had never had full capacity, and so their proxies had to base their decision on their knowledge of these men – what they liked, disliked, or were able to do – and the proxy's own views and attitudes about the research. The extent to which the proxies' perceptions of our research influenced their decision to give permission for their relatives to be approached is unknown; however, it can be speculated that their reasons were not always straightforward. All the family carers that we approached had themselves taken part, were very pro research, and extremely keen to help us not only by participating themselves, but also by facilitating the inclusion of men with ID. Given that some of the participants in the pilot study, in particular, were clearly uncomfortable during the interviews we have wondered to what extent their consent was voluntary and felt that, in some cases, family carers may have been a little over-enthusiastic about their relatives' participation.

Many people with ID have limited capacity and, thus, are able to give consent to research participation for themselves. However, while involving this group in the decision-making process is aimed at maintaining their autonomy, it can present problems for researchers, not least because it may be difficult to assess their decision-making competence accurately (Wong *et al.* 2000, and Chapter Nine by Bielby in this book). Indeed, this may, in part, account for some of our unease about the present study, for although we approached the less disabled men following consultation with their relatives, and they appeared to give their consent, as the study progressed we were less certain that they were really clear about what was expected of them. Indeed, the fact that we had to frequently abandon the interview schedule and discuss more familiar, but unrelated, topics with these men suggested to us that many of these men had been unaware of what our research entailed when they had consented to take part. Thus, we questioned the validity of their consent and it was this that led us to modify our protocol and not ask others from this subgroup to participate.

It is accepted that it is unethical to carry out research without consent (Nuremberg Code 1949), but is it unethical to decide not to continue with research after consent has been obtained? As was noted in the introduction to this chapter, despite what our dealings with RECs and IRBs may sometimes lead us to believe, consent is more than obtaining a signature on a form or research participants' verbal permission to include them. Valid consent to research participation must necessarily be voluntary and informed (Nuremberg Code 1949; World Medical Association 2004). Moreover, as the Declaration of Helsinki makes clear, it is the researchers' responsibility to ensure that consent is not only valid at the outset, but remains valid throughout the life of the project. In the case of clinical trials, there is always a clause in the information that is given to would-be participants which explains that the trial may be stopped at any time for safety reasons or if new information indicates that the trial is no longer needed. Indeed, one of the main purposes of data monitoring committees is to make sure that clinical research can obtain its objectives (the primary and secondary endpoints); if this should cease to be the case, then the data monitoring committee will stop the trial prematurely. In line with how we would normally conduct an interview study such as this, we gave no such warning to our participants. It was apparent after the pilot study that the interviews might provide very little, if any, data so we made the decision to only recruit more able men during the main part of the research. Even though we did this, we felt that the interviews that took place were of little use. However, we also felt it was difficult to tell the men with ID whom we had already recruited that they would not be needed. In retrospect, should we have warned the men in advance that they might not be required for an interview? That would be different from how research would normally be conducted and furthermore, we would have felt uneasy about rejecting their offer of participation once given in case the 'rejection' caused further upset or left the men feeling stigmatized.

In Chapter Nine of this volume, Bielby discusses whether consent is always sufficient and, using the example of consensual cannibalism, concludes that there are times when consent does not justify something going ahead if it is clearly wrong. The Mental Capacity Act (2005) dictates that research with individuals who lack capacity must be either to generate new knowledge or to be of benefit to those who take part. Arguably, including the men with ID in our study was not *wrong* per se, for we assumed that they might contribute to knowledge about this group's views on participation in genetic research. However, it became clear that interviews with these men were not providing information that could be used, and, more importantly, may have caused them minor psychological discomfort or embarrassment. At this point, it seemed more ethical to stop recruiting new interviewees with ID. With the benefit of hindsight, we now regret that we did not follow our original decision not to include the men with ID in our research.

10.10 Conclusion

In the field of ID research, participatory and emancipatory research designs have been used as tools for improving the lives of disabled people, enabling them to be active participants in research (Ramcharan *et al.* 2004). Unlike research in most fields, an important aim of these participatory studies is that research participation should be a positive experience for the disabled participants. We included men with ID in our interview study of family members' experiences of participating in molecular genetic research (the GOLD study) in response to the criticisms raised by a referee of our initial research proposal. Unlike the majority of ID studies, which focus on perceptions of ID services or quality of life, our research focused upon an area of life – taking part in scientific research – that the men with ID might be less familiar with. Unfortunately, for practical reasons, we were unable to adapt the study to make it more user-friendly for this group, and hence we had to include the men with ID on the same terms (with a few minor modifications) as those without ID.

With the luxury of hindsight, we feel that including the subgroup men with ID in our interview study was not necessary. Moreover, we feel that had we been less experienced interviewers, then the potential to cause harm or distress to these participants would have been greater. Originally we had decided not to include men with ID in the family study because although they had donated blood for testing in the GOLD study, we felt that they were unlikely to provide useable data in interviews. We now believe we were unwise to be persuaded by our funders to include them. We did this to counter criticism that we might be inappropriately discriminating against people with ID by not including them, but, arguably, this was not a good enough reason to have done so.

However, in saying that we should not have included the men with ID in this particular study, we are not advocating a return to the paternalistic practices of the past, in which vulnerable populations were excluded from research for 'their own good'. We believe when research questions are of direct relevance to people with ID or, as is the case with emancipatory research (Ramcharan *et al.* 2004), when people with ID have helped to formulate the research questions, then of course it is right, and arguably, necessary, to include them. However, if the topic is one that they are unfamiliar with or do not understand, and participation could make them uncomfortable, then we would question whether it is ethical to include them just because the research topic is (tangentially) related to ID.

In conclusion, ethical research practice is not only dependent upon following the rules outlined by research ethics committees but by researchers taking responsibility for the wellbeing of their research participants. In some studies, this may mean making a judgement call and overruling a consent given by a relative or an individual and sometimes this may have the result that the researchers are seen as discriminating against people with ID by excluding them from a research study. In such cases, we believe that exclusion should be seen not as discrimination or being overly paternalistic or protectionist, but as ethical research practice.

Acknowledgements

We would like to thank all the families who took part in our study; the Fragile X Society and Dr Lucy Raymond, and Jenny Moon for facilitating access to families who were part of the GOLD study. Our research was supported by the Wellcome Trust [grant number 068438].

References

Appelbaum, P.S., Roth, L.H., and Lidz, C. (1982). The therapeutic misconception: informed consent in psychiatric research. *International Journal of Law and Psychiatry*, **5**, 319–29.

Callahan, D. (1994). 'Bioethics: private choice and common good.' *The Hastings Center Report*, **24**, no. 3, 28–31.

Corrigan, O. (2003). Empty ethics: the problem with informed consent. *Sociology of Health and Illness*, **25**, 768–92.

Faden, R. and Beauchamp, T. (1986). *A History and Theory of Informed Consent.* New York: Oxford University Press.

The National Commission for the Protection of Human Subjects of Biomedical and Behavioral Research (1979). *Belmont Report: Ethical Principles and Guidelines for the Protection of Human Subjects of Research.* www.hhs.gov/ohrp/humansubjects/guidance/belmonts.htm

Nuremberg Code (1949). http://www.ushmm.org/research/doctors/Nuremberg_Code.htm

Ponder, M., Statham, H., Hallowell, N., Moon, J., Richards, M.P.M., and Raymond, F.L. (2008). Genetic research on rare familial disorders: consent and the blurred boundaries between clinical service and research. *Journal of Medical Ethics*, **34**, 690–94.

Ramcharan, P., Grant, G., and Flynn, M. (2004). Emancipatory and participatory research: how far have we come? In *The International Handbook of Applied Research in Intellectual Disabilities*, edited by E. Emerson, C. Hatton, T. Thompson and T. R. Parmenter. Chichester: John Wiley and Sons Ltd.

Raymond, F.L. (2006). X linked mental retardation: a clinical guide. *Journal of Medical Genetics*, **43**, 193–200.

Scottish Executive (2001). Adults with Incapacity (Scotland).

Ward, L., Howarth, J., and Rodgers, J. (2002). Difference and choice: exploring prenatal testing and the use of genetic information with people with learning difficulties. *British Journal of Learning Disabilities*, **30**, 50–5.

Wong, J.G., Clare, I.C.H., Holland, A.J., Watson, P.C., and Gunn, M. (2000). The capacity of people with a 'mental disability' to make a health care decision. *Psychological Medicine*, **30**, 295–306.

World Medical Association (2004). Declaration of Helsinki: Ethical Principles for Medical Research Involving Human Subjects. Available at http://www.wma.net/e/policy/63.htm

Chapter 11

Consent to genetic testing: a family affair?

Nina Hallowell

11.1 First things first

This chapter will explore the extent to which the familial nature of genetic information creates an ethical problem for our current conceptions of informed consent in the context of genetic testing. First, I will look at current understanding of the role of informed consent in research and clinical practice, and briefly outline the philosophical assumptions underpinning this concept. Second, I will sketch out and assess arguments that suggest that the new genetic technologies are subtly influencing the meaning (i.e., use) of *family*. The third section takes an empirical turn, and I will describe some of the findings of recent research that has explored individuals' motivations for undergoing genetic testing. Finally, I will endeavour to bring these differing strands together to argue that, as it stands, the accepted view of informed consent which is based upon an individualistic model of the person may be inadequate when it comes to genetic testing. In the closing section I will suggest an alternative approach that merits consideration. What I do not intend to do is to look at the issue of privacy, confidentiality, and the duty to warn in the context of genetic testing, except in passing. These issues are covered by other commentators elsewhere (e.g., Nuffield Council of Bioethics 1993; Knoppers 1998; Sommerville and English 1999).

Before I proceed, I think it is appropriate to add a rider to this chapter. The focus of this collection is informed consent within the context of medical research; however, the research I will draw upon in the latter part of the chapter is not about individuals' experiences of taking part in genetic research per se, but of having predictive or diagnostic DNA testing in a clinical context. My reason for focusing on genetic testing in a clinical rather than research context is as follows.

As many authors have observed, there is a degree of confusion about the status of many 'genetics activities' in the UK at the present time (Newson and Ashcroft 2004), such that is not always clear whether DNA testing is taking place in a clinical or research context. Indeed, as Parker *et al.* (2004) note, in the case of rare genetic disorders it is particularly difficult to distinguish clinical investigation to provide a diagnosis, and research undertaken to characterize a set of mutations for scientific purposes – which will also potentially supply research participants with a diagnosis. This scenario is illustrated by the GOLD (the Genetics of Learning Disability) study (Tarpey *et al.* 2004); an exploratory genetic study involving the sequencing of the

X chromosome in families who have a history of learning disabilities in males. The aim of this research project is to characterize genetic mutations that may be involved in the aetiology of learning disabilities. As a by-product of this research, some participants will receive a genetic diagnosis of their child(ren)'s learning disabilities and other female family members may learn they are potential carriers of an X-linked disorder.

In other cases, where the boundary between research and clinical practice is more clearly demarcated, the status of research-based testing still remains ambiguous (e.g., the Anglian Breast Cancer study: a genetic epidemiological project which included clinical feedback of research results), not only because research results are used for diagnostic purposes, but also because research participation may be implicitly encouraged in order to obtain a diagnosis. Thus, although genetic testing for hereditary ovarian, colorectal, and breast cancers is currently available as a clinical service in the UK, it is widely acknowledged that DNA testing may be accessed more quickly through research protocols. For example, there is currently a large backlog of samples awaiting *BRCA1/2* testing for hereditary breast and ovarian cancer; thus, in an effort to cut waiting lists, patients may be recruited to the exploratory *BRCA3* study, in which they will be tested to exclude the possibility that their cancer was caused by *BRCA1/2* mutations. Study participation in this instance, enables patients to, as it were, 'jump the queue' and have a test they might otherwise have to wait several months for. As these examples illustrate, the route through which patients access DNA testing is not straightforward, and may be dependent on their clinician's involvement in clinical research and/or the availability of local clinical/NHS facilities. What is quite clear in the case of the *BRCA3*, Anglian Breast Cancer, and GOLD studies is that clinical research, which is 'technically' non-therapeutic, may have a clinical benefit for those participants who are actively seeking a diagnosis. Whether the patients who participate in such projects are aware of this anomalous situation and, if so, whether they care, are empirical questions, which are the subject of ongoing investigations.[1]

To summarize, the decision to fail to differentiate genetic testing that takes place in research and clinical contexts in the current chapter is based upon the observation that the boundary between clinical practice and research in the field of medical genetics is fluid and highly ambiguous.

11.2 Informed consent: familiar perspectives in research and clinical practice

The model of informed consent used within clinical research is justified on the basis of respect for autonomy. Informed consent procedures exist to protect the

---

[1] Hallowell, N., M. Parker, and A. Lucassen, 'Cancer genetics – Research or clinical care? Lay and professional understanding of cancer genetics activities in the UK.' Project grant Cancer Research UK, 2005–7. Richards, M.P.M., N. Hallowell, H. Statham, and L. Raymond, 'Psychosocial effects of molecular genetic diagnosis: the case of X-linked learning disability.' Project grant Wellcome Trust, 2002–7.

individual's right to self-determination or self-governance; more specifically, their right to voluntarily accept or refuse research participation and be informed of the benefits/risks that they may incur through their participation (Beauchamp and Childress, 1994).

As many authors including Corrigan, McMillan, and Weijer (in the Introduction to this volume) have noted, the privileging of subjects' autonomy in clinical research, as codified in the Declaration of Helsinki (e.g., Articles 10–12, 2000), has arisen in response to the involuntary experimentation carried out in the Nazi concentration camps and other infamous instances of human subject experimentation, such as the Tuskegee study of syphilis in the US.

The 20th century also witnessed an increasing focus upon patient autonomy in clinical practice; a trend that was particularly pronounced within clinical genetics. This subspeciality of medicine is based upon an ethos of non-directiveness, which emphasizes the need for clinician/counsellor neutrality in all dealings with patients/clients (Clarke 1997). Thus, ideally, clinicians/counsellors should provide value-neutral information (objective 'facts') about genetic risks and the risks/benefits of genetic testing, while patients/clients interpret this information in the light of their pre-existing values and make an informed and uninfluenced decision about how to manage their risk – including whether to proceed with genetic testing or not. As Shiloh (1996) notes, the task of the clinician/genetic counsellor is not to direct the patient/client to make wise decisions, but to enable them to choose between the options wisely (see also Wang *et al.* 2004).

According to Huibers and van 't Spijker (1998), autonomous decision-making about genetic testing must satisfy the following conditions:

1. **voluntariness** – the patient/counsellee can choose otherwise (weak voluntariness) or there is absence of external coercion/pressure/influence (strong voluntariness)

2. **alternativity** – there are at least two available options

3. **adequate information** – the patient/counsellee is provided with as much information about the risks and benefits as a 'reasonable person' needs on which to base their decision

4. **competence** – the patient/counsellee is capable of gaining a comprehensive view of the options and their consequences.

Likewise, Beauchamp and Childress (1994) define autonomous decision-making in medical encounters as: (i) intentional, (ii) based upon understanding, and (iii) not subject to controlling influences.

Both of these definitions assume an individualistic conception of autonomy, in which, as was noted above, autonomy is seen as the individual's capacity for self-governance. But whilst autonomous decision-making and, thus, informed consent, may be reliant on a number of factors, arguably the defining feature of **autonomous** decisions is that they are uncoerced or free of influence (see O'Neill 2002, 2003). Indeed, delegating the responsibility for testing decisions or consent to patients/research participants, that is, requiring them to determine which course of action is in their best interests, given the available information, can be seen as all-important, for it enables clinical geneticists/researchers to distance themselves from some eugenic practices of the past.

However, while grounding consent on an individualistic conception of autonomy may appear to protect freedom of choice (see O'Neill 2002, 2003 for a critique of this conception of autonomy), as will be demonstrated below, it can be argued that such a model fails to take into account the fact that all decisions are contextualized and that this context may undermine individuals' capacity for self-determination and, thus, the notion of informed consent.

11.3 Genetics: a family affair?

Biological relationships are at the heart of clinical genetics and, thus, can be seen as the *raison d'etre* of genetic testing. By revealing the biological similarities and differences that exist between individuals and their descendants and antecedents, and relating these to particular phenotypes, genetic testing reveals information about individuals'[2] future health risks. It has been argued that this prescient quality of genetic testing has profound implications for the ways in which we conceive of family and kinship.

Finkler (2001) claims that by promising us a glimpse of potential futures that we may use to our own and other family members' advantage, genetic testing has transformed the way in which we view family relationships. According to Finkler, the introduction of genetic testing in the latter half of the 20th century has resulted in the medicalization of family and kinship. She argues that genetic technologies, by prioritizing biological relatedness, present a challenge to post-modern conceptions of 'family' which see family connections as grounded in socio-emotional ties rather than biological similarities. Finkler sees the medicalization of kinship or the rise of the 'biogenetic' family as characterized by an increasing focus on biological rather than social relationships, which, she claims, can be discerned in the emphasis on family history in medical consultations and a growing determination on the part of individuals to trace members of their biological kinship and familiarize themselves with their family history of disease (Finkler 2000, 2005). Indeed, it could be argued that the biologization of family relationships has also entered into the realm of public policy in the United Kingdom; for example, the Child Support Agency's use of DNA testing to resolve paternity disputes and the recent moves to remove donor anonymity in the case of gamete donation (see Richards 2006; Freeman and Richards 2006.)

However, while Finkler may be correct in noting a change in the ways in which we, as a society, conceptualize family relationships in the public domain, Richards (2001), amongst others, has argued that she may have overstated the extent to which the new genetic technologies have biologized family and kinship in the private sphere. In contrast to Finkler, Richards observes that lay views about the inheritance of disease and biological relatedness have a long history, which predate the discovery of DNA and the advent of molecular genetic testing. Thus, he comments that the biogenetic model of kinship is not a new phenomenon, as Finkler suggests, and points out that

---

[2] Predictive or diagnostic DNA testing identifies family members as mutation carriers/non-carriers and, thus, categorizes them as affected/unaffected by disease or at-risk/not-at-risk of disease.

biological relationships are just one way, amongst many, of conceptualizing *family* that exist within society.

Following Richards, it can be argued that what Finkler fails to acknowledge is that while the advent of DNA testing may, indeed, have resulted in the reification of biological relationships in certain contexts or circumstances, those persons who undergo genetic testing perceive themselves as related to others in a social and emotional as well as a biological sense. As the next section will demonstrate, recent research suggests that genetic testing decisions are frequently framed in terms of social responsibilities, responsibilities that emerge from, and are grounded within, the social relationships which exist between family members (Hallowell *et al.* 2003, 2005; Burgess and d'Agincourt Canning 2001; Downing 2001).

11.4 **Informed consent to genetic testing: familial perspectives**

Empirical studies of decision-making about genetic testing suggest that one of the major factors influencing individuals' decisions to proceed with testing, or attend genetic counselling, is to generate information about other family members' risks (Goelen *et al.* 1999), most frequently their offspring (Liede *et al.* 2000; Lodder *et al.* 2001; Daly *et al.* 2003; Biesecker *et al.* 2000). Indeed, many studies suggest that most individuals regard their relatives as having an interest in the information they receive from DNA testing or genetic counselling (Hallowell 1999; d'Agincourt-Canning 2001; Hallowell *et al.* 2003, 2005).

In recent years, I have worked on two studies that have looked at individuals' experiences of genetic testing for breast and ovarian cancer. Study I focused on (former) breast cancer patients who had undergone diagnostic genetic testing (*BRCA1/2* mutation searching[3]). Study II involved high-risk men who had predictive *BRCA1/2* testing[4] and also included their partners (primarily wives) and adult daughters.

---

[3] *BRCA1/2* mutation searching has one of two outcomes. A **confirmatory** result – that is, the patient is confirmed as a mutation carrier and, therefore, deemed to be at increased risk of developing other primary carcinomas of the breast/ovary – or an **inconclusive** result – that is, the patient does not carry a known *BRCA1/2* mutation. The latter result is less informative because it does not exclude the possibility that their cancer is caused by either an unknown mutation or a mutation in another unknown gene. These test results have different implications for (male and female) offspring. In the case of the former, the risks of children carrying a *BRCA1/2* mutation rise to 50%; in the case of the latter, children's risks of carrying a susceptibility mutation remain at 25%.

[4] Predictive *BRCA1/2* testing has one of two outcomes. Tested individuals may be found to be mutation **positive** or mutation **negative**. The former confirms risks of developing breast and ovarian cancers in women and breast, colorectal, and prostate cancers in men. Predictive DNA testing also confirms the risk status of offspring. Mutation carriers' children have a 50% risk of inheriting a mutation and, thus, an increased risk of developing cancer, while non-carriers' children are no longer at risk of carrying a mutation and, therefore, are not at increased risk of developing these cancers.

Although these two studies contained different groups of patients – men and women who were identified as mutation positive, at-risk women awaiting test results, at-risk women who received an inconclusive (i.e., uninformative) test result, and men who were confirmed mutation negative – their views on genetic testing were striking in their similarity.

When asked about their motivations for undergoing genetic testing all of those who had undergone testing described their actions as influenced by their perceptions of other family members' needs. For example, Mary, a breast cancer patient in Study I, said she had undergone testing because she would:

> ... do anything to help my children, and that's the way I look at it very selfish, I know, but in the full spectrum it helps other people, I would help other people, but the thing that concerns me is my family. ... I think in the testing there's nothing for me to be gained from it, other than as I say, for my family.

> *(at-risk with an inconclusive result)*

Likewise Angela, who was awaiting her DNA test results when I interviewed her, cited her feelings of responsibility for her brothers' children as influencing her decision to proceed with testing:

> I've got two nieces and obviously I felt a responsibility to, towards them and to their parents. So I thought for them also it would be useful and that I should do my bit really.

> *(at-risk)*

Finally, Deirdre, a gene carrier who had just completed adjuvant therapy for ovarian cancer, said that she had no personal interest in her test results and had undergone testing primarily to generate information for other family members. She reflected:

> ... it's [testing] not really made a huge difference to me at all. I suppose it, I feel sort of that I have done something for the rest of my family in helping them, going through the test so that's quite a nice feeling, but nobody in my family appreciates that I have done it.

> *(mutation positive)*

Genetic testing reveals risk information about oneself and related family members. In Study I receiving a mutation positive result not only confirmed the presence of a mutation within the family, thus confirming the at-risk status of biological kin, but also provided information about the women's risks of developing another primary breast/ovarian cancer. As I have noted elsewhere (Hallowell *et al.* 2004), very few of the women in Study I expressed an interest in having their cancer risks confirmed by testing, indeed, some had undergone testing even though they would have preferred to remain in ignorance of their health risks. The majority of women in this study saw their family's need for genetic information as greater than their own need to know, or not know,[5] their genetic status and, thus, made a decision about testing with others' needs in mind.

---

[5] See Andorno (2004) for a discussion of the right to not know genetic information about oneself.

However, while the knowledge that they had acted in, what they assumed were, others' best interests was regarded as paramount, the women also talked about the anxieties and dilemmas generated by genetic testing. Thus, for some being confirmed as a carrier resulted in feelings of existential anxiety – they reported feeling very anxious about their risks of developing other cancers and worried about the risks to their children – others commented that they felt unprepared for the responsibility of disclosing this information to other at-risk family members. A task which was described as raising ethical dilemmas they had not anticipated, such as: who to tell, when to tell them, how to tell them, and what they should do if others did not want to know. Thus, although genetic testing was seen as offering these women the chance to act responsibly, it was also experienced as ethically contentious in ways they had neither imagined nor expected.

Like the women in Study I, the men in Study II were also in the position of being able to establish their own risks of developing cancer from genetic testing, and as in Study I, this motivation was seen as much less important than establishing the risks to children. All the men said they had accessed predictive testing primarily to ascertain information that their children could use. Information they believed their children had an interest in knowing, and that they, as parents, had a responsibility to provide. Thus, Kevin said he had undergone testing because he was worried about his sons' risks, and felt he had a responsibility to determine his carrier status for their sakes:

> I was concerned about the future of my sons, because obviously if I carried the gene there was a chance that they would. So obviously I needed, it was a responsibility to them as well.

> *(mutation negative)*

Similarly, Mike, another non-carrier father of three young daughters, said he was less interested in finding about his own risks than determining the risks to his children:

> The risk to me wasn't that big, that would affect my health and me that much. I just wanted to know for the benefit of others.

> *(mutation negative)*

Finally Tom, who had been confirmed as a carrier, said the decision to undergo testing required little deliberation, for he knew that he had to have testing for his family's sake.

> I just looked at it – I didn't even think about it. I mean I knew that if it was going to help the family, I had to have it done ...

> *(mutation negative)*

Like the women in Study I, the men in Study II regarded their decision to undergo genetic testing as other-oriented rather than egocentrically motivated. In consenting to testing, they saw themselves as acting for the benefit of their children – people they cared about and/or cared for. However, although testing may have been motivated by beneficent intentions, that did not mean that it was necessarily undertaken voluntarily: many of the men in this study described how other people, namely their partners, had been instrumental in the testing decision. For example, John had been persuaded by his wife to undergo testing, despite his worries that confirmation of their risk status might increase his daughters' anxieties about developing cancer:

> I was a little hesitant about whether it was a good idea or a bad idea, because it seemed to me you could sort of argue that if it turned out bad [mutation positive] that would simply increase the level of worry for my children.

(mutation positive)

Indeed, many of the men in this study acknowledged their partner's interests in the test results and, as noted above, their partner's right (as the mother of their children, in most cases) to be involved in making testing decisions. These sentiments were echoed by many of the partners interviewed in this study, who said they felt they had a right to be involved in decision-making about testing because test results had implications for their children (Hallowell *et al.* 2005). Such observations confirm the view that social relationships and their associated responsibilities influence testing decisions. Finally, the (adult) children interviewed in Study II said they felt that they also had a role to play in their father's testing decision. In two cases, daughters described their distress upon learning that their father had proceeded with testing without informing them. These young women, who had been confirmed as non-carriers as a result, said they felt that in failing to consult them their father had undermined their right to determine when and whether they had their risk status confirmed by DNA testing.

Thus, Study II, like Study I, suggested that genetic testing is perceived as a family matter. These women and men described themselves as either having a responsibility to undergo testing to generate information for their kin or, alternatively, constructed their reticence to take a test as born out of a responsibility to relatives who they thought might be harmed by gaining information about their risk status (see also Burgess and d'Agincourt Canning 2001) – thus, other family members (biological and married-in kin) were seen as playing an implicit role in their testing decisions. In Study II, and to a lesser extent in Study I, there was also evidence of a more explicit form of familial influence on patients' testing decisions; insofar as other family members expressed the opinion that they had a right to be involved in their partner's/father's decision to take a genetic test (see also Donchin 2000, 245).

The data collected in Studies I and II and some other research in this area (e.g., Burgess and d'Agincourt Canning 2001; Downing 2001) suggest that in reality, genetic testing has come to be constructed as a manifestation of familial responsibility, in some instances, rather than an individual choice.[6] As the participants in these

----

[6] It must be noted that whilst the current studies and other research on *BRCA1/2* testing and predictive testing for Huntington's disease (HD) suggest that other family members (in)directly influence testing decisions, these observations may be disease-specific. First, testing decisions may be less egocentrically motivated in the case of *BRCA1/2* and HD because no effective or easily implemented prevention strategy exists (to counteract the risks of breast/ovarian cancer or HD – although risk-reducing surgery has recently been demonstrated to decrease morbidity in the case of breast/ovarian cancer).

studies acknowledged, because one's descendants and antecedents are necessarily implicated by genetic test results and, thus, may benefit from, or be harmed by, this knowledge, other family members, both biological and non-biological relatives, have an important, if implicit, role to play in genetic testing decisions. In both of these studies those who had undergone testing constructed testing decisions as benefiting self **and/or** others and thus, as being subject to relational (i.e., social) influences. As such, it is difficult to describe consent to genetic testing in these cases as an autonomous act or a demonstration of the participants' 'individual independence' (O'Neill 2003).

At this point one can ask whether consent to genetic testing should be seen as an expression of individual autonomy.[7] Clearly, I do not advocate that at-risk individuals undergo genetic testing against their will, but, given the familial nature of genetic information, is it really realistic to require that consent to genetic testing is an independent action[8] that is completely free of external influence?[9]

The research described above suggests that while the actual process of consenting to testing may be regarded as an exercise of individual autonomy – for after all, it is the individual who voluntarily signs the consent form or allows blood to be drawn from their arm – the decision to undergo testing is not autonomous, in the sense that it is based upon isolated self-interest, in every case. These observations suggest that we may need to consider an alternative approach to consent in the context of genetic testing; one which recognizes that human beings, as social beings, exist within a network of relationships that is structured by responsibilities. Arguably, we need to acknowledge that these 'relational responsibilities' (Burgess and d'Agincourt-Canning 2001) may have a direct and/or indirect influence on the choices individuals make about genetic testing and, thus, are implicated in consent.

To summarize, the empirical research suggests that the decision to undergo or forego genetic testing may be less about self-determination and fostering one's autonomy than acting responsibly towards others (Hallowell *et al.* 2003; Hallowell 1999; Burgess and d'Agincourt Canning 2001). In the final section, I will look at the implications of these findings for informed consent in the context of genetic testing.

....

[7] As Donchin (2000) notes, contrary to their followers and, indeed, the contemporary debate, Beauchamp and Childress (1994) were aware of the problems inherent in postulating a strongly individualistic view of autonomy, in which persons are seen as independent selves (see also Hallowell *et al.* 2003). Donchin argues that insofar as Beauchamp and Childress acknowledge that society and relationships provide a background against which self develops, they postulate, what she terms, 'a weak relational' view of autonomy. However, as Donchin points out, their view of autonomy can be seen as inadequate because they fail to acknowledge that relationships are constitutive of self-hood, that is, selves are defined in terms of the relationships they have with others.

[8] See Dawson and Kass (2005) who describe similar tensions arising when undertaking research in communities in which the concepts of individual autonomy and individual decision-making are seen as culturally inappropriate.

[9] It should be taken as read that all actions are potentially influenced or constrained by structural inequalities, arising from socio-economic, gendered, and ethnic differences, to name but a few.

11.5 **Conceptualizing consent to genetic testing: familial or familiar issues?**

Empirical research on decision-making about genetic testing suggests that, in some instances, testing is seen as an issue for the family not just the individual patient, an observation that raises questions about the suitability of regarding consent primarily in relation to individual autonomy. While I am not claiming that we can reach conclusions about what consent to genetic testing should be on the basis of these empirical observations, the data collected in a growing number of studies suggest that we may need to consider an alternative approach. Such an approach would take into account the social nature of human beings and explicitly acknowledge that their actions and choices are often influenced by virtue of the fact that they exist within a network of social relationships. In this final section of the chapter, I will assess an approach to consent in genetic testing that champions the adoption of a more contextualized and experiential or lived ethic, as encapsulated in the concept of 'relational responsibility' (Burgess and d'Agincourt-Canning 2001).

Burgess and d'Agincourt Canning (2001) call for the adoption of an experienced-based ethical approach to informed consent in the context of genetic testing, rather than one based upon an abstract idea of duty and obligation (see John, Chapter Seven in this volume). While recognizing the need to protect individual patient choice, they argue that if we are to facilitate informed consent in an ethical manner, then we need to acknowledge that individuals' choices are framed and moulded by their social experiences. As noted above, they observe that the choices that people make about genetic testing are influenced by their commitments or responsibilities to specific others. These relational responsibilities are regarded as 'central to the choices we make' (p. 363). According to Burgess and d'Agincourt-Canning (2001), relational responsibilities derive from specific life experiences and, thus, pertain to particular relationships (e.g., my physician–me, my mother–me) in particular circumstances. They argue that as relational responsibility is an emergent property of particular relationships, it is dynamic and ever-changing and, thus, contrasts with the abstract role-based responsibilities (e.g., doctor–patient, parent–child) imposed by society, which are static and maintained by social expectations and associated sanctions.

So what are the implications of the adoption of the concept of relational responsibility for informed consent to genetic testing? Burgess and d'Agincourt Canning (2001) note that focusing upon the relational responsibilities individuals have towards each other may enhance the consent process: primarily because relational responsibilities derive from particular circumstances, they are seen as voluntary rather than externally imposed. Thus, while they may influence individuals' choices – to have or reject a test – they do not constitute an externally imposed constraint on choice, in contrast to role-based responsibilities or, indeed, abstract duties (John, Chapter Seven in this volume), which impose abstract requirements to behave in certain ways. In practical terms, this would involve counsellors encouraging patients to focus upon the relational aspects of their lives and acknowledge the ways in which they may influence their choices. Thus, counselling would emphasize the notion of 'family' as a relational network connected by shifting responsibilities, rather than focusing upon 'family' as a collection of individuals bound by biological ties and pre-determined duties and rights.

However, as Burgess and d'Agincourt-Canning (2001) note, while a focus on relational responsibility may emphasize the social nature of individual agency in many situations including genetic testing, the adoption of such an approach is not unproblematic. As they observe, in many cases relational and role-based responsibilities may co-exist, and this may undermine the voluntary nature of relational responsibility, which may in turn potentially threaten the voluntary nature of informed consent. As they note, we need 'to consider who is being assigned responsibility, for what and by whom' (p. 370). Thus, while it may be the case that the relational responsibility may be an emergent property of particular relationships, it can be argued that there are few relationships which are completely voluntary.

Indeed, as Donchin (2000, 241) notes, many of the most significant relations we have – such as family relationships – are non-voluntary and bring with them pre-assigned role-responsibilities over which we, as individuals, have little control. Indeed, such observations seem very pertinent in the case of genetic testing. For if Finkler's observations about the changing conceptualization of 'family' are correct, and family relationships are increasingly seen as imposed by nature (or at least, society's prioritizing of nature) rather than as voluntary social arrangements, then perhaps the commitments emerging from such relationships may come to be regarded as similarly pre-determined or non-voluntary. If this is the case, then it could be argued that the decision to undergo a genetic test may come to be seen as less to do with acting responsibly towards certain significant others, than fulfilling one's duties to one's biological kin. In other words, if family is seen as primarily a biological category rather than a social network of interpersonal dependencies and responsibilities, then the decision to undergo testing may be seen as less of a 'choice' than it appears.

In conclusion, in this chapter I have argued that genetic testing is ultimately about relationships – biological and social relationships. I have suggested, following Burgess and d'Agincourt-Canning (2001), that if we are to make sense of the consent in this context, then we need to adopt a different view, one that stresses less the individuality of consent and instead emphasizes the implicitly social nature of genetic testing decisions. A view of consent that is particularized not universal, that acknowledges that others' needs are intimately involved in genetic testing decisions, that prioritizes the social context in which testing decisions are taken and choices are made.

It is widely accepted that one of the most important aspects of consent is that it is non-coerced or freely given (O'Neill 2002). However, if genetic testing decisions are to be seen as truly free or uncoerced, then individuals not only need to be able to say 'yes', but also must be able to refuse genetic testing. If we are to enable them to exercise this choice, then we need to give them the opportunity to reflect upon the impact that any decision may have upon their relationships with particular others. Genetic testing does not take place within a social vacuum and, as the empirical research outlined above suggests, genetic testing decisions are not perceived as morally neutral choices. Consent procedures need to emphasize these things, not sweep them under a carpet of information about abstract risks and benefits.

Acknowledgements

I would like to thank all of the women and men who took part in these studies and my collaborators and colleagues who were involved both directly and indirectly in this research: Sue Davolls, Claire Foster, Clare Moynihan, Audrey Ardern-Jones, Ros Eeles, Vicky Murday, Anneke Lucassen, Fiona Lennard, and Maggie Watson. The empirical research described in this chapter was carried out while I was employed at the Institute of Cancer Research in London. The research was funded by grants awarded to Maggie Watson from Cancer Research UK. Finally, I would like to thank the editors of this collection, particularly Oonagh Corrigan, for inviting me to contribute.

References

Andorno, R. (2004). The right not to know: an autonomy based approach. *Journal of Medical Ethics*, **30**, 435–9.

Beauchamp, T.L. and Childress, J.F. (1994). *Principles of Biomedical Ethics*. New York: Oxford University Press.

Biesecker, B.B., Ishibe, N., Hadley, D.W., *et al.* (2000). Psychosocial factors predicting BRCA1/BRCA2 testing decisions in members of hereditary breast and ovarian cancer families. *American Journal of Medical Genetics*, **93**, 257–342.

Burgess, M. and d'Agincourt-Canning, L. (2001). Genetic testing for hereditary disease: attending to relational responsibility. *The Journal of Clinical Ethics*, **12**, 361–72.

Clarke, A. (1997). The process of genetic counselling: beyond non-directiveness. In *Genetics, Society and Clinical Practice*, edited by P.S. Harper and A.J. Clarke. Oxford: Bios.

Donchin, A. (2000). Autonomy and interdependence: quandaries in genetic decision-making. In Mackenzie, C and Stolja N. eds. *Relational Autonomy: Feminist-perspectives on Autonomy, Agency and the Social Self*. Oxford: Oxford University Press. 236–258

d'Agincourt-Canning, L. (2001). Experiences of genetic risk: disclosure and the gendering of responsibility. *Bioethics*, **15**, 231–47.

Daly, P.A., Nolan, C., Green, A., *et al.* (2003). Predictive testing for BRCA1 and 2 mutations: a male contribution. *Annals of Oncology*, **14**, 549–53.

Dawson, L. and Kass, N.E. (2005). Views of US researchers about informed consent in international collaborative research. *Social Science and Medicine*, **61**, 1211–22.

Downing, C. (2001). *Reproductive Decision-Making in Families Facing the Risk for Huntington's Disease: Perceptions of Responsibility*. PhD Thesis, University of Cambridge.

Finkler, K. (2000). *Experiencing the New Genetics*. **61**, 1059–71 Philadelphia: University of Pennsylvania Press.

Freeman, T. and Richards, M. (2006). DNA testing and kinship: paternity geneology and the search for the 'truth' of genetic origins. In Ebtehaj, F., Lindley B., and Richards, M. (eds). *Kinship Matters*. 67–95. Oxford: Hard Publishing.

–ibid.– (2001). The kin in the gene: the medicalisation of family and kinship in American society. *Current Anthropology*, **42**, 235–63.

–ibid.– (2005). Family, kinship, memory and temporality in the age of the new genetics. *Social Science and Medicine*, **61**, 1059–71. http://www.sciencedirect.com/science accessed 15/03/2005.

Goelen, G., Rigo, A., Bonduelle, and De Greve, J. (1999). Moral concerns of different types of patients in clinical BRCA1/2 gene mutation testing. *Journal of Clinical Oncology,* **17,** 1595.

Hallowell, N. (1999). Doing the right thing: genetic risk and responsibility. *Sociology of Health and Illness,* **21,** 597–621.

Hallowell, N., Ardern-Jones, A., Eeles R., *et al.* (2005). Men's decision-making about predictive BRCA1/2 testing: the role of family. *Journal of Genetic Counseling,* **14,** 207–17.

Hallowell, N., Foster, C., Eeles, R., Ardern-Jones, A., Murday, V., and Watson, M. (2003). Balancing autonomy and responsibility: the ethics of generating and disclosing genetic information. *Journal of Medical Ethics,* **29,** 74–9.

Hallowell, N., Foster, C., Eeles, R., Ardern-Jones, A., and Watson, M. (2004). Accommodating risk: women's responses to BRCA1/2 genetic testing following a cancer diagnosis. *Social Science and Medicine,* **59,** 553–65.

Huibers, A.K. and van't Spijker, A. (1998). The autonomy paradox: predictive genetic testing and autonomy: three essential problems. *Patient Education and Counseling,* **35,** 53–62.

Knoppers, B. (1998). Towards a reconstruction of the 'genetic family' new principles? *International Digest of Health Legislation,* **49,** 241–53.

Liede, A., Metcalfe, K., Hanna, D., *et al.* (2000). Evaluation of the needs of male carriers of mutations in BRCA1 or BRCA2 who have undergone genetic counseling. *American Journal of Human Genetics,* **67,** 1494–504.

Lodder, L., Frets, P.G., Trijsburg, R.W., *et al.* (2001). Men at risk of being a mutation carrier for hereditary breast/ovarian cancer: an exploration of attitudes and psychological functioning during genetic testing. *European Journal of Human Genetics,* **9,** 492–500.

Newson, A. and Ashcroft, R. (2004). Time to untangle ethical review of genetic research. *Bionews* http://www.bionews.org.uk/new.lasso?storyid=2280

Nuffield Council on Bioethics (1993). *Genetic Screening: Ethical Issues.* London: Nuffield Council on Bioethics.

O'Neill, O. (2002). *Autonomy and Trust in Bioethics.* Cambridge: Cambridge University Press.

–*ibid.–* (2003). Some limits of informed consent. *Journal of Medical Ethics,* **29,** 4–7.

Parker, M., Ashcroft, R., Wilkie, A.O.M., and Kent, A. (2004). Ethical review of research into rare genetic disorders. *British Medical Journal,* **329,** 288–9.

Richards, M.P.M. (2001). Commentary on K Finkler's 'The kin in the gene'. *Current Anthropology,* **42,** 255–6.

Richards, M.P.M. (2006). Genes, geneologies and paremity: making babies in the twenty-first century. In *Freedom and Responsibility in Reproductive Choice,* edited by J. Spencer and A. Perdain. Oxford: Hart Publishing.

Shiloh, S. (1996). Decision-making in the context of genetic risk. In *The Troubled Helix: Social and Psychological Implications of the New Human Genetics,* edited by T. Marteau and M.P.M. Richards. Cambridge: Cambridge University Press.

Sommerville, A. and English, V. (1999). Genetic privacy: orthodoxy or oxymoron. *Journal of Medical Ethics,* **25,** 144–50.

Tarpey, P,. Parnau, J., Blow, M., *et al.* (2004). Mutations in the DLG3 gene cause nonsyndromic X-linked mental retardation. *American Journal of Human Genetics,* **75,** 318–324.

Wang, C., Gonzalez, R., and Merajver, S.D. (2004). Assessment of genetic testing and related counseling services: current research and future directions. *Social Science and Medicine,* **58,** 1427–42.

Chapter 12

Cultural authority of informed consent: indigenous participation in biobanking and salmon genomics focus groups

Michael Burgess and James Tansey

12.1 Introduction

The literature on ethics of research involving indigenous people emphasizes the inadequacy of individual informed consent, the importance of collaborative research design, and the importance of securing the permission of the group being researched (cf. Brunger and Weijer 2005; Burgess and Brunger 2001; Glass and Kaufert 2001; Kaufert *et al.*; Kaufert and Lavoie 2003; Weijer 1999, Weijer *et al.*, 1999; Weijer and Emanuel 2000). These concerns apply across the spectrum of health and social research, reflecting the concern to avoid further colonization of indigenous people through making them, their lives, and their knowledge simply objects to be studied (cf. Indigenous Peoples Council on Biocolonialism 2000). Central to these discussions is the critique of informed consent as an individualist model that cannot authorize research and the associated benefits and risks that are borne by groups. Community consent or the acceptability of research to the community or its authorized leaders is gaining wide acceptance as a new ethical principle in health and social research, as reflected in some of the ethical codes produced by governmental agencies or indigenous organizations (cf. Freeman 1998; Freeman and Romero 2002; Indigenous Peoples Council on Biocolonialism 2000; National Aboriginal Health Organization 2003; National Institutes of Health 2004; World Health Organization 2001).

   The clear message is that the goal of involving indigenous people in research must address or even give priority to their collective interests. This ethical emphasis is a response to the global history of colonization and within particular jurisdictions is reinforced by indigenous people's legal status. Although it is beyond the scope of this chapter, the substantive basis for extending protection to populations with common identity may extend beyond indigenous people to include those of common genomic, social, or geographical heritage (e.g., ethno-cultural groups or persons with disabilities). Research may bring harms or benefits via this group identity (Burgess and Brunger, 2001); a point that has been recognized in identity politics and deliberative democracy (cf. Williams 2000). Informed consent simply is an inadequate mechanism to assess and regulate the effects of research on groups.

Recent research experience has led us to reflect on the extent to which the historical and social significance of informed consent and its promotion of individual autonomy in mainstream health care and research have been integrated into some indigenous cultures. The intent of this exploration is to assess how to most respectfully and completely engage indigenous and non-indigenous people in public discussions and democratic approaches to designing public policy and dialogue related to biotechnology. Current sensitivity in research ethics and in other areas of indigenous knowledge emphasize the collective interests of indigenous people. Our research suggests that indigenous participation related to biobanks and human health issues was more inclusive of individual as well as collective interests than for research related to salmon genomics. But discussions of social and environmental risks of biotechnology that are not specific to indigenous people also tend to emphasize effects that are collective and cumulative in nature in contrast to individualist or consumer-based interests. The implication of our reflections may be more relevant to distinguishing the need for different approaches when engaging any population on issues of human health compared to environmental and food systems topics that more readily support consideration of collective interests.

Our project, Democracy, Ethics and Genomics,[1] was organized to compare across human and non-human genomics, using the examples of biobanking and salmon genomics. Both human biobanking and salmon genomics and aquaculture have been publicly acknowledged as having serious consequences for indigenous people. We were able to recruit First Nations' participants to participate in focus groups related to human biobanking, but not salmon genomics and aquaculture. This differential response suggests that some members of indigenous groups may find it less objectionable to be asked to participate in social research for health-related topics than for salmon genomics with its more immediately political and environmental aspects. This may not distinguish indigenous participants from non-indigenous participants as much as highlight an important feature of public engagement on health-related issues compared to food and environment – individuals may generally be more capable of distinguishing personal and collective interests in health and health services than in food systems and environmental issues. For issues related to the more politicized topic of salmon genomics and aquaculture, the individualist orientation was less powerful and concerns related to collective perspectives and acceptability may have reduced willingness to participate in the design of research or in focus groups.

---

[1] Funded by Genome Canada and Genome BC as part of a program of support for 'Genomics Ethics, Environment, Economics, Law and Society'. More information available at http://www.genomecanada.ca/

12.2 **Research ethics involving indigenous perspectives**

Recent scholarship and practical experience related to the ethics of research involving indigenous people, particularly in Canada and the US, has four themes:

1. The research objectives and activities should be co-created by the researchers and the indigenous community.

2. The research should provide benefits to the indigenous community studied.

3. The research activities should involve capacity building of the members of the community.

4. The research should be reviewed and approved by elders, or by a body established to provide ethical review from an indigenous perspective (this might be a regular ethics committee with indigenous representation or a committee of the community).

The terms 'community consent' or 'collective acceptability' have been used to characterize the mechanism whereby a community's representatives, ethics committee or agent reviews and approves the research (Weijer and Emanuel 2000; Brunger and Weijer 2005; Burgess and Brunger 2000).

The values on which ethical guidelines for research involving indigenous people are based seem to share a common commitment to trust, reciprocity, and respect for local knowledge, sometimes with reference to the 'OCAP' principles, or 'Ownership, Control, Access, and Possession' (Kaufert *et al.*, nd; Code of Research Ethics 1997; Snarch 2004).

12.3 **Seeking indigenous participants**

The consultations in our project were not initially designed to involve indigenous people; instead they were designed to examine how to construct consultations related to genomics that were adequately inclusive (Burgess 2003). The intent was to include and evaluate a diverse range of perspectives (Burgess 2004). The project goal of identifying diverse perspectives would be enhanced through indigenous involvement.

We approached individual tribal offices, personal contacts, indigenous members of Canadian research ethics boards (REBs), and advisory groups for Aboriginal interests. We offered three approaches. First Nations' people could participate in a mixed public focus group, form their own focus group using our facilitator, or they could use a group or meeting format that was traditional or appropriate for their community. In the latter case, they could structure our involvement or provide information from the group as they considered appropriate.[2]

The engagement related to salmon genomics did not result in a research activity, although the negotiation and follow-up led to several interviews and collaboration with the British Columbia Aboriginal Fisheries Commission (BCAFC) on the problem of consultation in this area. Interviews raised themes of negotiation about

---

[2] We are now building collaborative relationships with Aboriginal researchers.

fisheries, concerns about the effect of fish farms and hatcheries on wild stock, and the environment. We also learned that government sponsored groups have initiated 'consultations' with First Nations that often led to conclusions on topics that participants did not realize was the objective at the outset. There was, therefore, distrust of activities presented as 'consultation'. Consequently, despite our willingness to collaborate on the design of research contributions and process, our use of the term 'consultation' to designate collaboration was unfortunate, and may have undermined our objective.

As a result of our extended contacts and efforts, we did manage to organize a focus group involving First Nations, participants. The executive director of a 'Native Health Society' placed posters in the Society office, a friendship Centre, and at the local University. The Centre provides health services and health-related counselling for all bands and tribes in area. When posters failed to stimulate interest, the assistant to the executive director personally contacted participants who were at the Centre. The focus groups consisted of one staff member and clients or their supporters. The nine participants came from the local urban area and the outlying communities.

It is possible that the recruitment for biobanks was more successful than for the salmon topics simply due to good fortune and contact with a very helpful associate. But it is not at all clear that a small discussion group on salmon genomics involving First Nations' participants would ever be convened.

Both salmon genomics and aquaculture as well as biobanking have received media coverage in British Columbia (BC), including their serious implications for indigenous communities. Salmon is particularly important to West Coast First Nations, people for the following reasons:

♦ Salmon fisheries and the role of a Native fishery is a contentious and current political issue, involving civil disobedience by both Native and non-Native commercial fishers.

♦ Salmon is an important cultural symbol for most West Coast First Nations, with historical and spiritual significance.

♦ Aquaculture is a controversial practice that has implications for wild Pacific salmon stocks and the environment. Although there are a few First Nations groups that work in aquaculture, most are opposed.

♦ The field of salmon genomics research is not well known outside of scientific audiences, but in other focus groups, participants made up of randomly recruited members of the public usually expressed concern that financial benefits would lead to applications to create transgenic salmon, and it is a reasonable observation that other fisheries-related initiatives are perceived by First Nations, people to have had negative effects on natural resources and Aboriginal interests.

It is also important to realize that the anti-salmon aquaculture movement in the province has a strong consumer choice focus, encouraging individuals to eat only wild salmon because wild salmon 'don't do drugs' and are presented as healthier, more flavourful, and better for the environment than the aquaculture salmon.

Aboriginal participation in genetic testing and biobanks has also had a recent negative public profile. There has recently been considerable public attention paid to biobanks, and in BC to the Nuu-chah-nulth tribe's discovery that bloods taken for arthritis research was being used for anthropological studies without consent or tribal approval and (Baird Henderson 2001; Tymchuk 2000). Canadian research ethics bodies convened discussions with Aboriginal people and an international audience, about how to assure that research involving Aboriginal people is appropriately reviewed and conducted (cf. Glass and Kaufert 2001; Kaufert *et al.* 1999). The views of the focus group participants reflected the broader literature and social context expressing the following concerns about health research and biobanks:

- Health research should provide direct benefits to participants or their community
- Individual consent does not adequately signify that research is appropriate to the community
- Elders should be involved in approving research involving Aboriginal people
- Review and design of research should involve Aboriginal people
- Researchers have erroneously generalized to communities based on research involving a few individuals
- Individual participation by members of an ethnic group can lead to stigmatization of the entire group.

If knowledge about the collective basis for concern about salmon undermined our attempts to secure participation in the salmon-based research, then why were we able to secure participation related to biobanks despite concerns about the collective effects of health research?

The salmon genomics and aquaculture example contrast so well in the case of Canadian West Coast First Nations because in both cases the collective nature of political, economic, and cultural interests is widely understood. In contrast, non-Aboriginal participants did not differ in their participation in biobanks and salmon focus groups, and participants did not hesitate to discuss the collective interests related to salmon stocks, salmon wellbeing, culture, environmental impact, and economics. First Nations' participants understood the collective effects of biobanking research on Aboriginal interests. Participants were concerned that their views would not be taken as representative, but they were willing to articulate them.

This expression of individual perspectives in the context of health applications may be a product of the individualizing tendency in health care. Although it is beyond the scope of this chapter, the emphasis on the individual in health care ethics has been thoroughly articulated in relation to informed consent, standards of disclosure, compliance, diagnosis, and medicalization (cf. Corrigan, 2003). But the extent to which the individualizing influence of health and consent may undermine collective action is made visible by comparison to the salmon case. If it is even possible to assess cultural appropriateness, only indigenous individuals and communities can legitimately make that assessment. But the distinction between individual and collective effects of health research may 'enable' individual participants to feel it is appropriate to participate in the focus group. There is also evidence in the focus group discussion of the individual/collective effects on health distinction, and of the relationship between legitimate personal voice and collective representation.

12.4 **Consent and community in an indigenous group on biobanks**

The participants in the focus group reflected on Aboriginal interests related to biobanks and the focus group research itself. The focus group was recruited and facilitated by a professional facilitator, based on our research objectives and design and a facilitator's guide produced in collaboration with our research team. The focus group ran just over two hours. The participants were asked to describe how they understood biobanking, associated benefits, what concerns they had, and finally by whom and how they thought biobanks should be regulated or governed.

At the inception of the discussion of concerns, the participants revealed their knowledge of the Nuu-chah-nulth case and expressed a basic distrust of the extent to which researchers adhere to the conditions described in consent forms. Then one participant considered whether individual informed consent might authorize undisclosed uses of collected information.

> V4[3] I guess, I look at this consent form, here, I mean, what guarantee do I have that this information that you gather here today is not going to end up in – Switzerland somewhere. I've heard of stuff happening like that, I know that Nuu-chah-nulth people, that happened to them, that, a researcher came in, drew blood from the whole community, saying it was going to be used for this, and it ended up in Iceland, or something, that they were using that blood for something else.
>
> ...
>
> V3 If this information goes further than where it's supposed to go, maybe that's where it's supposed to go, as long as it benefits and helps somebody along the way, that's all my real concern. If it helps somebody and betters somebody else's life, that's good ... it all goes back to, kind of like, respect about people. We've been stabbed and stuck from, pushed aside, ignored, put on death's door for so long, it becomes natural to accept that what's going to happen. But time to put our foot down and say, 'No, we've had enough, it ain't going to do no more, you want any information, you must ask us.' I know for me, myself, anybody asks me I'd be more than willing to help in any way that I can. But if they just come and they take something then that offends me, and violates me as a human being. And how would they feel if I violated them?

Note that V4 is referring to the consent form related to participation in the focus groups when considering where the information might actually end up (is it relevant that neither she nor the researchers have anticipated the invitation to present this research at the Cambridge conference that led to this volume?). V3 objects to the presumptuousness and disrespectful approach of past research, but is quite willing to give individual consent if she receives an explanation of the good the extension of research might do. This is consistent with the hypothesis that participation in the biobanking focus group was acceptable on the model of individual consent.

Moments later the same participants raise another set of concerns – that they cannot be taken to be representative of 'Aboriginal perspectives'.

---

[3] Participants were coded 'V' for voice and numbered. The moderator is represented by 'M'.

V4 There's another question I wrote here.[4] Whose perspective should we include? Because you have to remember that, yes, we are Aboriginal people, but we all come from different nations.

M Okay.

V4 And that we're not speaking for all Aboriginal people.

…

V3 Not a representative of my people. In other words, representative of me.

So although these two participants recognize that they are speaking from an Aboriginal perspective, they also realize that they are not representative of any group. Yet they are willing to participate in the focus groups and air their views, whereas no-one was willing to go this far in the salmon genomics and aquaculture study.

Yet the biobanking focus groups did come under critique:

V6 Mm-hmm. One of the things I thought about was the assumption that could come out of this stuff, around it, and, one of the concerns I have is, what is the outcome going to be? I mean, is it just going to be, just an outcome?

M Now, again, are you talking specifically about this project, or about genetic

V6 I'm talking about this project, yeah.

…

V8 I think if Aboriginal people are going to be involved, they better be involved step by step, through the whole process. Because it's just like education, at the local agreement, compared to what the school districts – look at the school. I can say well, this is the way it is. I would hope that, you know, the Aboriginal people are a big component of what's happening.

M (responds with an explanation of the analysis of the focus groups)

V7 How many other communities have been done where there's been Aboriginals gathered together like this?

…

V5 Why did you choose (location) for an Aboriginal focus group?

V5 You should go – you should go to (another location).

Although the participants clearly wanted to know how the information would be used to see the design be more collaborative and the representation more broadly based, they did not refuse to participate. This suggests that there is nothing about the collective effects of health-related research that precludes individuals from consenting to participate, although they do so as individuals and not representatives, and can articulate the general concerns related to indigenous involvement in research. This would have been unremarkable if we had not run into a more definite refusal to participate as individuals in the research related to salmon genomics and aquaculture.

The final category on the facilitator's guide was about regulation and governance of biobanks. The group generated a list and then the moderator took them through the list to identify governance-related roles. When discussing the role of the federal government, some participants introduced the possibility of community-based governance.

[4] At the beginning of the discussion of hopes and then concerns, participants were first asked to write down their ideas.

V4 I don't know. Do we have a choice about it? I mean, why do you, why do we just say federal or provincial government, does it have to be a government thing?

V2 Well, I don't think it should be. I think they should be involved, but I think it should be in conjunction with the groups whose blood is being genetically banked.

The discussion then moved into detail on government inefficiency, the moderator redirects to consider a non-governmental organization, and the participants raise the topic of public representation.

M Is there an organization that you can think of, or one that could be created? If there was an organization, that was ultimately responsible for the regulations, the monitoring, making sure that the public's interest was represented, what would that body be, who would be in that body?

V3 Who would be in the body? The general layman. Just ordinary, everyday, John or Joan Doe in society. Not an educated person, not somebody that has some fancy degree, not somebody that's a doctor or a psychiatrist, somebody that is just an everyday –

M Representative of the public.

V3 Yeah.

M Maybe someone like you.

V2 I think maybe a cross-section of people.

M And – so what other kinds of people, what kinds of professions?

V1 I think people from health professions, from legal professions, to the people who are gathered in this room, people from different minority groups.

It is interesting to note that when it came to a discussion of the governance of biobanks and public participation the Aboriginal participants did not self-identify as having unique interests and identity. Following a discussion of the possible use of biobanks to investigate criminals, the roles of health researchers, scientists, universities, geneticists, social workers, and the military, the moderator reminded the group that they had listed communities.

V1 Well, they'd have to definitely be involved. I mean, from whoever, the entire community, like whether they want to, they have to have a group find out who wants to do this, who wants to be participants, who should be participants, and how come this community should be, whatever reason, and they've got to look at that. Like maybe this community has a high risk of diabetes, well that's what they should be looking at, and in that community. Not, you know, some other crap, that they don't have anything to do with, right?

Once again, the unique position of indigenous people is far less explicit than we would have expected if the topic were salmon genomics and aquaculture.

The role of elders is raised only in the final round of wrap-up questions. One by one, the moderator asks each person if they have anything to add. After discussion of what biobanking will look like in 40 years, the group's improved understanding of biobanks, the politics of biobanks and a wish to be better informed before the discussion, the topic of elders was raised.

V4 I had no idea what I was going into [when she agreed to participate in the focus group]. It's not like we have this conversation around the dinner table about genetics. I think one thing I would like more comment with, I would have loved to see maybe an elder involved here. That would have been nice to hear from their perspective. Yeah. And I think I do have a lot of questions regarding genetic banking. I'm hoping that I'll be able to see answers in black and white.

M   Okay. Thank you. V5?

V5   I didn't know what the hell I was doing. Why did I sign my name for this? It should be a lot longer, not only for a couple of hours, it should be a couple of days. An elder, like she was saying. And someone that is – someone that has an illness, like a diabetic, kidney disease, or something like that. That would be more interesting. But a lot longer. Two days. Longer hours …[5]

Perhaps once the group had understood what biobanking entails they were more concerned to seek the view of their elders and deliberate more fully. This demonstrates the collective and ambiguous nature of the benefits and risks, stimulating more of a concern to carefully assess the collective effects of biobanks.

The last participant in the wrap-up reiterates the hope for individual and family benefit from biobanks.

V7   Yeah. I found this quite interesting. Hopefully it will relate to some of my kids – like you know I said my husband and I both had cancer and they lost their dad to heart failure so – hopefully they'll find some answers for them, you know. So in that way, you know, I am glad I am here.

Concerns about collective interests and the perspectives of the elders co-exist with the desire to derive benefit for oneself and one's family. The topic of health care and research permits both elements of this tension to be articulated.

12.5 **Conclusion**

The use of informed consent in the focus group paints a picture of the legitimacy of individual agreement to discuss hopes and concerns related to biobanks. The group identified many of the issues listed in the research ethics literature as concerns that affect Aboriginal people as a group and informed consent was often posed as a partial or complete response. Often there was reference to the need to be involved early in research design, to control how and where research results were used, and to benefit directly from the research. This tracks much of the research ethics literature.

The contrast between participation in biobank – compared to salmon – focus groups might demonstrate that individuals consider that it is culturally acceptable to speak about collective effects in health but not salmon. Independent of cultural background, it may be that the context or 'culture' of health is distinguished by the extent to which individual interests and perspectives are perceived as more legitimate than in other areas that embody collective interests. This does not mean that there is

---

[5]   The shift from uncertainty about what participants could contribute to wanting more time and information has been consistent for most of our focus groups. Our next research project integrates face-to-face methods with online approaches that will enable ongoing information sharing and interaction.

homogeneity of interests related to salmon genomics and aquaculture. It is just that the collective interests apparently overwhelm the desire or willingness to discuss personal or non-representative perspectives. In biobanking, the structure of individual choice as reflected in the dominance of informed consent probably enables individuals to live more explicitly with the tension between collective interests and individual perspectives.

The absence of similar evidence in a First Nations group on salmon genomics and aquaculture does not equate to evidence of the rejection of the liberty of expression for individuals on salmon topics. This analysis depends on the refusal to participate and our subsequent efforts to understand that refusal. It is also possible that we failed to provide sufficient opportunity to recruit indigenous participants to salmon genomics and aquaculture on an individual basis, but all contacts with indigenous leaders and advisors suggested that would be inappropriate.

The 'so what?' question begs for a response. What is the significance of the context of health research supporting a cultural norm of individual benefit and consent even when collective benefits and risks are also strongly emphasized? Both the research ethics literature and the participants in the biobanking focus groups recognize the usefulness of evaluating collective acceptability, community consent, a 'visa' by elders, or through culturally appropriate deliberation. The participants manifested a tension between individual participation and evaluation of benefits for themselves against the concern to be representative and to consider effects on the community. This tension is explicit in the focus groups because we were able to initiate the discussion. In other areas of policy that involve more explicitly collective stakes such as salmon, this tension is more difficult to tease out. Any approach to the ethics of research involving indigenous peoples that does not explicitly address the tension between individual and collective participation will only provide a partial account of their perspectives.

Research on the ethics of involving indigenous people in research must try to find both the authoritative voice and the heterogeneity of perspectives within the broader community. There is always the hazard of the swinging pendulum, where the emphasis on community consent or collective acceptability risks obscuring the heterogeneity of indigenous communities. Indigenous communities have long histories of approaching the tension between individual and collective interests. It is in the interest of indigenous and other ethno-cultural communities to assess how best to promote their collective interests while recognizing and expressing the inevitable heterogeneity within their group. The tension between collective interests and individual variation within a collective is not unique to indigenous and ethno-cultural communities, but manifests in all of social life and is particularly salient in research related to governance, democracy, and biotechnology.

There may also be an implication for research ethics involving indigenous people. Brunger and Weijer (2005) explain that the task of determining the responsible parties and appropriate methods for collective approval of research depends on the social significance of the research in this particular point in history.

The question of which stakeholder communities should be consulted and which should give consent to research, is entirely dependent on the meanings of risk and the politics of risk, given the nature of a particular research project in a particular context.

From this perspective, the biobanking research, situated as it is in the context of health research, might more appropriately recruit participants to focus groups on the basis of individual consent. For the salmon genomics, our inability to find formal routes to constitute a focus group or other approach probably means that individual consent to the focus groups would have been inappropriate.[6]

The overall goal of the Democracy, Ethics and Genomics project was to contrast the different approaches to public engagement in order to tease out their strengths and weaknesses. Focus groups conducted without significant education on the issues avoided marginalizing and obscuring participants' initial responses, and provided the opportunity for more reflective responses stimulated by the discussion among the participants. Online surveys provide optional expert advisors and recorded Likert scale and qualitative responses.[7] This approach permitted participants to privately seek information and draw conclusions. Both social and private individual responses are likely to provide insight into the norms used by people when making decisions. This observation has led us to work on an integration of face-to-face and private online approaches. We hope to be able to characterize the tension between norms used in social contexts and private, individual decisions. Neither represents the 'real' or 'authentic' perspective, but together they describe a range of perspectives, informa-tion, and norms that constitute public dialogue informed by different approaches and information. The importance of accepting that there will important private and collective components of public engagement on all topics has been forcefully revealed to us by First Nations' participants in the biobanking focus group, as well as by their non-participation on the topic of salmon genomics and aquaculture.

References

Baird, L. and Henderson, H. (2001). Nuu-Chah-Nulth case history. In *Continuing the dialogue: Genetic Research with Aboriginal Individual and Communities*, edited by K.C. Glass and J.M. Kaufert.

B.C. ACADRE. (1997). Aboriginal Community Code of Research Ethics Template. UBC College fo Health Disciplines, Institute of Aboriginal Health BC ACADRE, Boston Bar First Nation. Available at http://www.health-disciplines.ubc.ca/iah/acadre/site-files/resources/templateRESEARCHCODEOFETHICS. pdf

Brunger, F. and Weijer, C. (2005). Politics, risk, and community in the Maya ICBG case. In *Ethical Issues in International Biomedical Research: a Case Book*, edited by J.V. Lavery, E. Wahl, C. Grady, E.J. Emanuel. New York: Oxford University Press.

Burgess, M.M. (2001). Beyond consent: ethical and social issues in genetic testing. *Nature Reviews: Genetics*, 2, 9–14.

---

[6] Indeed, there was a strategic decision taken in the project to work through official groups and avoid directly recruiting individuals.

[7] The current online survey on salmon is still available at http://www.yourviews.ubc.ca/?refer=017

–ibid.– (2003). *Starting on the Right Foot: Public Consultation to Inform Issue Definition in Genome Policy*. Electronic Working Papers Series. W. Maurice Young Centre for Applied Ethics, University of British Columbia at http://www.ethics.ubc.ca/workingpapers/deg/deg002.pdf.

–ibid.– (2004). Public consultation in ethics: an experiment in representative ethics. *Journal of Bioethical Inquiry*, **1**, 4–13.

Burgess, M.M. and Brunger, F. (2000). Negotiating collective acceptability of health research. In *The Governance of Health Research Involving Human Subjects*. Ottawa: Law Commission of Canada.

Corrigan, O. (2003). Empty ethics: the problem with informed consent. *Sociology of Health and Illness*, **25**, 768–92.

Freeman, M.M.R. (1998). Science and ethics in the North. *Arctic Medical Research*, **30**, 71–5.

Freeman, W.L. and Romero, F.C. (2002). Community consultation to evaluate group risk. In *Institutional Review Board: Management and Function*, edited by R.J. Amdur and E.A. Bankert Jones and Bartlett Publishers, MA: Sudbury.

Glass, K.C. and Kaufert, J.M. (eds) (2001). *Research involving Aboriginal Individuals and Communities: Genetics as a Focus*. ISBN 0–9688488–2-6.

Indigenous Peoples Council on Biocolonialism (2000). Indigenous Research Protection Act. http://www.ipbc.org/pub/irpaintro.html

Kaufert, J.M. (1999). Looking for solutions: recognizing communities in research ethics review. In *Research Involving Aboriginal Individuals and Communities: Genetics as a Focus*, edited by K.C. Glass and J.M. Kaufert. Ottawa: National Council on Ethics in Human Research.

Kaufert, J.M. and Lavoie, J.G. (2003). Comparative Canadian aboriginal perspectives on draft values and ethics in Aboriginal and Torres Strait Islander health research. *Monash Bioethics Review*, **22**, 31–7.

Kaufert, J.M., Commanda L., Elias, B., Grey, R., Young, T.K., and Masuzumi, B. (1999). Evolving participation of aboriginal communities in health research ethics review: the impact of the Inuvik Workshop (Conference Report 58/1999). *International Journal of Circumpolar Health*, 134–44.

Kaufert, J., Glass, K., and Freeman, W. (2004). Background paper on issues of group, community or First Nation consent in health research. (Unpublished working paper commissioned by the Aboriginal Ethics and Policy Development Project, supported as a joint undertaking of the Canadian Institutes of Health Research, Ethics Office and the Institute for Aboriginal Peoples Health, Sept., 2004.)

National Aboriginal Health Organization (2003). *Code of Ethics for First Nations Research (draft)*. Ottawa, Ontario.

National Institutes of Health (2004). Points to consider when planning a genetic study that involves members of named populations. Bioethics Resources on the Web. http://www.nih.gov/sigs/bioethics/named_populations.html

Snarch, B. (2004). Ownership, control access and possession (OCAP) or self-determination applied to research: a critical analysis of contemporary first nation research and some options for first nations communities. *Journal of Aboriginal Health*, **1**, 80–7.

Tymchuk, M. (2000). Bad blood: management and function. Canadian Broadcasting Company, National Radio.

Weijer, C. (1999). Protecting communities in research: philosophical and pragmatic challenges. *Cambridge Quarterly Review of Healthcare Ethics*, **8**, 501–3.

Weijer, C., Goldsand, G., and Emanuel, E.J. (1999). Protecting communities in research: current guidelines and limits of extrapolation. *Nature Genetics*, **23**, 275–9.

Weijer, C. and Emanuel, E.J. (2000). Protecting communities in biomedical research. *Science*, **289**, 1142–4.

Williams, M. (2000). The uneasy alliance of group representation and deliberative democracy. In *Citizenship in Diverse Societies*, edited by W. Kymlicka and W. Norman. New York: Oxford University Press.

World Health Organization (2001). International Decade of the World's Indigenous People (Report No. A54/33).

Consent and beyond:
some conclusions

Kathleen Liddell and Martin Richards

The preceding chapters have effectively emphasized that consent, as a regulatory touchstone, is in the ascendancy, and that the process of obtaining consent is widely perceived as a very important step in the legitimization of research. Indeed, it is widely claimed that research is ethically permissible only if the medical research subjects have given their informed consent to participate. Generally, the rationale is that people have a right to decide, which in turn is based, rather imprecisely, on assumptions about the importance of preserving individuals' autonomy. It is asserted that their bodies, and things intimately associated with their bodies such as tissue samples and personal data, should not be knowingly and intentionally exposed to risks or interference without their agreement because the desire for progress should not come at the expense of self-determination, privacy, dignity, or individual wellbeing. From this standpoint, some see consent as a stand-alone indicium of good research conduct; others see it as a procedure through which rights are waived and activities that would otherwise be impermissible are made lawful and ethical. But either way, they emphasize the importance of securing consent and avoiding a return to the post-war research values which grossly undervalued consent.

The authors contributing to this volume share these concerns but not the degree of emphasis with which they are pursued. This is because they also believe that there is a real and serious risk that consent can be over-valued in the governance of research. In this, they echo a point made by Beyleveld and Brownsword in 2007, who argued out that an over-valuation undermines the integrity of consent as much as under-valuation. It arises, they say,

> where consent is viewed as *the* key to ethical and legal justification, where – as Onora O'Neill put it in her Gifford Lectures – communities become 'fixated' with consent.' (O'Neill 2002) Left unchecked, 'a culture of consent [risks] being overtaken by a cult of consent.
>
> (Brownsword 2004).

The essayists in this volume have confirmed and shed light on this 'cult'. Importantly they have helped clarify the ways in which consent is over-valued, focusing on empirical evidence that demonstrates how consent practices rarely, if ever, live up to the lofty ideal. The authors also made bold attempts to outline constructive solutions to some of the problems identified. In this respect, the essays fall, roughly speaking, into three groups: several try to improve the practices of obtaining consent from potential research participants; some argue for better recognition of the situations in which consent is not necessary; and the majority emphasize the importance of recognizing that consent is rarely sufficient and must be governed within a wider network of procedural and cultural norms.

The over-valuation of consent

One of the books' central motifs is that the modern notion of consent is overly idealized. The idea that researchers can and should provide complete and rigorous information relevant to the cool-headed, rational research participant who then proceeds to analyse it competently, confidently, and sceptically is utopian.

In earlier work, Corrigan argues that the abstract accounts that pervade bioethical discussions do not reflect the experience of individuals in everyday research settings (Corrigan 2003). Social relationships of trust and role perception bear significantly upon the process of deciding whether or not to participate; perhaps more than the information presented to subjects in the process of seeking 'informed consent'. It is thus important not to get carried away with the idea that consent is a fundamental safe- guard against shoddy research.

Dawson (Chapter Six) claims that:

> we have good empirical evidence [extending 30 years] that many (perhaps even most) competent adults do not understand the information provided by researchers to the degree necessary to hold that they have given a fully informed consent.

He accordingly argues that consent is often 'unattainable' and it is a mistake to think it is a clear indicator of ethical research. To this we may add the not uncommon experience encountered by researchers when, having handed a would-be participant the (ethics committee approved) information sheet, the participant glances at it and only asks where a signature is required. Empirical research suggests that the issue is not so much misunderstanding as a different emphasis on the importance of the consent process. Unlike the insistence by bioethicists that the process of informing and being informed is fundamental to self-determination and dignity, participants put more emphasis on general beliefs and assumptions (especially concerning the benefits of medical research). They attach relatively little importance to the evaluation of specific information given at the time of recruitment. In practice, recruitment procedures may serve primarily as a signal that research is about to take place as distinct from diagnosis or treatment, though Holm and Madsen (Chapter One) in this volume say that even this purpose has been eroded by bundling consent to treatment and research together.

Snowdon et al.'s research (Chapter Four) adds a further concern. They suggest that attempts to gain consent for research are not simply pointless. The attempts can disturb and alienate already stressed individuals, some of whom find it very hard to deal with the idea that the doctor seeing them (and their child) is not exclusively engaged in trying to solve their personal and pressing clinical problems. That the doctor is also interested in conducting generalizable research, and wants them to make a considered, uninfluenced judgement about their willingness to assist, makes them feel isolated, and alone. Holm and Madsen (Chapter One) refer to this, poetically, as the loneliness of autonomy.

Hallowell (Chapter Eleven) highlights another limitation with the conventional individualistic model of a consenting person. In genetics practice and research, test results may have implications for other family members and, indeed, by collecting information about one person, researchers may also collect information about other individuals who did not consent. Consider for example a research proposal involving a predictive genetic test for an inherited condition which is presented to monozygotic ('identical') twins. One wants to participate, the other does not. Of course, the result of any genetic test on one twin will apply to both. So has the researcher obtained valid consent? Or does the decision of one twin not to know trump the decision of the other to participate? These kinds of situations are not confined to genetics but can arise, for instance, in research (and clinical practice) concerning infectious disease. Even the very basic task of a 'taking a family history' is at odds with the popular modern assumption that individuals have a right to control and determine how 'their' personal data is used. Hallowell further observed the significance of family members for participants choosing to take part in research. She states that, in some domains like genetic testing, consent is not 'an independent action free of external influence'. Is the agreement proffered by these participants unduly influenced? It is hard to say because the theoretical foundation of consent based on the autonomous, desert-island dwelling individual is an unrealistic fiction.

It seems consent is headed towards becoming an empty ritual – or 'empty ethics' as Corrigan (2003) has called it. Holm and Madsen take the view that current processes make it too much of a one-off event. The individual is asked whether they agree to a particular proposal; if they object to any proposed terms, their only choice is to refuse. In theory, this respects 'autonomy' but cheapens the individual's role and fails to promote a respectful, cooperative relationship between researcher and participant. The problem is exacerbated when clauses about research are bundled into consent forms for treatment. What is the individual to do? Refuse medical treatment because they are unhappy to allow tissue samples to be stored for research? Attempt to negotiate a tightly worded form? Holm and Madsen claim that this unnegotiable take it or leave it aspect of consent procedures could be likened to unfair contracts that have been prohibited in consumer law by the European Community. Perhaps they should also be prohibited in medical law.

The ritualistic approach crowds out other ethical issues. Liddell (Chapter Five) draws attention to this with a case study of the Human Tissue Act 2004. Despite the fact that civil servants had drafted a multi-faceted Act with several governance mechanisms, as far as the government spokespersons were concerned it was primarily and fundamentally about consent. Lobbyists seeking improvements struggled, often vainly, in the face of this rebarbative, unthinking, commitment to consent. In Liddell's view, it exemplified all too well the 'confused and confusing attitudes about consent that law and legal policymakers display'.

Bielby (Chapter Nine) points out that researchers are also at risk of adopting an overly regimented approach to consent. It can lead to a lack of sensitivity and imagination when conducting research with intellectually disabled people, or other cognitively vulnerable people. Often what is needed is not more forms and better information, but better support in the process of decision-making. Ponder *et al.* (Chapter Ten) point to another sort of issue, also involving the cognitively vulnerable. In their view research ethics committees and carers were blinkered by the epistemic proceduralism of consent and overlooked other indicators, which in hindsight suggest that the research interviews should not have taken place.

In short, we may have come to over-value and to fetishize consent as a stand-alone procedure involving ever rational individuals who live in a social vacuum.

Improving consent practices

If consent is flawed, what is to be done? An obvious response is to improve the quality and process of consent, and several contributors pursue this line of argument. Holm and Madsen suggest that a simple change would be to unbundle consent forms, so that separate forms deal with consent to treatment, consent to research intervention, and consent to storage of data and tissue for use in future research. Their comparison with the European Directive on unfair terms in consumer contracts (93/13/EEC) suggests that individuals should also be offered less rigidly standardized forms. This might mean having an opportunity to negotiate personal terms on which research takes place – a similar point is made by Hughes *et al.* (Chapter Eight). But unlike traders, researchers are not in a position to pass on the costs of personalized negotiations, which means they may not have the resources to offer anything other than a one-size-fits-all consent option. In this case, if research agreements are to be as fair as European consumer contracts, researchers should take care not to write terms that significantly imbalance the parties' rights and obligations; for example, consent forms should not inappropriately limit the legal rights of the research subject, irrevocably bind him to the terms of the agreement, or insist he complete his side of the bargain whilst leaving the researcher's contribution solely to his own will (see Article 3, 93/13/EEC).

Another reform would be to consider the amount of information and understanding that is required for genuine consent. In effect, the modern vision of consent, popular amongst bioethicists, would be regarded as merely aspirational, and a more realistic concept would be introduced in its place. Colloquially one might call this 'good enough' consent. Lawyers already use the term 'valid consent' and recognize that it must be sufficiently but not perfectly informed and voluntary. A quote from a US case, *Cobbs v. Grant* (Cal. 1972), illustrates this point:

> A physician violates his duty to his patient ... if he withholds any facts which are necessary to form the basis of an intelligent consent by the patient ... [but] ... the patient's interest in information does not extend to a lengthy polysyllabic discourse on all possible complications. A mini-course on medical science is not required ...

> (paras 43, 54).

The advantages of focusing on good enough consent are first that it is actually achievable (Dawson, Chapter Six), second that it reflects patients' and researchers' real desires and experiences in the governance of research, and third that it frees up time and resources for governance by other mechanisms (discussed below).

What are the indicia of good enough consent? This requires further research, empirical, legal, and ethical in nature but it would certainly be more than fictional 'implied' consent and less than utopian 'fully informed' consent. Guidance might be drawn from comparisons with other areas of life (untainted by bioethical hype about 'informed consent') in which individuals (and their families) are called upon to make decisions with far-reaching consequences: for example mortgage agreements, house purchases, marriage, voting, joining the army, motor vehicle repair work, or employment contracts.

A good starting point would be to differentiate between several different issues (Beyleveld and Brownsword 2007): (1) who can give consent; (2) the type of response that person must give in order for their response to constitute valid consent (this is a question of the explicitness of the signalling of consent); (3) the amount, type, and specificity of information that should be known to the individual for it to constitute valid consent; (4) the extent to which the obligation to assemble the information is the responsibility of the individual or the researcher or both; (5) the degree to which the individual must understand the information presented to him or her; (6) the degree to which the individual must be insulated from influences other than the risk information that affect whether or not they consent (e.g., is it permissible for families to encourage consent or refusal? Is it permissible for researchers to offer payments that reflect not only the inconvenience but also the risks undertaken? (Emanuel 2005; Anderson and Weijer 2001)); (7) principles for determining the scope of consent (a question of interpretation); (8) the conditions under which consent can be withdrawn.

As Manson and O'Neill (2007) insist, we are unlikely to understand informed consent unless we consider the sorts of communicative transactions it requires and the standards they must meet. The communicative transactions by which consent is sought, given or withheld are rationally evaluable social transactions between speech acts which are governed and constrained by a normative framework. By considering those norms, we may better understand the successful use of informed consent transactions to permit research interventions that would otherwise be unacceptable.

Another important step in improving consent practices is to recognize that they should be quite variable. This does not mean the principles underlying the integrity of consent should vary, but that differences in situational contexts affect their application. As Liddell notes (see Chapter Five),

> Although the *fact* of consent is all or nothing, the requirements for valid consent ... can [and should] vary according to the circumstances.

A problem, at present, is that such variation is made difficult by the forms used by ethics committees and the questions these pose. They imply that there are a standard set of requirements to be met and procedures to be followed by the researchers in all circumstances. They suggest that the process of seeking consent should be, by and large, the same for research involving possibly traumatized patients in an Accidents and Emergency department for a randomized, clinical trial of wound dressings, and an ethnographic study of an IVF clinic involving talking with clinical receptionists.

Several contributors to this volume described general categories of research which might be considered 'special' and, therefore, subject to qualitatively different consent procedures. Burgess and Tansey (Chapter Twelve) reminded us of the importance of collaborative research design when indigenous groups are being researched. This helps to avoid further colonization of indigenous people by not making them, their lives, and their knowledge simply objects to be studied, and undermining the group's identity and legal status. As others have argued, Burgess and Tansey suggested 'consent' to this sort of research might need to be reviewed and approved by elders or a body established to provide review from an indigenous perspective. 'Community consent' has already been recognized in some ethical codes produced by government and indigenous organizations. However, these codes deal mainly with research on environmental and agricultural systems, and Burgess and Tansey's research suggests alterations would be needed before the concept is suitable for health research affecting a population. Issues in environmental and agricultural policies involve more explicitly collective stakes. Indeed, 'community consent' could sometimes be taken to trump the refusal of an individual, for example, if indigenous societies were to approve certain types of salmon genomics and aquaculture, an individual's objection might be negated. (Burgess and Tansey suggest this might explain why the First Nation groups refused to discuss these issues with them.) In health care research (including biobanking), a 'mixed approach' may be more appropriate, perhaps involving group meetings or mixed focus groups. It is also important to be attuned to tensions between individuals and the community. The challenge with the involvement of indigenous people in research is to find an authoritative voice for the community whilst still respecting the heterogeneity of individual perspectives that make up that community.

Hallowell highlights another special case. In genetics research, information collected one person through genetic testing on may well have implications for other family members. It thus seems rather inappropriate to use standard consent forms that call simply for the consent of the individual who happens to be in the room with the researcher. But what is the alternative? Should the researcher (or clinician) seek individual consent from everyone in a family before enrolling an individual in genetic research? Or should we strive to develop procedures for 'family consent' along the lines suggested by Burgess and Tansey for 'community consent'? A third alternative might be that we continue to seek consent solely from the presenting individual but do more to make them aware of the potential implications for others. A further question is whether the individual should be held responsible if they fail to take reasonable steps to seek consent from affected family members?

The chapters by Bielby and Hughes *et al.* argue that consent practices might also be managed in distinctive ways for research involving the intellectually disabled and the elderly. Hughes *et al.* ask us to think of consent as an interactive process of communication grounded in relationships where the elderly take part in research, while Bielby argues that we should provide resources for 'supported decision-making' in research involving the cognitively impaired so that their capacity for autonomous decision-making is optimized through interaction and dialogue. With a 'helping relationship' (Rogers 1961), researchers can help to reduce power imbalances and can explain difficult ideas and concepts to potential participants whose understanding would otherwise be limited. The chapter by Ponder *et al.* adds a further point about the distinctive treatment of consent in the context of research with intellectually disabled people. Without opposing the points made by Bielby and Hughes *et al.*, they stress that in some situations 'consent' by intellectually disabled people and their carers should not be treated as being 'the same as' consent by other research participants. Drawing on a case history of a research project which involved men with significant cognitive impairment they argue that, at least in that project, the men should not have been included in the research despite consent ostensibly being given by the men and their carers.

These five chapters described several specific types of research – research involving populations, genetics, the intellectually disabled, and the elderly – but the analysis probably can be extended to some other types of research. Burgess and Tansey's points are relevant to some other kinds of social groups who share common interests (and risks). One example might be disease-related research for which groups representing patients have formed. Another example might be cluster trials involving groups of physicians, nurses, or other occupational groups (see MRC 2002, 9). Hallowell's argument is not confined to genetics research but applies also, for instance, to research (and clinical practice) concerning infectious disease. And the suggestions that particular consent procedures should be used in research involving the intellectually disabled and elderly are relevant to a much larger list of groups including children, severly sick or stressed patients, and those with communication difficulties. Special care might also be needed when seeking consent from prisoners, employees, and students (a point noted by the US Office of Human Research Protections).

Beyond consent

The essayists in this volume were not content with considering ways to improve our understanding of consent. They have argued that the limits of consent force us to look *beyond* consent when regulating medical research. In the main, they have explored the norms and practices that should complement consent to ensure research participants are properly protected (see next section). However, a few have also emphasized the importance of identifying when consent is unnecessary (as opposed to insufficient).

Recognizing situations where consent is unnecessary or unfair

One concern is that a strong culture of consent can create a climate of excessive caution that, all things considered, actually harms patients through hindering and even preventing vital research. Stereotypically, this sort of worry is attributed to utilitarians. Those who question the soundness of the utilitarian ethos then feel justified in ignoring it. However, the essayists in this volume (and the work they draw upon including that by Brownsword and O'Neill) argue that even if one rejects utilitarianism, there are reasons to be concerned that consent is (sometimes) insisted upon unnecessarily. Underlying this argument is the view that ethics does not guarantee a 'right to choose'. Some choices are decidedly unethical; for example, choices that are sadistic, selfish, unfair, hostile, and competitive (O'Neill 2002; Liddell, Chapter Five; Dawson, Chapter Six), and sometimes there is no reason to give more weight to one individual's view than another's. For example, Brownsword argues that an individual's consent is needed only when his or her right will be infringed upon.

John (Chapter Seven) gives this argument a twist. He suggests that rather than negate the requirement to seek consent or ignore refusals, we should instead regard some refusals as unfair and think creatively about the consequences that should follow. In particular, he argues that it is unfair for a citizen to decline to participate in research projects if the individual at the same time expects future access to state-provided health care. This would amount to free-riding whereby people enjoy some sort of 'health security' by virtue of widespread participation in research without undertaking similar risks themselves. The policy proposals that flow from this are interesting. John does not endorse the blunt, insensitive idea that people should be forced to participate in drug trials. Rather he argues that citizens have an obligation 'to be willing' to participate in research. Their decision to participate in research should be made against that background. This means they are not obliged to participate in every research project put to them or to participate if they are too ill to take part. Furthermore, the obligation would not be legally enforceable in any direct sense but would involve 'tracking who has participated in research, their rationale for refusing, and the availability of alternative research projects'.

The most controversial part of the proposal is in thinking about what to do with 'persistent refusers', or in other words, the free-riders who do not respect the obligation to be willing to participate in research. Does the policy have any teeth? John suggests the 'persistent refusers' might be denied some but not all health care privileges such as new drugs or a high queue position in a waiting list, and that those who agree to participate should receive special privileges. In effect, Hohn is suggesting a means to redistribute health care benefits, so that the free-riders cannot have it all their own way. An analogous social policy is the initiative in Australia which penalizes those who wait until old age to take out lifetime private hospital cover. For each year a resident remains uninsured after the age of 31, there is a penalty increase of 2% on top of the general premium up to a maximum of 70%, so that a resident who waits until the age of 50 could pay 40% more for cover. The purpose of the initiative is to encourage young people (who are likely to remain relatively healthy for some years) to contribute to the premium pool and to discourage older people (who are likely to develop health problems) from free-riding on other people's contributions (Department of Health and Ageing 2008). So although John's proposal sounds unusual, it is not without an analogous precedent.

Liddell put forward a different sort of proposal. She argued (Chapter 5) that the process of seeking consent was, and should be, bypassed in some research projects. One set of circumstances includes situations in which the participants' rights are not infringed upon. For example, where anonymized health records are used in research, it might be argued that no rights have been infringed. Against this it has been argued that anonymized data retains moral significance for an individual because it originated *from them*. If *their data* is used for a project for which they are vigorously opposed they might feel they have assisted an immoral exercise. The flaw in the counter-argument is that data is amorphous and should not be seen as *belonging* to an individual or having a discrete provenance. Provided the information is not about an indentifiable individual, it seems they have very little claim to control it or own it, and how it is used bears no relation to their moral character.

Liddell identifies a second set of circumstances in which the process of seeking consent jeopardizes the right of others to a good standard of health. This set, which essentially concerns rights in conflict, needs to be carefully evaluated. It is not simply a matter of the rights of the majority outweighing the rights of the minority. It is important to assess whether the risk of harm or infringement of rights is greater if one does, or does not, do the research. But it is equally important to ensure that if one proceeds with research without seeking consent, the injury or infringement of rights is minimized and proportionate. In addition, it is strongly arguable that the risks posed by involuntary research activities should not exceed a certain minimal threshold. Bearing this in mind, consent should very rarely be dispensed with. It might be ethical in some large-scale public health studies (e.g., 100,000+ people) based on health records or tissue samples where it is very costly to seek consent, there is no risk of physical injury, high levels of security are observed to ensure the data and tissue do not fall into the wrong hands, and steps are taken to minimize the interference in privacy (e.g., the data and tissue are anonymized swiftly by trained and accountable professionals and posters are used to notify people that they can opt out of the research). It is difficult to imagine that the conditions would be met in the case of clinical drug trials. It might also be ethical, subject to certain safeguards, to use patient records without the consent of individuals in order to identify those suitable to participate in research before they are approached for consent. Another situation in which research without consent is ethical is when incapacitated adults are involved in important research related to emergency treatment which cannot be carried out using competent patients and which it is impossible to delay until the individual's legal representative can be contacted (Liddell *et al.* 2006, 394–415).

Some people might find these proposals controversial, particularly as we are now so conditioned to think consent an absolute requirement for ethical research. However, there are analogies in other areas of life in which, as citizens of a community or members of a family, we are required against our will to shoulder certain risks, inconveniences, and even injuries for the benefit of others. For example, we may be called upon for jury service for the benefit of the criminal justice system even when it means our regular salary is foregone for the duration of the service. We may be called upon to pay taxes for the benefit of all manner of public services (cultural centres, Olympic games, and ministerial privileges) even when it means our own need for private health care, education, holidays, convenient travel, or comfortable accommodation are consequently thwarted. In our neighbourhoods, we may be expected to put up with the damage and risk to our home and person caused by vibrations, noise, smells, tree roots, unwanted correspondence, dangerous intersections, and buildings that block sunlight and views, simply because these things benefit other people. It is also worth noting that the framework Liddell outlines is broadly compatible with human rights and constitutional law.

A residual question is whether researchers should be allowed to self-police the decision to proceed without consent. Our risk-averse natures might persuade us that the decisions are best left to independent agencies. For example, researchers could be required to make applications to the Human Tissue Authority, the Information Commissioner, the Patient Information Advisory Group, or a Minister. But it is also worth questioning whether this bureaucracy is genuinely, or always, necessary. In the case of research using tissue and data, it is probably unnecessary. As a general rule, people are permitted to use and disclose confidential information for public interest purposes without first seeking permission from a regulatory body. They are expected to self-police whether their use or disclosure meets the legal conditions; if they reach the wrong conclusion, they are liable to pay compensation, to desist from further uses, and in some cases may be found guilty of a crime. So why single out researchers? Is there any reason to trust them less than bankers, teachers, auditors, bureaacrats, employers, insurers, shopkeepers, historians, or the media?

In the case of emergency research involving adults lacking decision making capacity, the risks associated with research might be considerably more serious, which would be a good reason for researchers to seek an independent opinion. However, in some situations this may be very difficult or impossible. Some countries insist on court orders or consent from legal representatives, but others have sensibly recognized tightly circumscribed exceptions whereby research can commence without consent, provided it is sought as soon as the emergency passes (Liddell *et al.* 2006, 399–406). The out-of-hospital PolyHeme trial in the US, which compared artificial blood with saline transfusions, and the TROICA trial in Europe, which compared a test drug for heart attack treatment and placebo, illustrate the importance of these exceptions (*ibid.*, 402–3).

Consent in context

Whilst the authors in this volume shared a common concern that the principle of informed consent is, quite frequently, over-valued, they also unanimously agreed that other mechanisms for protecting research participants should be given more weight. Taken in the round, the common theme was that consent should be seen as one regulatory tool amongst many. Another way of putting this is that consent should be seen in the wider context of research governance, and perhaps more prescriptively that bioethical research should be directed more often at other parts of the regulatory landscape.

To be regarded as ethical and legal, a research proposal must pass many standards and processes. Most notably, research proposals must pass ethics committee scrutiny. This is more than just a condition of law governing clinical trials. It is an NHS policy that patients and staff will not be permitted to participate in research without ethics committee approval. US Federal Regulations have instituted similarly strict standards stating that all projects involving human subjects research must apply for IRB approval (Chapter One). Most research funders also insist that projects be scrutinized by external ethics committees as a condition of funding. Some have also started to ask reviewers of the proposal explicitly about ethical issues and some have in-house ethics committees to consult on problematic issues. The publishers of many medical journals also now require evidence of appropriate ethics review before a paper is accepted for publication.

Liddell argues that these bodies may, at least potentially, have the ability to monitor some aspects of research more effectively than the individual participants or the researchers themselves. But as the experience described by Ponder *et al.* shows (Chapter Ten), these decision-makers do not always do a satisfactory job. It seems that research ethics committees and other ethical review bodies have become overly fixated on the process of obtaining informed consent (Kent 1997) and do not spend sufficient time on other issues such as assessing and monitoring study benefits and harms, refining procedures to minimize risk and inconvenience to participants, assessing the quality of facilities and the suitability of the investigating team, confirming the adequacy of insurance, assessing whether research burdens are being appropriately distributed, and assessing whether research results are being properly shared with participants and the community. It is also problematic that ethics committees focus their efforts on prospective review of research *plans* and spend little time analysing completed projects retrospectively. Although the US and Europe have instituted annual progress reviews, these are rudimentary and do little to check that conditions of ethical approval are obeyed, or that committees methodically improve their abilities to foresee and minimize ethical problems. There seems a strong case for some systematic empirical research into the current ethical review practice both by statutory research ethics committees and the in-house bodies set up by funders, publishers, and companies. How do they work, what types of monitoring could they practically implement (Heath 1979), and, more provocatively, what influence do they have on the processes and practices of research? Are they effective in their gatekeeper function?

Other layers of governance beyond research ethics committees may also be helpful in promoting ethical research. In areas of particular ethical controversy or public unease, we have special legislation regulating research practice. For example, under the UK's Human Fertilisation and Embryology Act 1990, an Authority was set up which licenses all research on human embryos and limits it to that which is 'necessary or desirable'. Researchers are also required to obtain a licence for storage of other types of tissue under the Human Tissue Act 2004, as a result of concerns following the large-scale storage of body parts at Alder Hey Royal Infirmary and elsewhere. Legislation also regulates research activities that involve adults who lack the capacity to consent (Mental Capacity Act 2005). It describes in general terms the maximum degree of risk to which individuals can be exposed in research activities as well as making it mandatory to consult with a carer (or similar).

The European Clinical Trials Directive 2001/20/EC is one of the broadest and most prescriptive pieces of legislation to govern research. In keeping with the current culture, it predominantly emphasizes the importance of consent, but alongside this it also sets out other regulatory initiatives including better monitoring of adverse reactions (pharmacovigilance), more explicit allocation of responsibilities to various parties (e.g., the sponsor, the investigator, the medicines authority), legal requirements for appropriate insurance or indemnity, a central database for recording clinical trial results, and standards about the manufacturing quality of drugs under investigation. In the main, these are described in general terms only. The detail is left to national legislation and agency policies.

Sometimes, where there are special issues of scale, novelty, complexity and/or public interest, independent advisory bodies are created. Examples include the Recombinant DNA Advisory Committee that has been reviewing US gene therapy studies since their inception and the UK Xenotransplantation Interim Regulatory Authority which reviewed proposals for animal to human transplants from 2000 to 2006. The Human Genetics Commission was also established in the UK to advise government on appropriate policies for human genetic technology, including research. A further example is the UK Biobank Ethics and Governance Council, which oversees a new and major research resource – known as UK Biobank – which will comprise the data and biological samples (including DNA) of some 500, 000 individuals aged 40–69. The proposal to recruit participants for UK Biobank went through the usual processes of research ethics committee review and a peer review by the funding bodies (Wellcome Trust, MRC, and the Department of Health). But, in addition, the funders established a special advisory body to design and monitor a dedicated ethics and governance framework for Biobank. As one would expect, the framework includes rules about informed consent, but consideration was also given to broader issues such as intellectual property rights, assessment of research priorities and on-going review. Interestingly, there have already been occasions when significant issues have arisen which were not foreseen in the initial research plans. For instance, participants were initially told at the point of recruitment that they would be free to withdraw from the project and their data and biological samples would then be removed from Biobank. However, it subsequently turned out that the nature of the data handling and security systems did not permit the removal of an individual's data from the system. The Ethics and Governance Council recommended that steps be taken to put the individuals' data 'beyond use' so that it could not be used in any subsequent data analysis and that recruits be informed accordingly. This underlines the need for continuing review rather than on–off prospective review of the kind undertaken by traditional ethics committees.

But perhaps this is not enough? Perhaps we also need better mechanisms to review the science and the assertions about the level of risk, especially for research involving healthy volunteers? And for patient volunteers, who checks that research arms are genuinely in a state of clinical equipoise? How closely do these people review the available evidence, and to what extent do they trust the assertions of the investigators? Who ensures the quality of research ethics committees' reasoning and the suitability of their members' expertise? Who checks that research is brought to a close as soon as reliable conclusions can be drawn that one treatment is more effective than another? Who checks that protocols are properly followed? Some of these tasks are the responsibility of the Medicines and Health Products Regulatory Agency and drug regulatory agencies in other countries. What sort of systems and resources have they devoted to the tasks?

The influential bioethicists, Miller and Brody, have argued (2003) that, in contrast to the clinical situation, physician-researchers do not have a duty of care to patient-subjects. Accordingly, they urge policymakers to re-consider existing restrictions on the use of placebo controlled trials, arguing they are not justified to the extent they are based on the presumption that physicians owe a duty of care to patient-subjects enrolled in randomized controlled trials. Furthermore they argue that clinical equipoise is fundamentally flawed to the extent that it represents an attempt to specify a duty that does not exist. Miller and Weijer (Chapter Two) convincingly undermine the key tenets of this position and clarify the nature of the relationship between patient-subject and physician-researcher which they hold is properly seen as one of trust in which the physician is subject to a range of moral and legal obligations, including a duty of loyalty, which extends beyond consent.

In Chapter Three, Miller and Johnston elaborate upon this, describing several layers of governance in the common law. They draw attention to three in particular: the law of negligence, the law of contract, and the law of fiduciary obligations. Under the law of negligence, a medical practitioner owes a duty to exercise reasonable skill and care in his treatment of a patient, even though no contract exists between them. Significantly, the content of the duty of care depends not upon informed consent, but upon the nature of the relationship. Only rarely will the patient's agreement to undergo the treatment negate the duty to provide professionally competent care. Miller and Johnston argue that although most case law concerns negligent clinical treatment, *researchers* are likely to owe a similar legal duty of care to research subjects. Potential liability in the field of contract law is rather different and, presently, uncertain. The first question is whether the participant has in fact entered a 'contract' when they agree to participate in research. A second question is to determine the terms of the contract. For example, was there any agreement that the researcher would provide a certain standard of care? A third concern is whether liability follows whenever a term of the contract is breached or only upon proof that the researcher acted negligently in breaching the term.

Miller and Johnston argue that liability for breach of fiduciary duty could potentially provide an extra degree of protection for research participants but, at the present time, its operation in this field is unclear. Whilst the Canadian courts have held that clinical doctors owe patients fiduciary duties, other jurisdictions have been more hesitant. Miller and Johnston recommend such a course of action, arguing that it would acknowledge the trust that research subjects place in researchers, while letting them make a variety of discretionary decisions that affect them. One consequence is that physician-researchers would owe special duties of care and loyalty to research participants, and would be legally required to exercise reasonable clinical judgement during the research and to privilege the interests of patients over the doctor's interests or the interests of others (e.g., research sponsors or future patients). The patient's consent would only rarely exclude liability for breach of fiduciary duty; and where it, did the effect would be diminished by the imposition of additional duties. This might offer greater protection for research subjects than is currently provided by laws of negligence and contract.

In addition to regulatory and legal protections, we should also be careful not to overlook the simplest of safeguards, namely the empathy of researchers. Indeed Hughes *et al.* referred to this explicitly in Chapter Eight and recommended we do more to build the right sort of character amongst researchers, one that is committed to protecting the wellbeing of their research participants as well as the pursuit of knowledge. In this they echo the perceptive words of Henry Beecher from 1970:

> An even greater safeguard for the patient than consent is the presence of an informed, able, conscientious, compassionate, responsible investigator, for it is recognized that patients can, when imperfectly informed, be induced to agree, unwisely, to many things ...

> (Beecher 1970 289-90)

A final word

Concluding with Beecher's words is salutary. It shows that this book is not so much about radical new ideas, but about repeating and developing wisdom from the past. As research ethics has matured, the concept of consent has become institutionalized and lost sight of its foundations. 'Consenting' the research subject is now so routine that it both trivializes and exaggerates the importance of consent. What this collection has helped to show is that, in fact, consent is usually (but not always) necessary and usually insufficient to justify medical research. Having failed to emphasize this, society is headed towards a highly problematic system of research governance; one that unduly stifles the activities of researchers and inadequately protects participants. The contributors to this volume have suggested several ways forward, the common link between them being a suggestion for more and better normative and empirical efforts to understand consent within the wider research regulatory context.

References

Anderson, J.A. and Weijer, C. (2001). The research subject as entrepreneur. *American Journal of Bioethics*, **1**, no. 2, 67–69.

Beecher H.K. 1970, *Research and the Individual*. Boston: Little, Brown and Co.

Beyleveld, B. and Brownsword, R. (2007). *Consent in the Law*. Oxford: Hart Publishing.

Brownsword, R. (2004). The cult of consent in fixation and fallacy. *King's College Law Journal*, **15**, 223–51.

Cobbs v. Grant, 502 P.2d 1 (Cal. 1972).

Corrigan, O. (2003). Empty ethics: the problem with informed consent. *Sociology of Health and Illness*, **25**, 768–92.

Department of Health and Ageing (May 2008). *Lifetime Health Cover*. (Australian Government.) http://www.health.gov.au/internet/main/publishing.nsf/Content/health-privatehealth-lhc-providers-general.htm. [Last accessed 21/5/08.]

Emanuel, E.J. (2005). Undue inducement: nonsense on stilts? *American Journal of Bioethics*, **5**, no. 5, 9–13. See also associated open peer commentary, 14–28.

Heath, E.J. (1979). The IRB's monitoring function: four concepts of monitoring. *IRB: A Review of Human Subjects Research*, **1**, no. 5, 1.

Kent, G. (1997). The views of members of local research ethics committees, researchers and members of the public toward the roles and functions of LRECS. *Journal of Medical Ethics*, **23**, 186–90.

Liddell, K., Bion, J., Chamberlain, D., Druml, C., Kompanje, E., Lemaire, F., Menon, D., Vhrovac, B., and Wiederman, C. (2006). Medical research involving incapacitated adults: implications of the EU Clinical Trials Directive 2001/20/EC. *Medical Law Review*, **14**, 367–417.

Manson, N.C. and O'Neill, O. (2007). *Rethinking Informed Consent in Bioethics*. Cambridge: Cambridge University Press.

Medical Research Council (2002). *Cluster Randomized Trials: Methodological and Ethical Considerations*. London: Medical Research Council.

Miller, F.G. and Brody, H. (2003). A critique of clinical equipoise: therapeutic misconceptions in the ethics of clinical trials. *Hastings Centre Report*, **33**, 19–82.

O'Neill, O. (2002). *Autonomy and Trust in Bioethics*. Cambridge: Cambridge University Press.

Rogers, C.R. (1961). *On Becoming a Person*. London: Constable.

Index

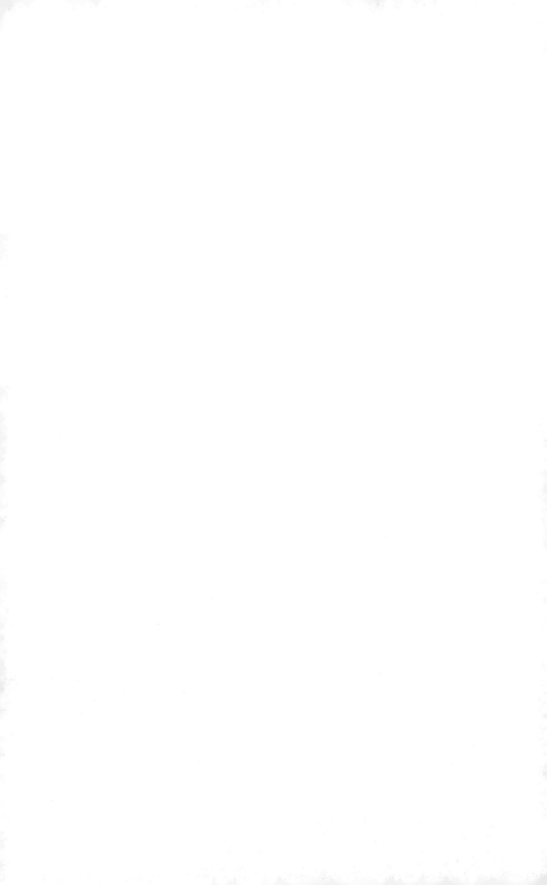